COVID-19: Current Challenges and Future Perspectives

COVID-19: Current Challenges and Future Perspectives

Editors

Peter A. Leggat
John Frean
Lucille Blumberg

MDPI • Basel • Beijing • Wuhan • Barcelona • Belgrade • Manchester • Tokyo • Cluj • Tianjin

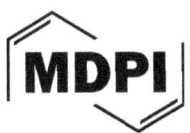

Editors

Peter A. Leggat
Professor and Co-Director,
World Health Organization
Collaborating Centre for
Vector-Borne and Neglected
Tropical Diseases,
College of Public Health,
Medical and Veterinary Sciences,
Division of Tropical Health
and Medicine,
James Cook University
Australia

John Frean
Deputy Director, Microbiology,
and Parasitology Reference
Laboratory, Centre for Emerging
Zoonotic and Parasitic Diseases,
National Institute for
Communicable Diseases,
University of the Witwatersrand
South Africa

Lucille Blumberg
Infectious Diseases Consultant,
Right to Care
Honorary Consultant,
National Institute for
Communicable Diseases
Associate Professor,
University of Stellenbosch
Honorary Lecturer, Faculty of
Veterinary Science,
University of Pretoria
South Africa

Editorial Office
MDPI
St. Alban-Anlage 66
4052 Basel, Switzerland

This is a reprint of articles from the Special Issue published online in the open access journal *Tropical Medicine and Infectious Disease* (ISSN 2414-6366) (available at: https://www.mdpi.com/journal/tropicalmed/special_issues/COVID-19_challenges_perspectives).

For citation purposes, cite each article independently as indicated on the article page online and as indicated below:

LastName, A.A.; LastName, B.B.; LastName, C.C. Article Title. *Journal Name* **Year**, *Volume Number*, Page Range.

ISBN 978-3-0365-3118-2 (Hbk)
ISBN 978-3-0365-3119-9 (PDF)

Cover image courtesy of Dr Monica Birkhead, EM Unit, NICD/NHLS.

© 2022 by the authors. Articles in this book are Open Access and distributed under the Creative Commons Attribution (CC BY) license, which allows users to download, copy and build upon published articles, as long as the author and publisher are properly credited, which ensures maximum dissemination and a wider impact of our publications.

The book as a whole is distributed by MDPI under the terms and conditions of the Creative Commons license CC BY-NC-ND.

Contents

About the Editors ix

Peter A. Leggat, John Frean and Lucille Blumberg
COVID-19: Current Challenges and Future Perspectives
Reprinted from: *Trop. Med. Infect. Dis.* **2021**, 7, 16, doi:10.3390/tropicalmed7020016 1

Anup Bastola, Sanjay Shrestha, Richa Nepal, Kijan Maharjan, Bikesh Shrestha, Bimal Sharma Chalise, Pratistha Thapa, Pujan Balla, Alisha Sapkota and Priyanka Shah
Clinical Mortality Review of COVID-19 Patients at Sukraraj Tropical and Infectious Disease Hospital, Nepal; A Retrospective Study
Reprinted from: *Trop. Med. Infect. Dis.* **2021**, 6, 137, doi:10.3390/tropicalmed6030137 5

Petros Ioannou, Stamatis Karakonstantis, Anna Mathioudaki, Angelos Sourris, Vasiliki Papakosta, Periklis Panagopoulos, Vasilis Petrakis, Dimitrios Papazoglou, Kostoula Arvaniti, Christina Maria Trakatelli, Evgenia Christodoulou, Garyfallia Poulakou, Konstantinos N. Syrigos, Vasiliki Rapti, Konstantinos Leontis, Dimitrios Karapiperis and Diamantis P. Kofteridis
Knowledge and Perceptions about COVID-19 among Health Care Workers: Evidence from COVID-19 Hospitals during the Second Pandemic Wave
Reprinted from: *Trop. Med. Infect. Dis.* **2021**, 6, 136, doi:10.3390/tropicalmed6030136 17

Carlos Henrique Alencar, Luciano Pamplona de Góes Cavalcanti, Magda Moura de Almeida, Patrícia Pereira Lima Barbosa, Kellyn Kessiene de Sousa Cavalcante, Débora Nunes de Melo, Bruno Cavalcante Fales de Brito Alves and Jorg Heukelbach
High Effectiveness of SARS-CoV-2 Vaccines in Reducing COVID-19-Related Deaths in over 75-Year-Olds, Ceará State, Brazil
Reprinted from: *Trop. Med. Infect. Dis.* **2021**, 6, 129, doi:10.3390/tropicalmed6030129 31

Anup Bastola, Richa Nepal, Bikesh Shrestha, Kijan Maharjan, Sanjay Shrestha, Bimal Sharma Chalise and Jenish Neupane
Persistent Symptoms in Post-COVID-19 Patients Attending Follow-Up OPD at Sukraraj Tropical and Infectious Disease Hospital (STIDH), Kathmandu, Nepal
Reprinted from: *Trop. Med. Infect. Dis.* **2021**, 6, 113, doi:10.3390/tropicalmed6030113 37

Anthony D. Harries, Pruthu Thekkur, Irene Mbithi, Jeremiah Muhwa Chakaya, Hannock Tweya, Kudakwashe C. Takarinda, Ajay M. V. Kumar, Srinath Satyanarayana, Selma Dar Berger, I. D. Rusen, Mohammed Khogali and Rony Zachariah
Real-Time Operational Research: Case Studies from the Field of Tuberculosis and Lessons Learnt
Reprinted from: *Trop. Med. Infect. Dis.* **2021**, 6, 97, doi:10.3390/tropicalmed6020097 47

Pruthu Thekkur, Kudakwashe C. Takarinda, Collins Timire, Charles Sandy, Tsitsi Apollo, Ajay M. V. Kumar, Srinath Satyanarayana, Hemant D. Shewade, Mohammed Khogali, Rony Zachariah, I. D. Rusen, Selma Dar Berger and Anthony D. Harries
Operational Research to Assess the Real-Time Impact of COVID-19 on TB and HIV Services: The Experience and Response from Health Facilities in Harare, Zimbabwe
Reprinted from: *Trop. Med. Infect. Dis.* **2021**, 6, 94, doi:10.3390/tropicalmed6020094 61

Pruthu Thekkur, Hannock Tweya, Sam Phiri, James Mpunga, Thokozani Kalua, Ajay M. V. Kumar, Srinath Satyanarayana, Hemant D. Shewade, Mohammed Khogali, Rony Zachariah, I. D. Rusen, Selma Dar Berger and Anthony D. Harries
Assessing the Impact of COVID-19 on TB and HIV Programme Services in Selected Health Facilities in Lilongwe, Malawi: Operational Research in Real Time
Reprinted from: *Trop. Med. Infect. Dis.* 2021, 6, 81, doi:10.3390/tropicalmed6020081 77

Irene Mbithi, Pruthu Thekkur, Jeremiah Muhwa Chakaya, Elizabeth Onyango, Philip Owiti, Ngugi Catherine Njeri, Ajay M.V. Kumar, Srinath Satyanarayana, Hemant D. Shewade, Mohammed Khogali, Rony Zachariah, I. D. Rusen, Selma Dar Berger and Anthony D. Harries
Assessing the Real-Time Impact of COVID-19 on TB and HIV Services: The Experience and Response from Selected Health Facilities in Nairobi, Kenya
Reprinted from: *Trop. Med. Infect. Dis.* 2021, 6, 74, doi:10.3390/tropicalmed6020074 93

Pritimoy Das, Syed M. Satter, Allen G. Ross, Zarin Abdullah, Arifa Nazneen, Rebeca Sultana, Nadia Ali Rimi, Kamal Chowdhury, Rashedul Alam, Shahana Parveen, Md Mahfuzur Rahman, Mohammad Enayet Hossain, Mohammed Ziaur Rahman, Razib Mazumder, Ahmed Abdullah, Mahmudur Rahman, Sayera Banu, Tahmeed Ahmed, John D. Clemens and Mustafizur Rahman
A Case Series Describing the Recurrence of COVID-19 in Patients Who Recovered from Initial Illness in Bangladesh
Reprinted from: *Trop. Med. Infect. Dis.* 2021, 6, 41, doi:10.3390/tropicalmed6020041 109

Johannes Jochum, Benno Kreuels, Egbert Tannich, Samuel Huber, Julian Schulze zur Wiesch, Stefan Schmiedel, Michael Ramharter and Marylyn M. Addo
Malaria in the Time of COVID-19: Do Not Miss the Real Cause of Illness
Reprinted from: *Trop. Med. Infect. Dis.* 2021, 6, 40, doi:10.3390/tropicalmed6020040 119

Kristal An Agrupis, Annavi Marie G. Villanueva, Ana Ria Sayo, Jezreel Lazaro, Su Myat Han, Alyannah C. Celis, Shuichi Suzuki, Ann Celestyn Uichanco, Jocelyn Sagurit, Rontgene Solante, Lay-Myint Yoshida, Koya Ariyoshi and Chris Smith
If Not COVID-19 What Is It? Analysis of COVID-19 versus Common Respiratory Viruses among Symptomatic Health Care Workers in a Tertiary Infectious Disease Referral Hospital in Manila, Philippines
Reprinted from: *Trop. Med. Infect. Dis.* 2021, 6, 39, doi:10.3390/tropicalmed6010039 123

Sarah Cristina Gozzi-Silva, Gil Benard, Ricardo Wesley Alberca, Tatiana Mina Yendo, Franciane Mouradian Emidio Teixeira, Luana de Mendonça Oliveira, Danielle Rosa Beserra, Anna Julia Pietrobon, Emily Araujo de Oliveira, Anna Cláudia Calvielli Castelo Branco, Milena Mary de Souza Andrade, Iara Grigoletto Fernandes, Nátalli Zanete Pereira, Yasmim Álefe Leuzzi Ramos, Julia Cataldo Lima, Bruna Provenci, Sandrigo Mangini, Alberto José da Silva Duarte and Maria Notomi Sato
SARS-CoV-2 Infection and CMV Dissemination in Transplant Recipients as a Treatment for Chagas Cardiomyopathy: A Case Report
Reprinted from: *Trop. Med. Infect. Dis.* 2021, 6, 22, doi:10.3390/tropicalmed6010022 129

Caterina Ledda, Flavia Carrasi, Maria Teresa Longombardo, Gianluca Paravizzini and Venerando Rapisarda
SARS-CoV-2 Seroprevalence Post-First Wave among Primary Care Physicians in Catania (Italy)
Reprinted from: *Trop. Med. Infect. Dis.* 2021, 6, 21, doi:10.3390/tropicalmed6010021 137

Graciela Mujica, Zane Sternberg, Jamie Solis, Taylor Wand, Peter Carrasco, Andrés F. Henao-Martínez and Carlos Franco-Paredes
Defusing COVID-19: Lessons Learned from a Century of Pandemics
Reprinted from: *Trop. Med. Infect. Dis.* **2020**, 5, 182, doi:10.3390/tropicalmed5040182 143

Saad Alhumaid, Abbas Al Mutair, Zainab Al Alawi, Naif Alhmeed, Abdul Rehman Zia Zaidi and Mansour Tobaiqy
Efficacy and Safety of Lopinavir/Ritonavir for Treatment of COVID-19: A Systematic Review and Meta-Analysis
Reprinted from: *Trop. Med. Infect. Dis.* **2020**, 5, 180, doi:10.3390/tropicalmed5040180 155

Mauro Giuffrè, Stefano Di Bella, Gianluca Sambataro, Verena Zerbato, Marco Cavallaro, Alessandro Agostino Occhipinti, Andrea Palermo, Anna Crescenti, Fabio Monica, Roberto Luzzati and Lory Saveria Crocè
COVID-19-Induced Thrombosis in Patients without Gastrointestinal Symptoms and Elevated Fecal Calprotectin: Hypothesis Regarding Mechanism of Intestinal Damage Associated with COVID-19
Reprinted from: *Trop. Med. Infect. Dis.* **2020**, 5, 147, doi:10.3390/tropicalmed5030147 179

Francesco Di Gennaro, Claudia Marotta, Pietro Locantore, Damiano Pizzol and Giovanni Putoto
Malaria and COVID-19: Common and Different Findings
Reprinted from: *Trop. Med. Infect. Dis.* **2020**, 5, 141, doi:10.3390/tropicalmed5030141 185

Kefyalew Addis Alene, Kinley Wangdi and Archie C A Clements
Impact of the COVID-19 Pandemic on Tuberculosis Control: An Overview
Reprinted from: *Trop. Med. Infect. Dis.* **2020**, 5, 123, doi:10.3390/tropicalmed5030123 195

Rony Zachariah, Selma Dar Berger, Pruthu Thekkur, Mohammed Khogali, Karapet Davtyan, Ajay M. V. Kumar, Srinath Satyanarayana, Francis Moses, Garry Aslanyan, Abraham Aseffa, Anthony D. Harries and John C. Reeder
Investing in Operational Research Capacity Building for Front-Line Health Workers Strengthens Countries' Resilience to Tackling the COVID-19 Pandemic
Reprinted from: *Trop. Med. Infect. Dis.* **2020**, 5, 118, doi:10.3390/tropicalmed5030118 203

Faryal Farooqi, Naveen Dhawan, Richard Morgan, John Dinh, Kester Nedd and George Yatzkan
Treatment of Severe COVID-19 with Tocilizumab Mitigates Cytokine Storm and Averts Mechanical Ventilation during Acute Respiratory Distress: A Case Report and Literature Review
Reprinted from: *Trop. Med. Infect. Dis.* **2020**, 5, 112, doi:10.3390/tropicalmed5030112 211

I.D. Rusen
Challenges in Tuberculosis Clinical Trials in the Face of the COVID-19 Pandemic: A Sponsor's Perspective
Reprinted from: *Trop. Med. Infect. Dis.* **2020**, 5, 86, doi:10.3390/tropicalmed5020086 233

Tope Oyelade, Jaber Alqahtani and Gabriele Canciani
Prognosis of COVID-19 in Patients with Liver and Kidney Diseases: An Early Systematic Review and Meta-Analysis
Reprinted from: *Trop. Med. Infect. Dis.* **2020**, 5, 80, doi:10.3390/tropicalmed5020080 239

About the Editors

Peter A. Leggat AM, ADC, is currently Professor and Co-Director of the World Health Organization (WHO) Collaborating Centre for Vector-borne and Neglected Tropical Diseases (AUS-131), College of Public Health, Medical and Veterinary Sciences, Division of Tropical Health and Medicine, James Cook University (JCU), Australia. He served as an elected staff member on the JCU Council from 2005 to 2018. He has served on JCU Academic Board since 2018 and is currently the Deputy Chairperson. Professor Leggat has more than three decades of experience in medicine and higher education in Australia and Internationally. He is a specialist in public health medicine and the President of the International Society of Travel Medicine and President of The Australasian College of Tropical Medicine. At JCU, throughout his academic career, he has been seconded for various senior academic positions, including Dean. A former Fulbright Scholar, Professor Leggat has published more than 500 journal papers; more than 100 chapters; and more than 35 books, directories and proceedings.

John Frean is qualified in medicine and pathology at the University of the Witwatersrand and holds postgraduate qualifications from South African, British and Australian institutions. He currently holds senior positions in the National Institute for Communicable Diseases (NICD); has a joint academic appointment in the Wits Research Institute for Malaria, University of the Witwatersrand; and is an Extraordinary Lecturer in the Faculty of Veterinary Science, University of Pretoria. His interest is in infectious diseases, particularly tropical, parasitic and zoonotic diseases.

Lucille Blumberg is currently a Consultant at Right to Care (RTC). She focuses on creating a One Health programme within RTC, especially for rabies, and on responding to health emergencies in South Africa and its surrounding region. Until 30 September 2021, she was the Deputy Director at the National Institute for Communicable Diseases (NICD) of the National Health Laboratory Service, and the founding head of the Division of Public Health Surveillance and Response. She is currently a Medical Consultant to the Division for Outbreak Preparedness and Response (incudes the Travel medicine Unit) and a Medical Consultant to the Centre for Emerging, Zoonotic and Parasitic Diseases, where her major focus is on malaria, rabies, viral haemorrhagic fevers, zoonotic diseases and travel-related infections. She has worked on a number of outbreaks including rabies, avian influenza, cholera, typhoid and the Lujo virus. She is a medical graduate of the University of the Witwatersrand; an Associate Professor in the Department of Medical Microbiology at the University of Stellenbosch; and a lecturer in the Faculty of Veterinary Medicine. University of Pretoria, South Africa. She has specialist qualifications in clinical microbiology, travel medicine and infectious diseases.

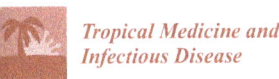

Editorial

COVID-19: Current Challenges and Future Perspectives

Peter A. Leggat [1,2,*], John Frean [3] and Lucille Blumberg [3]

1. World Health Organization Collaborating Centre for Vector-borne and Neglected Tropical Diseases, College of Public Health, Medical and Veterinary Sciences, James Cook University, Townsville, QLD 4811, Australia
2. School of Public Health, Faculty of Health Sciences, University of the Witwatersrand, Johannesburg 2000, South Africa
3. Centre for Emerging Zoonotic and Parasitic Diseases, National Institute for Communicable Diseases, Johannesburg 2131, South Africa; johnf@nicd.ac.za (J.F.); lucilleb@nicd.ac.za (L.B.)
* Correspondence: Peter.Leggat@jcu.edu.au; Tel.: +61-7-4781-6108

This Special Issue focuses on recent global research on the current coronavirus (COVID-19) pandemic. The disease is caused by a novel virus, severe acute respiratory syndrome coronavirus 2 (SARS-CoV-2) [1,2]. The International Committee on Taxonomy of Viruses (ICTV) named the virus SARS-CoV-2, as it is genetically related to the coronavirus responsible for the SARS outbreak of 2003 [2]. While related, the two viruses are quite different in their behaviour. At the time of submission for publication (7 January 2022), COVID-19, named by the World Health Organization (WHO) on 11 February 2020, had caused more than 296.5 million cases and over 5.5 million deaths with over 2.6 million new cases in the past 24 h [2]. The COVID-19 pandemic has greatly affected the capacity of health systems providing essential health care [1], but more than 9.195 billion vaccine doses have been administered as of 10 January 2021 [2]. There have been 22 papers published upon peer review acceptance in this Special Issue, including one editorial, twelve research papers [3–14], three review papers [15–17] and seven other papers [18–24], including one perspective, two case reports, one brief report, two viewpoints and one commentary. They each contribute to a much better understanding of COVID-19.

The contributions of these papers can be summarized as follows for the 12 research papers. The first of the research papers was a study of mortalities due to COVID-19 through a retrospective, observational study that included all inpatients from a major hospital in Nepal. Interestingly, 16% of patients also showed microbiological evidence of secondary infection [3]. The second of these studies was a cross-sectional survey exploring the knowledge and perceptions of healthcare workers (HCWs) regarding COVID-19 issues during the second wave of the pandemic, in four tertiary care hospitals in Greece. This study reveals some misconceptions and knowledge gaps in HCWs' everyday practice, especially regarding hand hygiene and antimicrobial use in COVID-19 patients [4]. The third study looked at COVID-19 vaccination in those aged 75 years and older in Brazil. COVID-19 vaccines were highly effective in reducing the number of COVID-19-related deaths in over 75-year-olds [5]. The fourth paper studied persistent symptoms in post-COVID-19 patients attending a follow-up clinic at a tertiary care hospital in Nepal. Of these, 97 (82.2%) patients reported that they had at least one persistent/new symptom beyond two weeks from the diagnosis of COVID-19, including dyspnoea, fatigue, chest heaviness, and cough, emphasizing the need to extend the monitoring of symptoms after discharge [6]. The fifth of these papers was a study to examine the impact of the COVID-19 pandemic on tuberculosis (TB) and human immunodeficiency virus (HIV) management in Zimbabwe. Impacts were demonstrated on the management of both diseases [7]. The sixth of these papers was a similar study conducted in Malawi, where there were similar impacts of the COVID-19 pandemic on TB and HIV management [8]. The seventh of these papers was a similar study conducted in Kenya, where there were similar impacts of the

Citation: Leggat, P.A.; Frean, J.; Blumberg, L. COVID-19: Current Challenges and Future Perspectives. *Trop. Med. Infect. Dis.* **2022**, *7*, 16. https://doi.org/10.3390/tropicalmed7020016

Received: 12 January 2022
Accepted: 19 January 2022
Published: 24 January 2022

Publisher's Note: MDPI stays neutral with regard to jurisdictional claims in published maps and institutional affiliations.

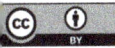

Copyright: © 2022 by the authors. Licensee MDPI, Basel, Switzerland. This article is an open access article distributed under the terms and conditions of the Creative Commons Attribution (CC BY) license (https://creativecommons.org/licenses/by/4.0/).

COVID-19 pandemic on TB and HIV management [9]. The eighth was a case series of five clinically- and laboratory-confirmed COVID-19 patients from Bangladesh, who suffered a second episode of COVID-19 illness after 70 symptom-free days. The study suggested the need for COVID-19 vaccination and continuation of other preventive measures to further mitigate the pandemic [10]. The ninth of these papers was a case of *Plasmodium falciparum* malaria in a patient asymptomatically co-infected with COVID-19, which reinforced the need not to miss the diagnosis of malaria infection [11]. The tenth of these papers was a study looking for common respiratory viruses amongst HCWs with upper and lower respiratory tract infection symptoms in a major hospital in Manila, Philippines. Of these, 38 (13%) identified positive for another viral etiologic agent, compared with seven (2%) who were positive for COVID-19 [12]. The eleventh of these papers sought to estimate the seroprevalence of COVID-19 in a cohort of general practitioners working in Catania, Italy, after the first wave of COVID-19, which was low (3%) [13]. The last paper was a survey by the WHO Special Programme for Research and Training in Tropical Disease (TDR) and collaborators of health workers trained through the Structured Operational Research and Training IniTiative (SORT IT). This survey was designed to determine whether they were contributing to the COVID-19 pandemic response and, if so, to map where and how they were applying their SORT IT skills. It showed that investing in training ahead of such public health emergencies is vital [14].

There were three review papers in this Special Issue. The first of these was a review of the literature on the influenza pandemics of the 20th century, and of the coronavirus and influenza pandemics of the 21st century. There are remarkable similarities among them and it was concluded that the public health response to the COVID-19 pandemic constitutes the basis for delineating best practices to confront future pandemics [15]. The second was a review of the efficacy and safety of lopinavir–ritonavir (LPV/RTV) in COVID-19. This review did not reveal any significant advantage in the efficacy of LPV/RTV for the treatment of COVID-19 over standard care [16]. The third review was an evaluation of severity and mortality in COVID-19 patients with underlying kidney and liver diseases. This study found an increased risk of severity and mortality in COVID-19 patients with liver diseases or chronic kidney disease [17]. There were seven other papers in this Special Issue. The first was a perspective, examining how operational research can improve the delivery of established health interventions and ensure the deployment of new interventions as they become available, irrespective of diseases [18]. The second was a case report of two cases of heart transplantation with concomitant infections with SARS-CoV-2, with rapid progression to death due to Chagas disease and cytomegalovirus dissemination [19]. The third was a brief report, which evaluated faecal calprotectin (FC) concentrations in 25 in-patients with COVID-19 pneumonia without gastrointestinal symptoms. Of these, 21 patients showed increased FC and a strong positive correlation between FC and D-dimer [20]. The fourth was a viewpoint providing an overview of common and different findings for both malaria and COVID-19, with possible mutual influences of one on the other, especially in countries with limited resources [21]. The fifth was also a viewpoint providing an overview of the potential impact of COVID-19 on TB programs and disease burden, as well as possible strategies that could help to mitigate the impact [22]. The sixth was a case report involving a patient with severe COVID-19, who was treated with a non-weight-based dosage of tocilizumab to prevent the onset of a cytokine storm. It was concluded that tocilizumab played a substantial role in his ability to avert clinical decline, particularly the need for mechanical ventilation [23]. The last was a commentary that looked at the challenges faced due to the pandemic, and the steps taken to protect the safety of trial participants and the integrity of the trial in the STREAM Clinical Trial, which is the largest trial for MDR-TB [24].

The diversity of papers, the depth of the topics and the relative geographical reach of the authors in this Special Issue confirm the continued collective major interest in COVID-19. There are 223 contributors to the 22 papers published in this Special Issue, with affiliations in Europe, Africa, North America, South America and Asia-Pacific. This wide-ranging open access collection contributes to a much better understanding on the epidemiology, presentation, diagnosis, treatment, prevention and control of COVID-19. As the editors of this Special Issue, we trust that you find the content useful, as the authors are pleased to share their knowledge with an international audience.

We currently have another opportunity to update advances in this field through a second Special Issue, "COVID-19: Current Status and Future Prospects". We encourage you to publish your work in, or propose a Special Issue for, *Tropical Medicine and Infectious Disease* (https://www.mdpi.com/journal/tropicalmed).

Funding: This research received no external funding.

Institutional Review Board Statement: Not applicable.

Informed Consent Statement: Not applicable.

Data Availability Statement: Not applicable.

Acknowledgments: The Special Issue editors acknowledge all the contributors to this Special Issue.

Conflicts of Interest: The authors declare no conflict of interest.

References

1. World Health Organization. Country and Technical Guidance–Coronavirus Disease (COVID-19). Available online: https://www.who.int/emergencies/diseases/novel-coronavirus-2019/technical-guidance (accessed on 10 January 2022).
2. World Health Organization. WHO Coronavirus Disease (COVID-19) Dashboard. Available online: https://covid19.who.int/ (accessed on 10 January 2022).
3. Bastola, A.; Shrestha, S.; Nepal, R.; Maharjan, K.; Shrestha, B.; Chalise, B.S.; Thapa, P.; Balla, P.; Sapkota, A.; Shah, P. Clinical Mortality Review of COVID-19 Patients at Sukraraj Tropical and Infectious Disease Hospital, Nepal; A Retrospective Study. *Trop. Med. Infect. Dis.* **2021**, *6*, 137. [CrossRef] [PubMed]
4. Ioannou, P.; Karakonstantis, S.; Mathioudaki, A.; Sourris, A.; Papakosta, V.; Panagopoulos, P.; Petrakis, V.; Papazoglou, D.; Arvaniti, K.; Trakatelli, C.M.; et al. Knowledge and Perceptions about COVID-19 among Health Care Workers: Evidence from COVID-19 Hospitals during the Second Pandemic Wave. *Trop. Med. Infect. Dis.* **2021**, *6*, 136. [CrossRef] [PubMed]
5. Alencar, C.H.; de Góes Cavalcanti, L.P.; de Almeida, M.M.; Barbosa, P.P.L.; de Sousa Cavalcante, K.K.; de Melo, D.N.; de Brito Alves, B.C.F.; Heukelbach, J. High Effectiveness of SARS-CoV-2 Vaccines in Reducing COVID-19-Related Deaths in over 75-Year-Olds, Ceará State, Brazil. *Trop. Med. Infect. Dis.* **2021**, *6*, 129. [CrossRef] [PubMed]
6. Bastola, A.; Nepal, R.; Shrestha, B.; Maharjan, K.; Shrestha, S.; Chalise, B.S.; Neupane, J. Persistent Symptoms in Post-COVID-19 Patients Attending Follow-Up OPD at Sukraraj Tropical and Infectious Disease Hospital (STIDH), Kathmandu, Nepal. *Trop. Med. Infect. Dis.* **2021**, *6*, 113. [CrossRef]
7. Thekkur, P.; Takarinda, K.C.; Timire, C.; Sandy, C.; Apollo, T.; Kumar, A.M.V.; Satyanarayana, S.; Shewade, H.D.; Khogali, M.; Zachariah, R.; et al. Operational Research to Assess the Real-Time Impact of COVID-19 on TB and HIV Services: The Experience and Response from Health Facilities in Harare, Zimbabwe. *Trop. Med. Infect. Dis.* **2021**, *6*, 94. [CrossRef]
8. Thekkur, P.; Tweya, H.; Phiri, S.; Mpunga, J.; Kalua, T.; Kumar, A.M.V.; Satyanarayana, S.; Shewade, H.D.; Khogali, M.; Zachariah, R.; et al. Assessing the Impact of COVID-19 on TB and HIV Programme Services in Selected Health Facilities in Lilongwe, Malawi: Operational Research in Real Time. *Trop. Med. Infect. Dis.* **2021**, *6*, 81. [CrossRef]
9. Mbithi, I.; Thekkur, P.; Chakaya, J.M.; Onyango, E.; Owiti, P.; Njeri, N.C.; Kumar, A.M.V.; Satyanarayana, S.; Shewade, H.D.; Khogali, M.; et al. Assessing the Real-Time Impact of COVID-19 on TB and HIV Services: The Experience and Response from Selected Health Facilities in Nairobi, Kenya. *Trop. Med. Infect. Dis.* **2021**, *6*, 74. [CrossRef]
10. Das, P.; Satter, S.M.; Ross, A.G.; Abdullah, Z.; Nazneen, A.; Sultana, R.; Rimi, N.A.; Chowdhury, K.; Alam, R.; Parveen, S.; et al. A Case Series Describing the Recurrence of COVID-19 in Patients Who Recovered from Initial Illness in Bangladesh. *Trop. Med. Infect. Dis.* **2021**, *6*, 41. [CrossRef]
11. Jochum, J.; Kreuels, B.; Tannich, E.; Huber, S.; zur Wiesch, J.S.; Schmiedel, S.; Ramharter, M.; Addo, M.M. Malaria in the Time of COVID-19: Do Not Miss the Real Cause of Illness. *Trop. Med. Infect. Dis.* **2021**, *6*, 40. [CrossRef] [PubMed]
12. Agrupis, K.A.; Villanueva, A.M.G.; Sayo, A.R.; Lazaro, J.; Han, S.M.; Celis, A.C.; Suzuki, S.; Uichanco, A.C.; Sagurit, J.; Solante, R.; et al. If Not COVID-19 What Is It? Analysis of COVID-19 versus Common Respiratory Viruses among Symptomatic Health Care Workers in a Tertiary Infectious Disease Referral Hospital in Manila, Philippines. *Trop. Med. Infect. Dis.* **2021**, *6*, 39. [CrossRef]
13. Ledda, C.; Carrasi, F.; Longombardo, M.T.; Paravizzini, G.; Rapisarda, V. SARS-CoV-2 Seroprevalence Post-First Wave among Primary Care Physicians in Catania (Italy). *Trop. Med. Infect. Dis.* **2021**, *6*, 21. [CrossRef] [PubMed]
14. Zachariah, R.; Dar Berger, S.; Thekkur, P.; Khogali, M.; Davtyan, K.; Kumar, A.M.V.; Satyanarayana, S.; Moses, F.; Aslanyan, G.; Aseffa, A.; et al. Investing in Operational Research Capacity Building for Front-Line Health Workers Strengthens Countries' Resilience to Tackling the COVID-19 Pandemic. *Trop. Med. Infect. Dis.* **2020**, *5*, 118. [CrossRef] [PubMed]

15. Mujica, G.; Sternberg, Z.; Solis, J.; Wand, T.; Carrasco, P.; Henao-Martínez, A.F.; Franco-Paredes, C. Defusing COVID-19: Lessons Learned from a Century of Pandemics. *Trop. Med. Infect. Dis.* **2020**, *5*, 182. [CrossRef] [PubMed]
16. Alhumaid, S.; Al Mutair, A.; Al Alawi, Z.; Alhmeed, N.; Zaidi, A.R.Z.; Tobaiqy, M. Efficacy and Safety of Lopinavir/Ritonavir for Treatment of COVID-19: A Systematic Review and Meta-Analysis. *Trop. Med. Infect. Dis.* **2020**, *5*, 180. [CrossRef] [PubMed]
17. Oyelade, T.; Alqahtani, J.; Canciani, G. Prognosis of COVID-19 in Patients with Liver and Kidney Diseases: An Early Systematic Review and Meta-Analysis. *Trop. Med. Infect. Dis.* **2020**, *5*, 80. [CrossRef] [PubMed]
18. Harries, A.D.; Thekkur, P.; Mbithi, I.; Chakaya, J.M.; Tweya, H.; Takarinda, K.C.; Kumar, A.M.V.; Satyanarayana, S.; Berger, S.D.; Rusen, I.D.; et al. Real-Time Operational Research: Case Studies from the Field of Tuberculosis and Lessons Learnt. *Trop. Med. Infect. Dis.* **2021**, *6*, 97. [CrossRef]
19. Gozzi-Silva, S.C.; Benard, G.; Alberca, R.W.; Yendo, T.M.; Teixeira, F.M.E.; de Mendonça Oliveira, L.; Beserra, D.R.; Pietrobon, A.J.; de Oliveira, E.A.; Branco, A.C.C.C.; et al. SARS-CoV-2 Infection and CMV Dissemination in Transplant Recipients as a Treatment for Chagas Cardiomyopathy: A Case Report. *Trop. Med. Infect. Dis.* **2021**, *6*, 22. [CrossRef]
20. Giuffrè, M.; Di Bella, S.; Sambataro, G.; Zerbato, V.; Cavallaro, M.; Occhipinti, A.A.; Palermo, A.; Crescenzi, A.; Monica, F.; Luzzati, R.; et al. COVID-19-Induced Thrombosis in Patients without Gastrointestinal Symptoms and Elevated Fecal Calprotectin: Hypothesis Regarding Mechanism of Intestinal Damage Associated with COVID-19. *Trop. Med. Infect. Dis.* **2020**, *5*, 147. [CrossRef]
21. Di Gennaro, F.; Marotta, C.; Locantore, P.; Pizzol, D.; Putoto, G. Malaria and COVID-19: Common and Different Findings. *Trop. Med. Infect. Dis.* **2020**, *5*, 141. [CrossRef]
22. Alene, K.A.; Wangdi, K.; Clements, A.C.A. Impact of the COVID-19 Pandemic on Tuberculosis Control: An Overview. *Trop. Med. Infect. Dis.* **2020**, *5*, 123. [CrossRef]
23. Farooqi, F.; Dhawan, N.; Morgan, R.; Dinh, J.; Nedd, K.; Yatzkan, G. Treatment of Severe COVID-19 with Tocilizumab Mitigates Cytokine Storm and Averts Mechanical Ventilation during Acute Respiratory Distress: A Case Report and Literature Review. *Trop. Med. Infect. Dis.* **2020**, *5*, 112. [CrossRef] [PubMed]
24. Rusen, I.D. Challenges in Tuberculosis Clinical Trials in the Face of the COVID-19 Pandemic: A Sponsor's Perspective. *Trop. Med. Infect. Dis.* **2020**, *5*, 86. [CrossRef] [PubMed]

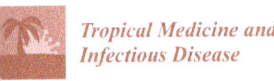

Article

Clinical Mortality Review of COVID-19 Patients at Sukraraj Tropical and Infectious Disease Hospital, Nepal; A Retrospective Study

Anup Bastola [1], Sanjay Shrestha [2,*], Richa Nepal [2], Kijan Maharjan [2], Bikesh Shrestha [2], Bimal Sharma Chalise [2], Pratistha Thapa [3], Pujan Balla [3], Alisha Sapkota [4] and Priyanka Shah [4]

1. Department of Tropical Medicine, Sukraraj Tropical and Infectious Disease Hospital, Kathmandu 44600, Nepal; docanup11@gmail.com
2. Department of Internal Medicine, Sukraraj Tropical and Infectious Disease Hospital, Kathmandu 44600, Nepal; nepaldeepika123@gmail.com (R.N.); kijan1069@gmail.com (K.M.); bkeshshrestha4@gmail.com (B.S.); bschalise@gmail.com (B.S.C.)
3. Department of Anesthesiology, Sukraraj Tropical and Infectious Disease Hospital, Kathmandu 44600, Nepal; prats.thapa@gmail.com (P.T.); pujanballa@gmail.com (P.B.)
4. Department of Internal Medicine, Nepal Medical College and Teaching Hospital, Kathmandu 44600, Nepal; alishasapkota@gmail.com (A.S.); shahpriyanka543@gmail.com (P.S.)
* Correspondence: shrestha834@gmail.com; Tel.: +977-9851214949

Abstract: Coronavirus Disease 2019 (COVID-19) has challenged the health system worldwide, including the low and middle income countries like Nepal. In view of the rising number of infections and prediction of multiple waves of this disease, mortalities due to COVID-19 need to be critically analyzed so that every possible effort could be made to prevent COVID-19 related mortalities in future. Main aim of this research was to study about the mortalities due to COVID-19 at a tertiary level hospital, in Nepal. This was a retrospective, observational study that included all inpatients from Sukraraj Tropical and Infectious Disease Hospital, who were reverse transcriptase polymerase chain reaction positive for SARS-COV-2 and died during hospital stay from January 2020 till January 2021. Medical records of the patients were evaluated. Out of 860 total admissions in a year, there were 50 mortalities in the study center. Out of 50 mortalities, majority were males (76%) with male to female ratio of 3.17:1. Most were above 65 years of age (72%) and had two or more comorbidities (64%). The most common comorbidities among the patients who had died during hospital stay were hypertension (58%) followed by diabetes mellitus (50%) and chronic obstructive airway disease (24%). The median duration from the symptom onset to death was 18 days, ranged from the minimum of 2 days till maximum of 39 days. D-dimer was found to be >1 mg/L in 58% cases and ferritin was >500 ng/ml in 42% patients at presentation. A total of 42% patients had thrombocytopenia, 80% patients had lymphocytopenia and 60% had Neutrophil to Lymphocyte ratio >11.75 with the mean NLR of 18.38. Of total mortalities, 16% patients also showed microbiological evidence of secondary infection; Male gender, age more than 65 years, multiple comorbidities with lymphocytopenia, elevated Neutrophil lymphocyte ratio and elevated inflammatory markers were risk factors found in majority of mortalities in our study. These findings could be utilized for early triage and risk assessment in COVID-19 patients so that aggressive treatment strategies could be employed at the earliest to reduce mortalities due to COVID-19 in future.

Keywords: COVID-19; mortality; Nepal

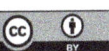

1. Introduction

Cases of pneumonia with unknown cause emerged in Wuhan, China, in December 2019 [1]. Epidemic investigation and gene sequencing revealed that a novel corona virus was the etiologic agent. The virus was tentatively named 2019-nCoV but officially named severe acute respiratory syndrome corona virus 2 (SARS-CoV-2) later by the Coronavirus

Study Group of the International Committee on Taxonomy of Viruses and the disease caused by this virus was named as COVID-19 by the World Health Organization [2,3]. Globally, as of 7 July 2021, there have been 184,324,026 confirmed cases of COVID-19, including 3,992,680 deaths, reported to WHO [4].

It has been one year since Nepal reported its first COVID-19 patient. Sukraraj Tropical and Infectious Disease Hospital (STIDH), the only central government infectious disease hospital of Nepal, was the first to diagnose and treat the first-ever patient infected with COVID-19 in the country [5]. As of 7 July 2021, there have been 650,162 confirmed cases of COVID-19, including 9291 deaths accounting 1.42% of cases, reported to Ministry of Health and Population, Nepal [6].

The demographics of inpatient mortalities in published studies show association with different factors, such as age >60 years, male gender and multiple co-morbidities [7,8]. However, mortality data in Nepalese context is lacking. This study describes the demographic characteristics of COVID-19 mortalities in STIDH and observation of risk factors that contributed to mortality. As a central tropical and infectious disease hospital in Nepal, experiences of mortality at STIDH during this pandemic could help describe situational awareness and guide interventional strategies and responses at community and national levels, especially for low and middle income countries like Nepal.

2. Materials and Methods

2.1. Study Design and Participants

This was a retrospective, observational study that included all inpatients from Sukraraj Tropical and Infectious Disease Hospital, who were reverse transcriptase polymerase chain reaction positive for SARS-COV-2 and died during the study period from January 2020 to January 2021.

Out of total 860 COVID-19 confirmed cases (reverse transcriptase polymerase chain reaction positive for SARS-COV-2) admitted at STIDH during the study duration, there were 50 mortalities, which were included in the study.

COVID-19 cases were categorized as asymptomatic or pre-symptomatic, mild, moderate, severe and critical and were defined as follows [9]:

- Asymptomatic or pre-symptomatic infection: Individuals who test positive for SARS-CoV-2 using a virologic test (i.e., a nucleic acid amplification test or an antigen test) but who have no symptoms that are consistent with COVID-19.
- Mild illness: Individuals who have any of the various signs and symptoms of COVID-19 (e.g., fever, cough, sore throat, malaise, headache, muscle pain, nausea, vomiting, diarrhea, loss of taste and smell) but who do not have shortness of breath, dyspnea, or abnormal chest imaging.
- Moderate illness: Individuals who show evidence of lower respiratory disease during clinical assessment or imaging and who have peripheral capillary saturation of oxygen (SpO_2) $\geq$ 94% on room air at sea level.
- Severe illness: Individuals who have SpO_2 < 94% on room air at sea level, a ratio of arterial partial pressure of oxygen to fraction of inspired oxygen (PaO_2/FiO_2) < 300, respiratory frequency >30 breaths/min, or lung infiltrates >50%.
- Critical illness: Individuals who have respiratory failure, septic shock and/or multiple organ dysfunctions.

The study was approved by the Ethical Review Board of Nepal Health Research Council prior to start of data collection (Reference number 169/2021P, date of approval—21 March 2021) and permission was taken from the hospital director to include medical records of the inpatients of STIDH. Since this was a retrospective study and the data were analyzed anonymously, the requirement for taking consent was waived off by the ethical review board.

2.2. Ethics and Data Collection

Demographic, clinical, laboratory, treatment and outcome data were extracted from medical records using a data collection form. Two experienced clinicians reviewed and abstracted the data. Data were entered into a computerized database and cross-checked.

2.3. Statistical Analysis

Statistical analyses were done using IBM Statistical Packages for Social Sciences (SPSS), version 20.0 (IBM Corp., IBM SPSS Statistics for Windows, Armonk, NY, USA). Continuous variables were directly expressed as median and interquartile range (IQR) values. Categorical variables were expressed as numbers and percentages (%). Pearson Chi-Square test and Fisher's exact test were used as appropriate, based on the distribution and p-values were tabulated with a level of significance set at <0.05.

3. Results

This section may be divided by subheadings. It should provide a concise and precise description of the experimental results, their interpretation, as well as the experimental conclusions that can be drawn.

3.1. Clinical Characteristics of Total Patients Admitted in STIDH

Out of total 860 COVID-19 patients admitted over the period of one year, 628 (73%) were males and 232 (27%) were females with the male to female ratio of 2.7:1. A total of 439 (51%) patients were ≤45 years, 165 (19.2%) were from age group 46–55 years, 103 (12.0%) were from age group 56–65 years, 83 (9.7%) were from age group 66–75 years and 70 (8.1%) patients were more than 75 years of age. Age and gender wise distribution of total admitted patients has been represented in Figure 1.

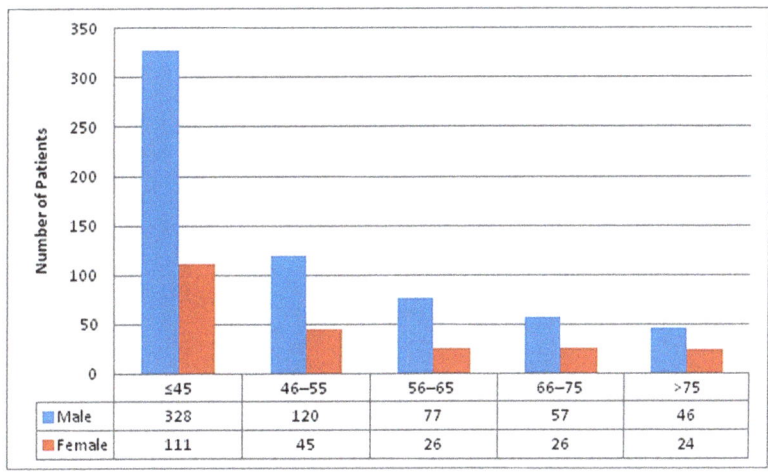

Figure 1. Age and Gender wise distribution of total COVID-19 patients admitted in STIDH (N = 860).

Out of total admitted patients, the majority (44.3%) had severe COVID-19, 16.7% had moderate COVID-19 and remaining 39% had mild COVID-19 (Figure 2).

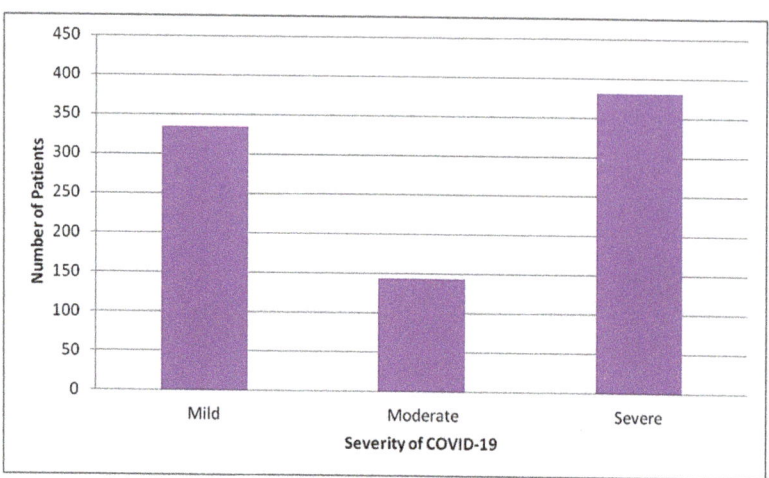

Figure 2. Distribution of total patients admitted in STIDH by severity of COVID-19 (N = 860).

Among 860 patients admitted in our facility, 50 (5.8%) patients had died whereas 25 (2.9%) patients had to be referred to other center either due to the need of mechanical ventilation which could not be made available to few patients at our center during the peak of pandemic or due to the need of multispecialty care which included dialysis or concomitant surgical care (Figure 3).

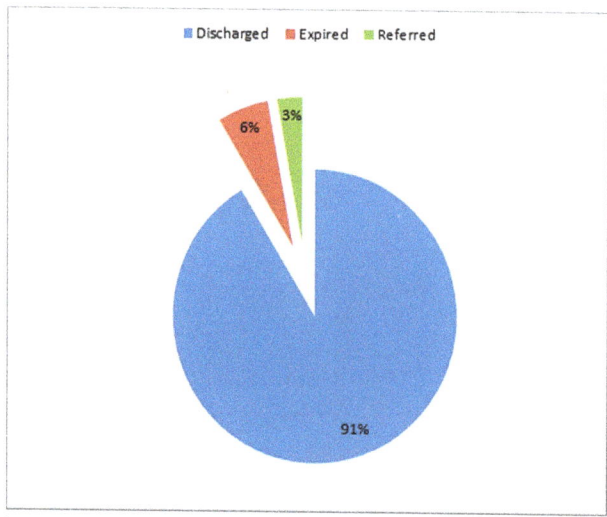

Figure 3. Outcome of total patients admitted in STIDH (N = 860).

3.2. Clinical Characteristics of the Mortalities in STIDH

3.2.1. Baseline Characteristics

Among 50 deaths recorded, 38 (76%) were males and 12 (24%) were females, with male to female ratio of 3.17:1. The median age was 72.5 years, ranging from 36 to 95 years. Most (21/50, 42%) patients were of the age group ≥76 years, followed by 66–75 years (15/50, 30%). Distribution of total mortalities by gender and age groups are shown in Figure 4.

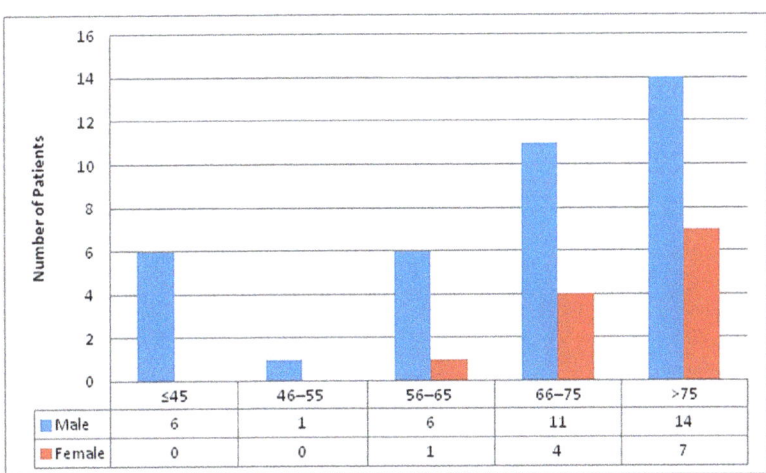

Figure 4. Age and gender wise distribution of mortalities in STIDH (n = 50).

41 patients (82%) who died of COVID-19 had underlying disease, the most common of which was hypertension (29/50, 58%), followed by diabetes (25/50, 50%), chronic obstructive pulmonary disease (12/50, 24%), obesity (9/50, 18%), heart disease (7/50, 14%), asthma (3/50, 6%), neoplastic disease (2/50, 4%) (One had carcinoma of gall bladder and the other had multiple myeloma) and chronic kidney disease (1/50, 2%) (Figure 5). A total of 33 (66%) patients who died during hospital stay had multiple (two or more than two) co-morbidities in our study.

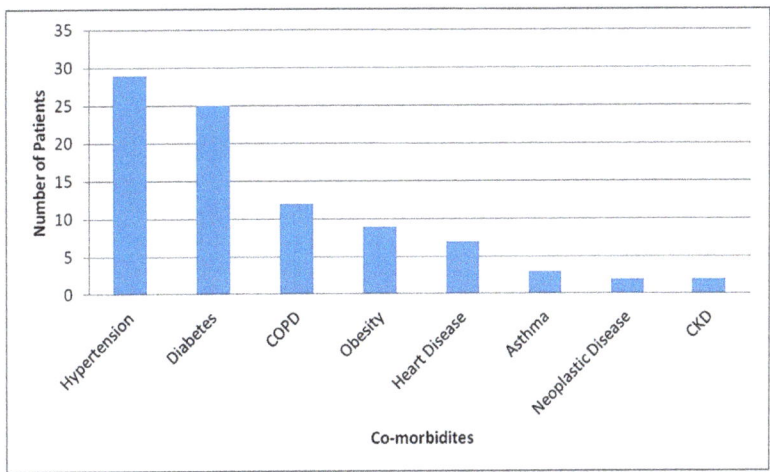

Figure 5. Distribution of co-morbidities among mortalities in STIDH (n = 50).

Multiple comorbidities (2 or more) were likely to be present in patients with increasing age with statistically significant association (Table 1).

Table 1. Age wise distribution of comorbidities among mortalities in STIDH (n = 50).

Age Group	Multiple (2 or More) Comorbidities		Total	p-Value
	Absent (n)	Present (n)		
≤45	5	1	6	
46–55	1	0	1	
56–65	5	2	7	0.001
66–75	4	11	15	
>75	2	19	21	
Total	17	33	50	

The presence of multiple comorbidities, however, did not seem to have a significant association with sex (Table 2).

Table 2. Sex wise distribution of multiple comorbidities among mortalities in STIDH (n = 50).

Sex	Multiple (2 or More) Comorbidities		Total	p-Value
	Absent (n)	Present (n)		
Female	3	9	12	
Male	14	24	38	0.510
Total	17	33	50	

3.2.2. Clinical Presentation

The median duration of symptoms prior to admission was 5 days, ranging from 1–20 days. The median duration of hospital stay was 10.5 days, ranging from 1–35 days. The median duration from the first symptom to death was 18 days, ranging from 2–39 days. For male patients, the median duration from the first symptom to death was 18.5 days and for female patients was 13.5 days. Most of the patients presented as severe disease (47/50, 94%), rest (3/50, 6%) presented as moderate disease and later progressed. Shortness of breath was the most common reported symptom among patients who eventually died (46/50, 92%), followed by cough (42/50, 84%), fever (37/50, 74%), body ache (13/37, 26%), headache (9/50, 18%) and diarrhea (2/50, 4%), as represented in Figure 6.

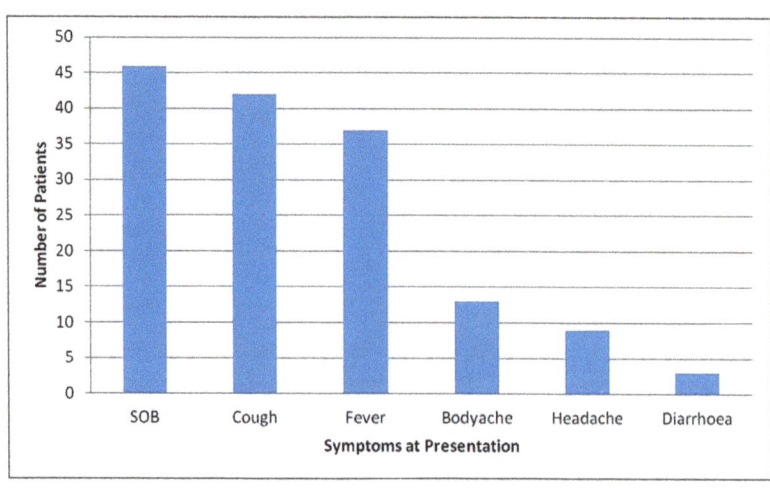

Figure 6. Distribution of symptoms at presentation among mortalities at STIDH (n = 50).

3.2.3. Biomarkers and Hematological Variables

C-reactive protein was positive in 42/50 (84%) cases. D-dimer was found to be >1 mg/L in 29/50 (58%) cases and ferritin was >500 ng/ml in 21/50 (42%) patients at presentation. A total of 14 patients had repeated D-dimer measurements, which showed increase in the level of D- dimer. A total of 23/50 (46%) patients were anemic with the mean hemoglobin level being 12.85 g/dL, ranging from 9.6 to 18.4 g/dL. A total of 21/50 (42%) patients had thrombocytopenia, while 4/50 (8%) had thrombocytosis at presentation. A total of 25/50 (50%) had normal platelet count. Of 21 patients with thrombocytopenia, 10 had moderate and 11 had mild thrombocytopenia. A total of 40/50 (80%) patients had lymphocytopenia (absolute lymphocyte count <1000 cells/µL) at presentation (Figure 7). Neutrophil to lymphocyte ratio was >11.75 in 30/50 (60%) patients, with the mean NLR being 18.38, ranged from 1.52 to 98. A total of 10/50 (20%) patients had renal impairment and 4/50 (8%) had transaminitis at presentation. A total of 29/50 (58%) developed acute kidney injury during hospital stay, while 10/50 (20%) developed hepatic impairment.

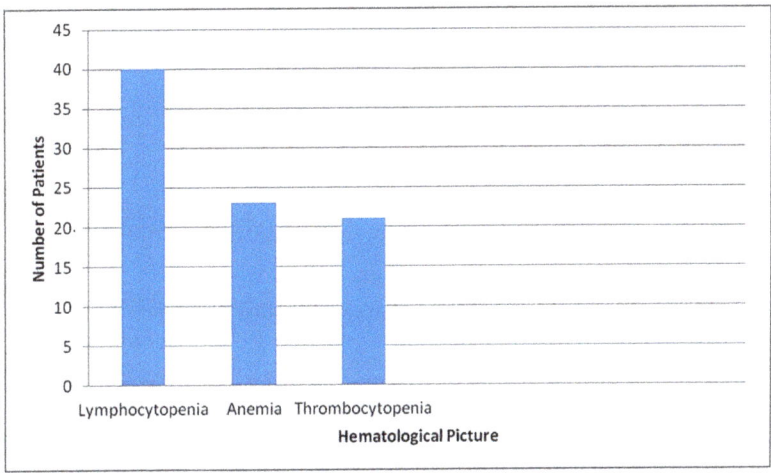

Figure 7. Distribution by hematological picture of the mortalities in STIDH (n = 50).

3.2.4. Microbiology

A total of 8/50 (16%) patients showed microbiological evidence of secondary infection, 6/50 (12%) patients had sputum culture positive for organisms and 2/50 (4%) had urine culture positivity. *Klebsiella pneumoniae* was the predominant organism in sputum culture (5/6, 83.3%) followed by *Escherichia coli* (1/6, 16.7%). A total of 2/50 (4%) patients had urine culture positive for *E. coli*.

3.2.5. Treatment

The antiviral drug remdesivir was used in 41/50 (82%) patients, while convalescent plasma transfusions were used in 17/50 (34%) patients (Figure 8). A total of 6/41 (14.6%) patients received remdesivir for 10 days, 27/41 (65.9%) received for 5 days. One patient received for 4 days, while 2 received for 3, 2 for 2 days and 2 for 1 day. Some died before completion of therapy and in some patients; the drug was stopped prematurely when they developed significant hepatic or renal impairment limiting the use of drug. A total of 31/50 (62%) patients received therapeutic anticoagulation with low molecular weight heparin (LMWH), whereas 19/50 (38%) patients had only received prophylactic anticoagulation with heparin. The highest level of oxygen delivery device used in most patients was non-invasive ventilation in 40/50 (80%) patients. Invasive ventilation was only used in 7/50 (14%) patients, followed by the use of reservoir mask in 2/50 (4%) patients and High Flow Nasal Cannula (HFNC) in 1/50 (2%) patient. The reason for inability to escalate respiratory support to invasive mechanical ventilation was due to the do not resuscitate status of patients as per the wishes of patient's party after knowing about grave prognosis and also due to logistic issues at our center.

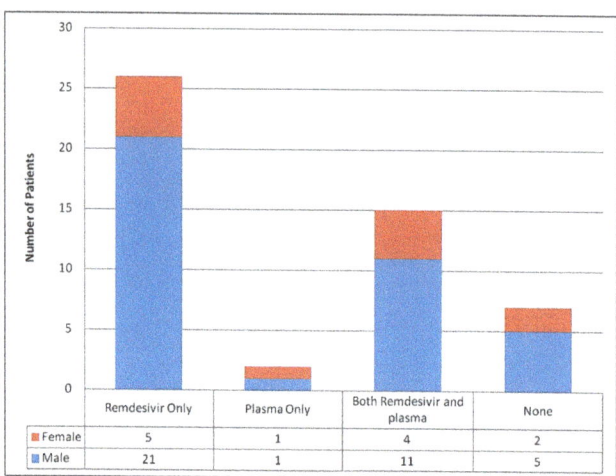

Figure 8. Treatment according to the gender of patients who died.

3.2.6. Cause of Death

A total of 40/50 (80%) deaths were due to type 1 respiratory failure, while 7/50 (14%) died of septic shock and 3/50 (6%) died of multiple organ dysfunction syndrome. The contributory cause was AKI in 20/50 (40%) patients and sepsis in 5/50 (10%) patients.

4. Discussion

This study represents a review of the COVID-19 deaths at Sukraraj Tropical and Infectious Disease Hospital during the first wave of coronavirus pandemic in Nepal from early 2020 till early 2021. Patients with underlying diseases and age over 65 years made up the majority of deaths, similar to demographics of COVID-19 deaths from other studies [10–13]. Du et al. performed a single center prospective cohort study to investigate the possible risk factors associated with the poorest clinical outcome (dying from COVID-19 pneumonia) and reported that age ≥65 years to be one of the predictors for mortality in COVID-19 [10]. The current study also suggested that old age was associated with deaths in patients with COVID-19. Age as a determinant for prognosis could be due to poor health and associated comorbidities. This signifies the need for aggressive monitoring and intensive treatment strategies to be employed at the earliest to limit deaths in older age population. Further, prophylactic treatments in anticipation of the disease in the elderly could involve natural repetitive stimulations of the heat shock response in the whole body through controlled intense physical exercise, sauna therapies and the regular maintenance of calorie-restricted diets containing minimal amounts of saturated lipids and cholesterol [14].

Recent studies revealed lymphocytopenia as an important characteristic of SARS-CoV-2 infection, especially in critically ill and deceased patients [11,12]. Huang et al. and Wang et al. showed an association between lymphocytopenia and need of intensive care unit [1,13]. Similarly, Wu et al. showed an association between lymphocytopenia and acute respiratory distress syndrome (ARDS) development [15]. In Singapore, Fan et al. found that patients requiring ICU support had significantly lower lymphocyte levels at baseline [16]. Similar to these studies, our study also showed that the majority (80%) of patients who died had lymphocytopenia at presentation. Thus, lymphocytopenia can be taken as one of the severity markers of COVID-19 and we need to be vigilant in patients presenting with lymphocytopenia.

A meta-analysis of nine studies suggested that thrombocytopenia is significantly associated with the severity of COVID-19 disease; a more sizeable drop in platelet counts was noted especially in non-survivors [17]. In our study, significant proportion (42%) of cases that died had thrombocytopenia at presentation. A systematic review and meta-analysis by Li et al. concluded that NLR has significant predictive value for disease severity and mortality in patients with COVID-19 infection [18]. Similarly, Liu Y et al. showed that NLR is an independent risk factor of the in-hospital mortality for COVID-19 patients [19]. A retrospective cross-sectional study done by Yan et al. showed that NLR more than 11.75 was significantly correlated with all-cause in-hospital mortality [20]. In our study, the majority of patients who died presented with NLR > 11.75. NLR evaluation can help clinicians identify potentially severe cases early, conduct early triage and initiate aggressive management at the earliest, which may reduce the overall mortality of COVID-19.

A retrospective, multi-center cohort study from Jinyintan Hospital and Wuhan Pulmonary Hospital (Wuhan, China) showed that older age, D-dimer levels greater than 1 µg/mL and higher SOFA score on admission were associated with higher odds of in-hospital death [21]. A meta-analysis done by Huang et al. also suggested that elevated serum C-reactive protein, procalcitonin, D-dimer and ferritin were associated with poor outcome in COVID-19. It showed that a D-dimer >0.5 mg/dL had 58% sensitivity and 69% specificity for severe disease [22]. In a retrospective study by Tang et al. encompassing data from 183 consecutive patients with COVID-19, non-survivors had significantly higher D-dimer ($p < 0.05$), fibrin degradation product (FDP) levels ($p < 0.05$), prolonged PT ($p < 0.05$) and APTT ($p < 0.05$) compared with survivors at initial evaluation [23]. In a multicenter retrospective cohort study from China by Wu et al, increased D-dimer levels (>1 µg/mL) were significantly associated with in-hospital death in the multivariable analysis [15]. Similarly, the same study also showed that higher serum ferritin was associated with ARDS development. Zhou et al. also supported an association between higher serum ferritin levels and death [21]. D-dimer was high (>1.0 mg/L) in 58% of our patients and high ferritin levels (>500 ng/ml) were present in 42% patients who had died at our center during the study duration. Follow-up D-dimer estimation in 14 patients showed increased levels. Thus, we conclude that the D-dimer dynamics can reflect the severity of disease and their increased levels are associated with adverse outcomes among patients with COVID-19.

Our study has some limitations. Since this was a single centered study, the results cannot be generalized. Secondly, being a retrospective study, laboratory tests of all the patients were not available, including quantitative CRP measurements, D-dimer and serum ferritin levels. Therefore, their role might have been underestimated in predicting the in-hospital deaths. Thirdly, some patients were transferred late in their illness to our hospital. Lack of early interventions and inadequate adherence to standard supportive therapy, might have also contributed to the poor clinical outcome in some patients. Fourthly, a significant number of critical patients were referred to centers due to multiple reasons. Follow up and outcome of those patients were not included in this study. Furthermore, data related to thromboembolism, which is a significant cause of COVID-19 related death, could not be investigated due to logistic limitation.

5. Conclusions

In summary, most of the COVID-19 deaths in our study were of older age, male gender and had multiple comorbidities. Hematologically, lymphocytopenia and increased neutrophil to lymphocyte ratio were found in the COVID-19 mortalities. Similarly, elevated D-dimer and ferritin at admission were risk factors for death of adult patients with COVID-19. Evaluation of these factors during admission might help us for risk assessment and early triage of potential severe COVID-19 cases so that every possible effort can be made for the prompt management of COVID-19 and avoidance of deaths.

Author Contributions: Conceptualization, A.B., S.S., R.N., B.S.C.; methodology, S.S., A.B., R.N.; validation, A.B., B.S.C.; formal analysis, A.B., S.S.; investigation, R.N., K.M.; resources, K.M., B.S., B.S.C., P.T., P.B.; data curation, S.S., A.S., P.S.; writing—original draft preparation, S.S., R.N.; writing— review and editing, A.B., S.S., R.N., B.S., K.M., B.S.C., P.B., P.T., A.S., P.S.; supervision, A.B., B.S.C.; project administration, A.B., S.S., B.S.C. All authors have read and agreed to the published version of the manuscript.

Funding: This research received no external funding.

Institutional Review Board Statement: The study was conducted according to the guidelines of the Declaration of Helsinki and approved by the Institutional Review Board (or Ethics Committee) of Nepal Health Research Council (ERB Protocol registration No. 169/2021 P).

Informed Consent Statement: Not applicable. Hospital approval was taken for acquisition of medical records for conduction of research.

Data Availability Statement: Data will be made available from the corresponding author on request.

Acknowledgments: The authors would like to thank all the staffs of Sukraraj tropical and Infectious Disease Hospital for administrative and technical supports.

Conflicts of Interest: The authors declare no conflict of interest.

References

1. Huang, C.; Wang, Y.; Li, X.; Ren, L.; Zhao, J.; Hu, Y.; Zhang, L.; Fan, G.; Xu, J.; Gu, X. Clinical features of patients infected with 2019 novel coronavirus in Wuhan, China. *Lancet* **2020**, *395*, 497–506. [CrossRef]
2. Lu, R.; Zhao, X.; Li, J.; Niu, P.; Yang, B.; Wu, H.; Wang, W.; Song, H.; Huang, B.; Zhu, N. Genomic characterisation and epidemiology of 2019 novel coronavirus: Implications for virus origins and receptor binding. *Lancet* **2020**, *395*, 565–574. [CrossRef]
3. Zhu, N.; Zhang, D.; Wang, W.; Li, X.; Yang, B.; Song, J.; Zhao, X.; Huang, B.; Shi, W.; Lu, R. A novel coronavirus from patients with pneumonia in China, 2019. *N. Engl. J. Med.* **2020**, *382*, 727–733. [CrossRef] [PubMed]
4. WHO. Coronavirus (COVID-19) Dashboard | WHO Coronavirus (COVID-19) Dashboard with Vaccination Data. Available online: https://covid19.who.int/ (accessed on 7 July 2021).
5. Bastola, A.; Sah, R.; Rodriguez-Morales, A.J.; Lal, B.K.; Jha, R.; Ojha, H.C.; Shrestha, B.; Chu, D.K.; Poon, L.L.; Costello, A. The first 2019 novel coronavirus case in Nepal. *Lancet Infect. Dis.* **2020**, *20*, 279–280. [CrossRef]
6. CoVid19-Dashboard. Available online: https://covid19.mohp.gov.np/ (accessed on 7 July 2021).
7. Jarrett, M.P.; Schultz, S.F.; Lyall, J.S.; Wang, J.J.; Stier, L.; De Geronimo, M.; Nelson, K.L. Clinical Mortality Review in a Large COVID-19 Cohort. *medRxiv* **2020**. [CrossRef]
8. Yancy, C.W. COVID-19 and african americans. *JAMA* **2020**, *323*, 1891–1892. [CrossRef] [PubMed]
9. National Institutes of Health. COVID-19 Treatment Guidelines Panel. Coronavirus Disease 2019 (COVID-19) Treatment Guidelines. Available online: https://www.covid19treatmentguidelines.nih.gov/ (accessed on 7 July 2021).
10. Du, R.-H.; Liang, L.-R.; Yang, C.-Q.; Wang, W.; Cao, T.-Z.; Li, M.; Guo, G.-Y.; Du, J.; Zheng, C.-L.; Zhu, Q. Predictors of mortality for patients with COVID-19 pneumonia caused by SARS-CoV-2: A prospective cohort study. *Eur. Respir. J.* **2020**, *55*. [CrossRef] [PubMed]
11. Yang, X.; Yu, Y.; Xu, J.; Shu, H.; Liu, H.; Wu, Y.; Zhang, L.; Yu, Z.; Fang, M.; Yu, T. Clinical course and outcomes of critically ill patients with SARS-CoV-2 pneumonia in Wuhan, China: A single-centered, retrospective, observational study. *Lancet Respir. Med.* **2020**, *8*, 475–481. [CrossRef]
12. Chen, T.; Wu, D.; Chen, H.; Yan, W.; Yang, D.; Chen, G.; Ma, K.; Xu, D.; Yu, H.; Wang, H. Clinical characteristics of 113 deceased patients with coronavirus disease 2019: Retrospective study. *BMJ* **2020**, *368*. [CrossRef] [PubMed]
13. Wang, D.; Hu, B.; Hu, C.; Zhu, F.; Liu, X.; Zhang, J.; Wang, B.; Xiang, H.; Cheng, Z.; Xiong, Y. Clinical characteristics of 138 hospitalized patients with 2019 novel Coronavirus–Infected pneumonia in Wuhan, China. *JAMA* **2020**, *323*, 1061–1069. [CrossRef] [PubMed]
14. Guihur, A.; Rebeaud, M.E.; Fauvet, B.; Tiwari, S.; Weiss, Y.G.; Goloubinoff, P. Moderate Fever Cycles as a Potential Mechanism to Protect the Respiratory System in COVID-19 Patients. *Front. Med.* **2020**, *7*. [CrossRef] [PubMed]
15. Wu, C.; Chen, X.; Cai, Y.; Zhou, X.; Xu, S.; Huang, H.; Zhang, L.; Zhou, X.; Du, C.; Zhang, Y. Risk factors associated with acute respiratory distress syndrome and death in patients with coronavirus disease 2019 pneumonia in Wuhan, China. *JAMA Intern. Med.* **2020**, *180*, 934–943. [CrossRef] [PubMed]
16. Fan, B.E. Hematologic parameters in patients with COVID-19 infection: A reply. *Am. J. Hematol.* **2020**, *95*, E215. [CrossRef] [PubMed]
17. Lippi, G.; Plebani, M.; Henry, B.M. Thrombocytopenia is associated with severe coronavirus disease 2019 (COVID-19) infections: A Meta—Analysis. *Clin. Chim. Acta* **2020**, *506*, 145–148. [CrossRef] [PubMed]
18. Li, X.; Liu, C.; Mao, Z.; Xiao, M.; Wang, L.; Qi, S.; Zhou, F. Predictive values of neutrophil-to-lymphocyte ratio on disease severity and mortality in COVID-19 patients: A systematic review and meta-analysis. *Crit. Care* **2020**, *24*, 1–10. [CrossRef] [PubMed]

19. Liu, Y.; Du, X.; Chen, J.; Jin, Y.; Peng, L.; Wang, H.H.; Luo, M.; Chen, L.; Zhao, Y. Neutrophil-to-lymphocyte ratio as an independent risk factor for mortality in hospitalized patients with COVID-19. *J. Infect.* **2020**, *81*, e6–e12. [CrossRef] [PubMed]
20. Yan, X.; Li, F.; Wang, X.; Yan, J.; Zhu, F.; Tang, S.; Deng, Y.; Wang, H.; Chen, R.; Yu, Z. Neutrophil to lymphocyte ratio as prognostic and predictive factor in patients with coronavirus disease 2019: A retrospective Cross—Sectional study. *J. Med. Virol.* **2020**, *92*, 2573–2581. [CrossRef]
21. Zhou, F.; Yu, T.; Du, R.; Fan, G.; Liu, Y.; Liu, Z.; Xiang, J.; Wang, Y.; Song, B.; Gu, X. Clinical course and risk factors for mortality of adult inpatients with COVID-19 in Wuhan, China: A retrospective cohort study. *Lancet* **2020**, *395*, 1054–1062. [CrossRef]
22. Huang, I.; Pranata, R.; Lim, M.A.; Oehadian, A.; Alisjahbana, B. C-reactive protein, procalcitonin, D-dimer, and ferritin in severe coronavirus disease-2019: A meta-analysis. *Ther. Adv. Respir. Dis.* **2020**, *14*, 1753466620937175. [CrossRef]
23. Tang, N.; Li, D.; Wang, X.; Sun, Z. Abnormal coagulation parameters are associated with poor prognosis in patients with novel coronavirus pneumonia. *J. Thromb. Haemost.* **2020**, *18*, 844–847. [CrossRef]

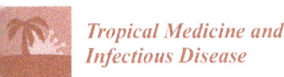

Article

Knowledge and Perceptions about COVID-19 among Health Care Workers: Evidence from COVID-19 Hospitals during the Second Pandemic Wave

Petros Ioannou [1], Stamatis Karakonstantis [1], Anna Mathioudaki [1], Angelos Sourris [1], Vasiliki Papakosta [1], Periklis Panagopoulos [2], Vasilis Petrakis [2], Dimitrios Papazoglou [2], Kostoula Arvaniti [3], Christina Maria Trakatelli [3], Evgenia Christodoulou [3], Garyfallia Poulakou [4], Konstantinos N. Syrigos [4], Vasiliki Rapti [4], Konstantinos Leontis [4], Dimitrios Karapiperis [5] and Diamantis P. Kofteridis [1,*]

1. Department of Internal Medicine and Infectious Diseases, University Hospital of Heraklion, 71110 Heraklion, Greece; p.ioannou@med.uoc.gr (P.I.); stamkar2003@gmail.com (S.K.); mathiouanna94@gmail.com (A.M.); angelosourris@gmail.com (A.S.); vasopapacosta@gmail.com (V.P.)
2. Department of Infectious Diseases, Second Department of Internal Medicine, University Hospital of Alexandroupoli, 68100 Alexandroupoli, Greece; ppanago@med.duth.gr (P.P.); vasilispetrakis1994@gmail.com (V.P.); dpapazog@med.duth.gr (D.P.)
3. Infection Control Unit, COVID-19 Coordinating Team, General Hospital Papageorgiou, 56403 Thessaloniki, Greece; arvanitik@hotmail.com (K.A.); cmtrakatelli@gmail.com (C.M.T.); eugenia1381@yahoo.gr (E.C.)
4. Third Department of Medicine, Thoracic Diseases General Hospital Sotiria, 11527 Athens, Greece; gpoulakou@gmail.com (G.P.); ksyrigos@med.uoa.gr (K.N.S.); vassiarapti@gmail.com (V.R.); kostas.leontis@hotmail.com (K.L.)
5. Department of Infectious Diseases, 424 General Military Teaching Hospital, 56429 Thessaloniki, Greece; dimkarapip@yahoo.gr
* Correspondence: kofteridisd@hotmail.com; Tel.: +302813405050

Abstract: Health care workers (HCWs) face a higher risk of infection, since they work at the front line of COVID-19 patients' management. Misinterpretations of current scientific evidence among HCWs may impact the delivery of appropriate care to COVID-19 patients and increase the risk of SARS-CoV-2 transmission in the hospital setting. Moreover, knowledge may affect HCWs perceptions depending on their broad beliefs and past experiences. The aim of this study was to explore the knowledge and perceptions of HCWs regarding COVID-19 issues during the second wave of the pandemic. A cross-sectional survey, involving a printed questionnaire, was conducted from 21 October 2020 to 31 January 2021 in four tertiary care hospitals located at four distant geographical regions in Greece. In total, 294 HCWs participated in this study. The majority of HCWs provided precise responses regarding general knowledge, perceptions, and practices concerning the COVID-19 pandemic. However, responses on hand hygiene and antimicrobial use in HCWs with COVID-19 were mistaken. This study reveals a certain degree of misconceptions and knowledge gaps in HCWs everyday practice, especially regarding hand hygiene and antimicrobial use in COVID-19 patients.

Keywords: COVID-19; SARS-CoV-2; healthcare workers; attitudes; perceptions; knowledge

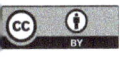

1. Introduction

Coronavirus-disease-19 (COVID-19), the disease caused by severe acute respiratory syndrome coronavirus-2 (SARS-CoV-2) has evolved into a pandemic with tremendous effects on public health, world economy, and quality of life of every individual [1]. The disease spreads from human to human primarily through droplet and direct contact and has an incubation period of 2 to 14 days [2]. Health care workers (HCWs) are in the front line of COVID-19 patients' management, thus, they are facing constantly higher risk of infection than the wider community [3]. On the other hand, COVID-19 has affected quality of life, psychological condition, and training of HCWs, as shown in recent studies [4–7]. Several recommendations have been published from national and international societies, such as the World Health Organization (WHO) regarding the prevention and control of COVID-19 for HCWs [8]. However, misunderstandings among HCWs may negatively impact the delivery of appropriate care to COVID-19 patients and increase the risk of transmission of the virus. Additionally, knowledge gaps may affect the perceptions of HCWs, certainly depending on their beliefs and past experiences [9,10]. Except of few studies performed during the first wave of the pandemic, the level and quality of knowledge and the global perceptions of HCWs regarding COVID-19 have not been extensively studied [11].

The aim of the study was to explore the knowledge and perceptions of HCWs in COVID-19 tertiary hospitals of distal geographical regions in Greece regarding COVID-19 issues during the second wave of the pandemic. In addition, we aimed to explore the beliefs and practices of HCWs concerning personal protection equipment matters.

2. Materials and Methods

2.1. Study Design

This is a cross-sectional survey conducted from 21 October 2020 to 31 January 2021 in four tertiary care COVID-19 hospitals in four metropolitan areas in Greece. All HCWs were eligible to participate.

A printed questionnaire was developed by a team of infectious disease specialists, fellows, and internists. It consisted of 36 items, including close-ended, multiple choice, and Likert-scale questions, divided as follows: 6 on demographics and practice-related information, 4 regarding knowledge on COVID-19, 7 regarding personal beliefs on COVID-19, 7 regarding infection control measures, 3 regarding daily practice for COVID-19 patients and issues, 2 regarding COVID-19 vaccination, and 7 regarding medical evidence on COVID-19. The questionnaire is available as Supplementary Material.

2.2. Participation and Ethical Approval

Participation was voluntary, anonymous, and without compensation. Invitation to participate was through direct contact with a study investigator. Informed consent was distributed concomitantly with the questionnaire. The study was approved by the Ethical Committee of the University Hospital of Heraklion.

2.3. Statistics

Descriptive statistics were performed with GraphPad Prism 6.0 (GraphPad Software, Inc., San Diego, CA, USA). Qualitative data were presented as counts and percentages. Continuous variables (age) were initially assessed for normality with the D'Agostino and Pearson omnibus normality test and were then presented as means with standard deviation, as they were normally distributed. Statistical analysis of quantitative data was performed through contingency analysis with chi-square test, while, a $p < 0.05$ was considered to be statistically significant.

3. Results

In total, 294 HCWs participated in this study. Among them, 164 (55.8%) were nurses, 114 (38.8%) medical doctors (MDs), 14 (4.8%) paramedical staff, 1 (0.3%) employee of the technical service, and 1 (0.3%) participant did not report his profession. Median age was 42 years (interquartile range: 22 to 66 years), and 103 (35%) of the participants were male. Participants' characteristics are shown in Table 1. The questionnaire used in this study is shown in Document S1.

In terms of the source of participants' information, 171 (69%) responded that the main information sources were academic journals and specialized COVID-19 websites, while 40 (16.1%) stated that their main source of information were the media. When asked about the causative agent of COVID-19, 291 (99.3%) participants stated that it is a virus. Regarding the origin of the causative agent of COVID-19, 199 (70.1%) stated it is a virus that occurred as a result of natural mutation in China, however, 76 (26.8%) answered it is a virus that was created in a Chinese laboratory. In terms of transmission, 210 (75.3%) of the responders believe COVID-19 is transmitted through aerosol, while 62 (22.2%) believe it is transmitted through droplets. When asked about the most common symptoms of COVID-19, most HCWs (252 (92.3%)) replied the disease causes fever and respiratory symptoms (Figure 1).

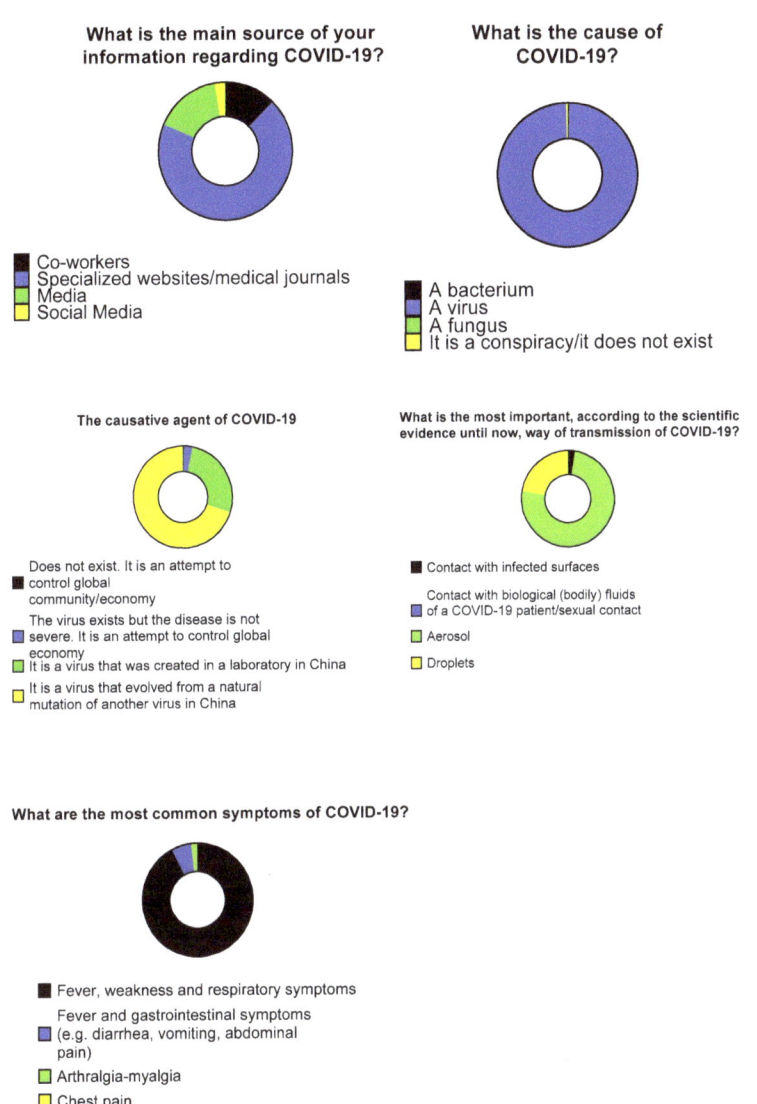

Figure 1. Knowledge of healthcare workers on COVID-19.

Among the participants HCWs, 104 (35.5%) believe the preparedness of their hospital is high, 52 (17.7%) believe it is very high, while 91 (31.1%) believe it is adequate. The majority of the responders were not significantly afraid of developing COVID-19, 97 (33.1%) and 84 (28.7%) HCWs were moderately or slightly afraid, respectively, while the rates of fear of having a close relative developing COVID-19 were 91 (31%) and 66 (22.4%), respectively. The majority of the HCWs was slightly satisfied from the personal protective equipment provided from their hospital, whereas, 89 (30.3%) and 79 (26.9%) were moderately and significantly satisfied, respectively (Figure 2).

Table 1. Participants' characteristics. NR: not reported; SD: standard deviation.

Characteristic	Value
Gender (male), n (%)	103 (35)
Age, mean (SD)	41.8 (8.6)
HCW category	
Nurse, n (%)	164 (55.8)
Medical Doctor, n (%)	114 (38.8)
Paramedical, n (%)	14 (4.8)
Technical staff, n (%)	1 (0.3)
NR, n (%)	1 (0.3)

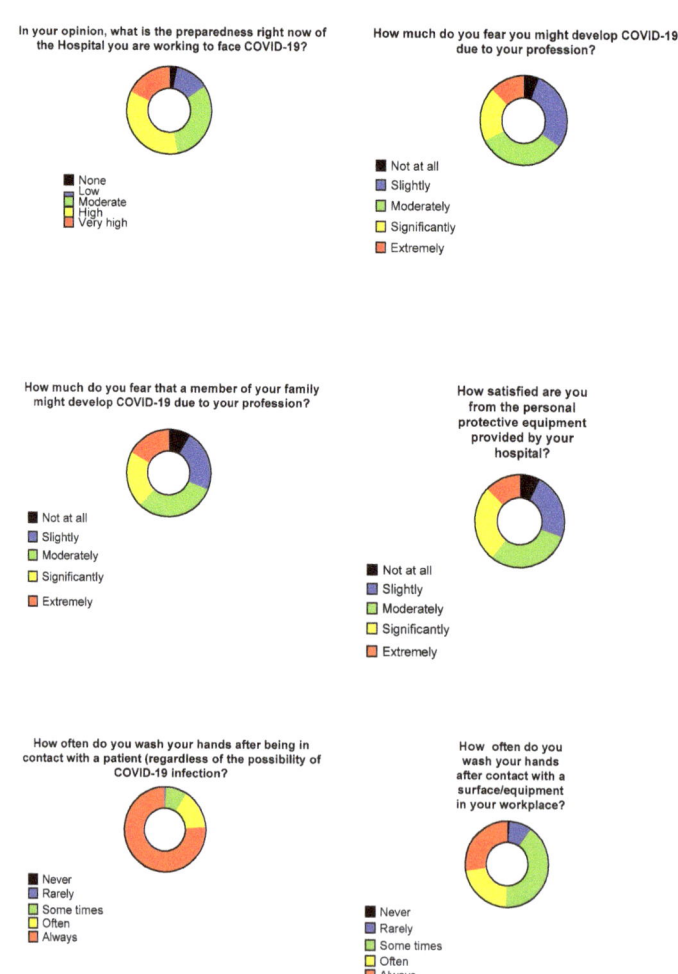

Figure 2. Personal perceptions regarding COVID-19 and hand-wash practices of healthcare workers.

The vast majority (222, 76%) of the participants stated they always perform hand hygiene after contact with a patient, regardless of COVID-19 suspicion. On the other hand, 114 (40.7%) HCWs stated they do not always perform hand hygiene after contacting a surface or equipment in their workplace (Figure 2).

Regarding knowledge on disinfection and room ventilation guidance, 246 (85.4%) responded correctly regarding the reduction in infectivity in a room with active ventilation system, while 214 (74%) responded correctly regarding the reduction in infectivity by purely fresh air ventilation. When questioned on how much aeration of closed spaces contributes to prevention of SARS-CoV-2 hospital spread, 146 (49.7%) and 88 (29.9%) thought they contribute extremely, and significantly, respectively. When asked about the most effective method of HCWs protection against COVID-19, 149 (84.7%) answered the combination of appropriate use of surgical mask and appropriate application of hand hygiene yielded the maximum protection. Twelve responders (6.8%) believed that use of higher-protection masks (FFP2/FFP3) is most important (Figure 3).

Regarding the knowledge on hand washing 80 (47.9%) HCWs responded correctly for the appropriate practice. Notably, 46 (27.5%) responders stated that hands should only be washed when visibly dirty, and an alcoholic antiseptic solution should be used in other instances. Thirty six (21.6%) HCWs stated that hand hygiene with alcoholic antiseptics should be used in every occasion instead of hand washing. In total, 216 (73.5%) HCWs answered they know the five steps of hand hygiene and they applied them all whenever indicated, while 47 (16%) stated they know them but do not always perform them due to lack of time during their daily shifts. Female HCWs replied more often that they knew the five steps and that they always applied them compared to men. HCWs stated they were performing aerosol-producing activities in patients with possible COVID-19, 62 (32.3%) among them stated they are performing such acts with adequate preventive measures, 38 (19.8%) were performing such acts and were, also, trying to avoid them, while 49 (25.5%) were trying to avoid them most of the times (Figure 3).

When asked on the duration of isolation before returning to work in the case of COVID-19 acquisition (provided no immunosuppression and not working in a department with high-risk patients), 106 (36.6%) responded that the isolation should be 7 days, while 102 (35.2%) responded that it should be 14 days. A total of 75 (25.9%) HCWs mentioned that they were not aware, but they would consult the Hospital Infection Control Committee or the Greek National Public Health Organization. More female HCWs responded that it should be 14 days, or that they should contact the Hospital Infection Control Committee or the Greek National Public Health Organization compared to men.

When asked regarding their actions after close contact with an asymptomatic COVID-19 patient (both wearing surgical masks), 115 (40.5%) responded they would consult the Hospital Infection Control Committee or the Greek National Public Health Organization, 113 (39.9%) would stay at work with appropriate personal protection equipment and 14 days maintenance of high level awareness for the development of any COVID-19 symptoms and 43 (15.1%) responded they should be isolated for 14 days along with maintaining high level 14 days awareness for the development of any COVID-19 symptoms. When asked about their intention to be vaccinated against SARS-CoV-2, 208 (71.2%) responded positively, 65 (22.3%) responded that they had not decided so far, and 19 (6.5%) responded negatively. Regarding the perceptions of the HCWs on flu vaccination, 135 (47.5%) replied it only protects from flu, 31 (10.8%) replied it also protects against COVID-19, 88 (31%) replied it should be compulsory for all HCWs, and 22 (7.7%) replied it should be compulsory for the whole population (Figure 4).

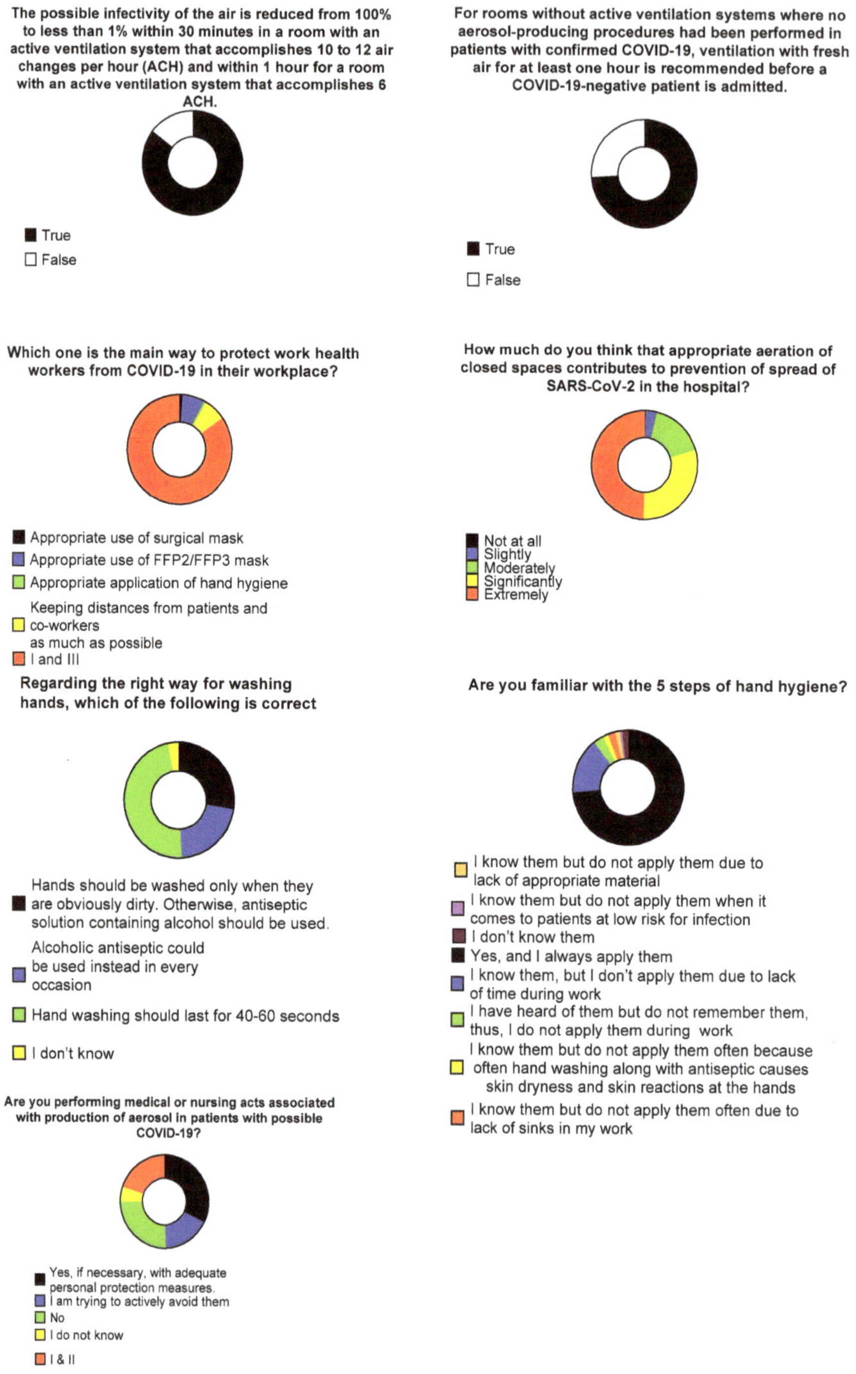

Figure 3. Healthcare workers' opinions on aeration and hand-hygiene practices.

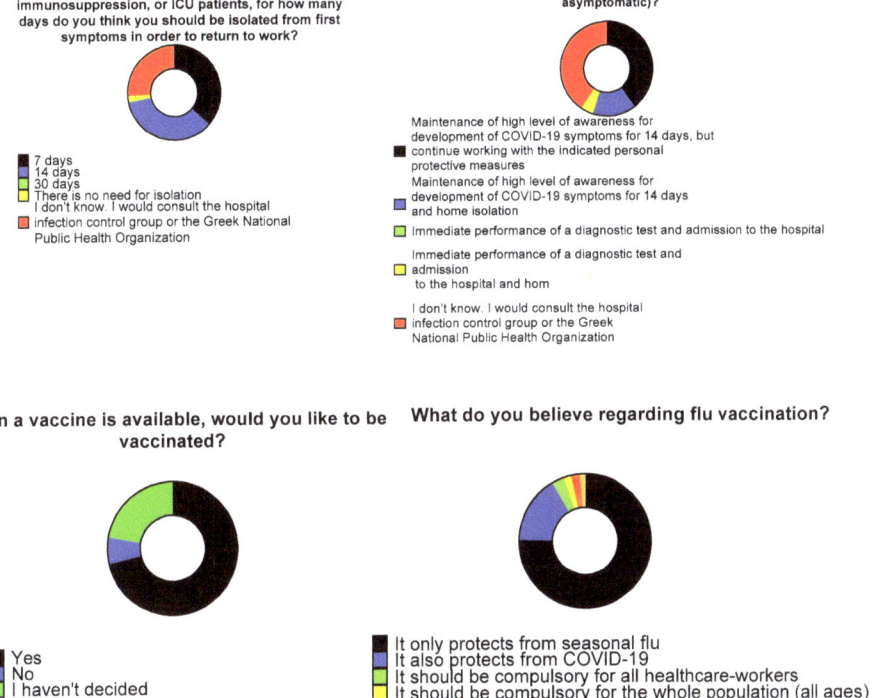

Figure 4. Healthcare workers' opinions regarding isolation and vaccination.

Among physicians, 98/114 (86%) stated their specialty, and the most common specialties were internal medicine, surgery, pulmonary medicine, and hematology in 18 (18.4%), 15 (15.3%), 11 (11.2%) and 9 (9.2%), respectively (Table S1). Overall, 50 (51.5%) physicians were attendings or consultants, and 47 (48.5%) were residents. Clinical experience was less than 5 years in 45 (44.6%), 5–10 years, and >10 years in 28 (27.7%) each. When asked about the most appropriate testing for COVID-19 diagnosis, 91 (92.9%) considered rhinopharyngeal RT-PCR as the most sensitive test, while 6 (6.1%) replied oropharyngeal RT-PCR is the most sensitive. Female HCWs were more likely to respond that oropharyngeal RT-PCR was the most sensitive. When asked about whether antimicrobials are a first line treatment for COVID-19 patients, 85 (86.7%) replied negatively and 11 (11.2%) positively. Among physicians that replied to the question whether there are specific criteria for antimicrobial prescription in COVID-19 patients, 79 (80.6%) replied positively, 9 (9.2%) negatively, and 10 (10.2%) replied they did not know. When asked regarding the most appropriate indication for starting antimicrobial treatment in COVID-19 patients, 57 (59.4%) replied all of the following are useful: procalcitonin measurement, PCR for respiratory pathogens, sputum and blood cultures, chest X-ray, and computerized tomography. Among physicians, 35 (36.1%) replied they did know what percentage of COVID-19 patients presents with co-infection by other pathogens, while 33 (34%) and 26 (28.8%), respectively, answered the percentage is 1–10% and 30–50%, respectively.

Regarding the termination of isolation for mildly symptomatic COVID-19 patients, 53 (53.5%) replied isolation should be terminated after 14 days after symptoms' initiation (along with 3 days of defervescence), while 25 (25.3%) replied isolation should be terminated 10 days post symptoms' initiation (along with 3 days of defervescence). When asked on the isolation period for asymptomatic patients, 60 (61.2%) replied isolation should be terminated after 14 days after the first positive test, while 30 (30.6%) said that isolation should be terminated after 10 days after the first positive test (Figure 5).

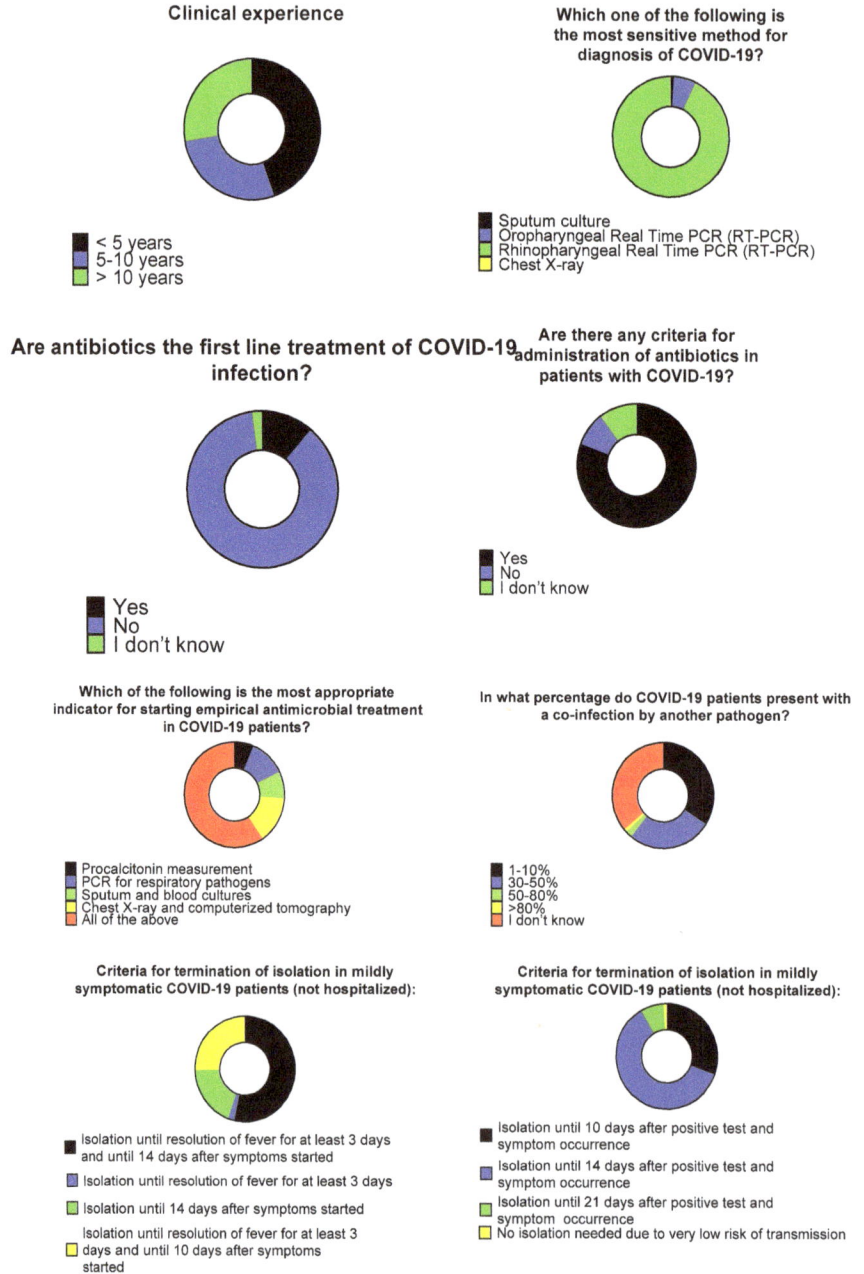

Figure 5. Medical doctors' opinions and knowledge regarding antimicrobial use and isolation.

A sub-analysis of the responses was performed in order to compare the knowledge, perceptions and attitudes among physicians and non-physicians, and revealed several differences in the responses of most of the provided questions. Physicians were more likely to be informed from specialized websites and medical journals, were more likely to believe that the virus evolved from a natural mutation of another virus in China, they were more likely to respond correctly to the questions on disinfection, they were less afraid being infected by the virus in their workspace, they were less satisfied from the protective equipment of their hospital, they were more likely to wash their hands after contact with a surface or equipment in their workplace, they were more likely to know the five steps of hand hygiene, while, on the other hand, they were more knowledgeable regarding COVID-19 symptoms and isolation guidelines. Finally, physicians had a higher intention to be vaccinated when a vaccine was available. Another sub-analysis of the data in regards to the hospital revealed that HCWs from the University Hospital of Heraklion and the General Hospital Papageorgiou of Thessaloniki were slightly less afraid of being infected, or of contracting the virus, compared to their relatives.

4. Discussion

The present study examines the perceptions, attitudes, and practices of healthcare workers related to the COVID-19 pandemic in four major COVID-19 hospitals in Greece. The study reveals some misconceptions and knowledge gaps in everyday practice that allow for further improvement, especially in terms of hand hygiene and antimicrobial use in COVID-19 patients.

In the fight against infectious diseases, knowledge, attitudes, and practices towards these diseases can be very important, since they can affect the extent of their spread, the severity of the disease, as well as, the overall mortality rates [11–13]. Thus, it is important to evaluate the knowledge, perceptions, and practices of HCWs during a pandemic, in order to recognize early any misconceptions in HCWs and elaborate targeted educational initiatives and preventive interventions [14].

Female participants were twice as male participants in this study sample, while, most participants were nurses, followed by physicians. The majority of the participants had chosen scientific websites and medical journals as their main source of information regarding COVID-19, with media being the second most prevalent source. Knowledge regarding the causal pathogen, transmissibility, and COVID-19 symptoms was adequate, with most participants replying correctly to the questions. Compared to other studies evaluating the knowledge and perceptions of HCWs on COVID-19 that were performed earlier during the pandemic, our study shows superior overall knowledge of COVID-19 transmissibility and symptoms [11,15]. Similarly to our results, a recent study that was performed in Turkey, showed adequate knowledge and correct perceptions among HCWs on COVID-19 matters in the hospital setting [16].

Interestingly, a significant proportion of HCWs doubts about the preparedness of their hospital to face COVID-19 second wave, while another significant proportion is afraid about the possibility of contracting the virus and spreading the disease to their family. This is a very important finding, since anxiety and fear of acquiring COVID-19 may affect the level of provided healthcare and contribute to reduced willingness of HCWs to accept new admissions, even though their fear was associated with appropriate infection prevention practices [17]. Furthermore, fear and anxiety, in conjunction to long working hours due to increasing demands during the COVID-19 pandemic may lead to the development of mental disorders in HCWs, such as depression, suggesting that psychosocial interventions could be developed in order to support the staff [18]. We found significant compliance to infection control measures, especially in terms of hand hygiene after contact with patients, irrespective of their COVID-19 status. On the other hand, hand hygiene was not adequately performed after a contact with the patient's surrounding environment. Misconceptions regarding the proper use of antiseptic solutions and indications for hand washing were observed in a small proportion of HCWs. This could serve as alarming issue and guide the Hospital Infection Control Committees of the participating hospitals to enhanced educational programs during the pandemic. The knowledge of HCWs regarding the hospital aeration was adequate.

Knowledge regarding isolation after exposure to a COVID-19 patient was inadequate and diverged between HCWs of the same hospital and between the participating hospitals. Interestingly, the expressed willingness for COVID-19 vaccination was around 71%, in accordance with other European studies [19,20], but was higher compared to other studies performed in healthcare professionals, that show a willingness for vaccination of about 50% [21].

Physicians, even though aware of criteria for antimicrobial prescription in COVID-19 patients, overestimated the percentage of COVID-19 patients with bacterial co-infection. As previously shown, only a minority of physicians recognized that co-infections at the time of COVID-19 diagnosis are evident in less than 10% of patients [22,23]. This could help initiate educational efforts towards antimicrobial stewardship in the pandemic era. Additionally, physicians provided diverse responses regarding the isolation guidance for patients tested positive for COVID-19, either with or without symptoms, which represents a need for focused actions towards better education, based on the local guidelines by the National Public Health Organization.

There were slight differences in the responses of male and female HCWs, with female HCWs more often stating that they know and always apply the five steps of hand hygiene, slightly more often responding that oropharyngeal RT-PCR is the most reliable means of COVID-19 diagnosis, and by supporting in a higher proportion that isolation period for HCWs exposed to SARS-CoV-2 is 14 days, or that they would consult the hospital infection control group or the Greek National Public Health Organization in the case of such exposure. This is partially in line with the literature, where female gender is associated with better hand-washing practices during the COVID-19 pandemic [24–26].

Responses from HCWs from different hospitals differed slightly, with the most obvious difference being the significantly, less fear noted in HCWs working in the University Hospital of Heraklion and the General Hospital Papageorgiou, Thessaloniki regarding the possibility of suffering from COVID-19, or contracting it to their relatives. This, suggests that, in general, there are no important specific local factors affecting knowledge and perceptions regarding COVID-19 infection, as most responses did not differ significantly. However, different levels of preparedness of different hospitals, factors regarding epidemiology and geographic distribution of COVID-19 cases in Greece or other factors may have influenced the perceived fear by HCWs of being infected by SARS-CoV-2. Thus, in areas with higher burden of COVID-19 cases, and lower preparedness due to financial or political reasons, perceived fear of exposure to SARS-CoV-2 may be higher. This suggests that targeted interventions to hospitals with higher burden of COVID-19 could positively affect the psychology and perceptions of HCWs, leading to improvement of their well-being, and, as a consequence, to an improvement in the healthcare provided. To that end, this study shows that centrally controlled initiatives (for example, directed from the Ministry of Health or the Greek National Public Health Organization) involving questionnaires like the one used in the present study, or audits, could help identify gaps in knowledge and practice of HCWs during the pandemic both in general, as well as more specific gaps that have to do with specific areas and hospitals. This more individualized approach could allow for interventions, such as educational activities towards the groups that require them the most, in order to improve infection control practices and increase knowledge regarding COVID-19. Interestingly, the less fear of being infected by SARS-CoV-2 in the hospitals of Heraklion and Thessaloniki does not correlate to the local trends of the pandemic, since, the second wave of the pandemic (during which, this study was performed), involved the northern part of Greece, including Thessaloniki [27–29].

Physicians were found in this study to be more knowledgeable regarding COVID-19, disinfection and hand-washing practices. On the other hand, they were less satisfied with the protective equipment provided by their hospital, but were also less afraid of being infected by the virus. This shows that not all HCWs share the same beliefs, or knowledge regarding COVID-19, as their education regarding healthcare in general, and COVID-19 in particular, differs. This also underlies the need for an individualized approach towards targeted interventions in order to increase awareness regarding COVID-19 and infection control practices (such as hand hygiene and disinfection). Furthermore, the increased willingness of physicians to be vaccinated suggests, as probably expected, that approval of vaccination will vary depending on the social status, the profession and other factors. This suggests that, in order to increase the approval of vaccination, HCWs and the society in general should be approached also in a structured and individualized manner, through political decisions regarding educational interventions in the workplace, media coverage, and maybe societal benefits for vaccinated individuals [30–32].

This study has limitations that should be mentioned. First, the exact number of persons asked to participate in the study could not have been recorded due to the nature of the questionnaire (paper-based), even though, it is estimated that the response rate was about 50% which is close to the rate noted in other studies [33,34]. Second, this is a study conducted in four tertiary COVID-19 hospitals, and the results cannot be generalized until additional data are collected from multiple hospital settings in other countries. Finally, the questionnaire reflects the perceptions, attitudes, and knowledge at the specific time period the study was conducted, as such, one cannot predict what the perceptions and attitudes of the HCWs would be in other instances, for example in times of COVID-19 vaccination generalization or in countries not experiencing a pandemic wave as the one we were experiencing in Greece at the time the study was performed.

5. Conclusions

To conclude, this study presented the perceptions, attitudes and practices of healthcare workers related to the COVID-19 pandemic in four COVID-19 Greek hospitals. HCWs were adequately knowledgeable regarding COVID-19 and infection control measures. Certain misconceptions and knowledge gaps in everyday practice were revealed which could promote future interventions, especially in terms of repeated education on hand hygiene and antimicrobial use in COVID-19 patients.

Supplementary Materials: The following are available online at https://www.mdpi.com/2414-6366/6/3/136/s1, Table S1: Medical doctors' specialties, Document S1: Questionnaire regarding knowledge, perceptions, and practice in regards to the COVID-19 pandemic.

Author Contributions: Conceptualization, D.P.K.; methodology, P.I., S.K., A.M. and D.P.K.; software, P.I.; validation, P.I., P.P., K.A., G.P. and D.P.K.; formal analysis, P.I.; investigation, A.M., A.S., V.P. (Vasiliki Papakosta), P.P., V.P. (Vasilis Petrakis), D.P., K.A., C.M.T., E.C., G.P., K.N.S., V.R., D.K. and K.L.; resources, D.P.K., G.P., P.P., K.A., D.K. and K.N.S.; data curation, P.I.; writing—original draft preparation, P.I., S.K. and D.P.K.; writing—review and editing, A.M., A.S., V.P. (Vasiliki Papakosta), P.P., V.P. (Vasilis Petrakis), D.P., K.A., C.M.T., E.C., G.P., K.N.S., V.R., D.K. and K.L; visualization, D.P.K.; supervision, D.P.K., P.P., K.A., G.P.; project administration, D.P.K. All authors have read and agreed to the published version of the manuscript.

Funding: This research received no external funding.

Institutional Review Board Statement: The study was conducted according to the guidelines of the Declaration of Helsinki, and approved by the Institutional Review Board of University Hospital of Heraklion (protocol code 25/07-10-2020).

Informed Consent Statement: Informed consent was obtained from all subjects involved in the study.

Data Availability Statement: The data presented in this study are available on request from the corresponding author.

Conflicts of Interest: The authors declare no conflict of interest.

References

1. Nicola, M.; Alsafi, Z.; Sohrabi, C.; Kerwan, A.; Al-Jabir, A.; Iosifidis, C.; Agha, M.; Agha, R. The socio-economic implications of the coronavirus pandemic (COVID-19): A review. *Int. J. Surg.* **2020**, *78*, 185–193. [CrossRef]
2. Backer, J.A.; Klinkenberg, D.; Wallinga, J. Incubation period of 2019 novel coronavirus (2019-nCoV) infections among travellers from Wuhan, China, 20–28 January 2020. *Eurosurveillance* **2020**, *25*, 2000062. [CrossRef] [PubMed]
3. Iversen, K.; Bundgaard, H.; Hasselbalch, R.B.; Kristensen, J.H.; Nielsen, P.B.; Pries-Heje, M.M.; Knudsen, A.D.; Christensen, C.E.; Fogh, K.; Norsk, J.B.; et al. Risk of COVID-19 in healthcare workers in Denmark: An observational cohort study. *Lancet Infect. Dis.* **2020**, *20*, 1401–1408. [CrossRef]
4. Ungureanu, B.S.; Vladut, C.; Bende, F.; Sandru, V.; Tocia, C.; Turcu-Stiolica, R.-A.; Groza, A.; Balan, G.G.; Turcu-Stiolica, A. Impact of the COVID-19 Pandemic on Health-Related Quality of Life, Anxiety, and Training Among Young Gastroenterologists in Romania. *Front. Psychol.* **2020**, *11*, 579177. [CrossRef] [PubMed]
5. Marasco, G.; Nardone, O.M.; Maida, M.; Boskoski, I.; Pastorelli, L.; Scaldaferri, F.; Italian Association of Young Gastroenterologist and Endoscopist (AGGEI). Impact of COVID-19 outbreak on clinical practice and training of young gastroenterologists: A European survey. *Dig. Liver Dis.* **2020**, *52*, 1396–1402. [CrossRef] [PubMed]
6. Anand, S.; Baishya, M.; Singh, A.; Khanna, P. Effect of awake prone positioning in COVID-19 patients—A systematic review. *Trends Anaesth. Crit. Care* **2021**, *36*, 17–22. [CrossRef]
7. Marcoux, J.T. Training Residents during the COVID-19 Pandemic. *J. Foot Ankle Surg.* **2020**, *59*, 881. [CrossRef]
8. World Health Organization 2020. [30-10-2020]. Prevention, Identification and Management of Health Worker Infection in the Context of COVID-19. Available online: https://www.who.int/publications/i/item/10665-336265 (accessed on 30 May 2021).
9. Oppenheim, B.; Lidow, N.; Ayscue, P.; Saylors, K.; Mbala, P.; Kumakamba, C.; Kleinman, M. Knowledge and beliefs about Ebola virus in a conflict-affected area: Early evidence from the North Kivu outbreak. *J. Glob. Health* **2019**, *9*, 020311. [CrossRef]
10. Vinck, P.; Pham, P.N.; Bindu, K.K.; Bedford, J.; Nilles, E. Institutional trust and misinformation in the response to the 2018–19 Ebola outbreak in North Kivu, DR Congo: A population-based survey. *Lancet Infect. Dis.* **2019**, *19*, 529–536. [CrossRef]
11. Bhagavathula, A.S.; AlDhaleei, W.A.; Rahmani, J.; Mahabadi, M.A.; Bandari, D.K. Knowledge and Perceptions of COVID-19 Among Health Care Workers: Cross-Sectional Study. *JMIR Public Health Surveill.* **2020**, *6*, e19160. [CrossRef]
12. Kim, J.-S.; Choi, J.S. Middle East respiratory syndrome-related knowledge, preventive behaviours and risk perception among nursing students during outbreak. *J. Clin. Nurs.* **2016**, *25*, 2542–2549. [CrossRef] [PubMed]
13. Khan, M.U.; Shah, S.; Ahmad, A.; Fatokun, O. Knowledge and attitude of healthcare workers about middle east respiratory syndrome in multispecialty hospitals of Qassim, Saudi Arabia. *BMC Public Health* **2014**, *14*, 1281. [CrossRef] [PubMed]
14. Al-Shammary, A.A.; Hassan, S.U.-N.; Zahra, A.; Algahtani, F.B.Z.; Suleiman, S. Role of community-based measures in adherence to self-protective behaviors during first wave of COVID-19 pandemic in Saudi Arabia. *Health Promot. Perspect.* **2021**, *11*, 69–79. [CrossRef] [PubMed]
15. Zhang, M.; Zhou, M.; Tang, F.; Wang, Y.; Nie, H.; Zhang, L.; You, G. Knowledge, attitude, and practice regarding COVID-19 among healthcare workers in Henan, China. *J. Hosp. Infect.* **2020**, *105*, 183–187. [CrossRef]
16. Arslanca, T.; Fidan, C.; Daggez, M.; Dursun, P. Knowledge, preventive behaviors and risk perception of the COVID-19 pandemic: A cross-sectional study in Turkish health care workers. *PLoS ONE* **2021**, *16*, e0250017. [CrossRef] [PubMed]
17. Apisarnthanarak, A.; Apisarnthanarak, P.; Siripraparat, C.; Saengaram, P.; Leeprechanon, N.; Weber, D.J. Impact of anxiety and fear for COVID-19 toward infection control practices among Thai healthcare workers. *Infect. Control Hosp. Epidemiol.* **2020**, *41*, 1093–1094. [CrossRef] [PubMed]
18. Krammer, S.; Augstburger, R.; Haeck, M.; Maercker, A. Adjustment Disorder, Depression, Stress Symptoms, Corona Related Anxieties and Coping Strategies during the Corona Pandemic (COVID-19) in Swiss Medical Staff. *Psychother. Psychosom. Med. Psychol.* **2020**, *70*, 272–282. [CrossRef]
19. Verger, P.; Scronias, D.; Dauby, N.; Adedzi, K.A.; Gobert, C.; Bergeat, M.; Gagneur, A.; Dubé, E. Attitudes of healthcare workers towards COVID-19 vaccination: A survey in France and French-speaking parts of Belgium and Canada, 2020. *Eurosurveillance* **2021**, *26*, 2002047. [CrossRef]
20. Gagneux-Brunon, A.; Detoc, M.; Bruel, S.; Tardy, B.; Rozaire, O.; Frappe, P.; Botelho-Nevers, E. Intention to get vaccinations against COVID-19 in French healthcare workers during the first pandemic wave: A cross-sectional survey. *J. Hosp. Infect.* **2021**, *108*, 168–173. [CrossRef]
21. Turcu-Stiolica, A.; Bogdan, M.; Subtirelu, M.-S.; Meca, A.-D.; Taerel, A.-E.; Iaru, I.; Kamusheva, M.; Petrova, G. Influence of COVID-19 on Health-Related Quality of Life and the Perception of Being Vaccinated to Prevent COVID-19: An Approach for Community Pharmacists from Romania and Bulgaria. *J. Clin. Med.* **2021**, *10*, 864. [CrossRef]
22. Langford, B.J.; So, M.; Raybardhan, S.; Leung, V.; Westwood, D.; MacFadden, D.R.; Soucy, J.-P.R.; Daneman, N. Bacterial co-infection and secondary infection in patients with COVID-19: A living rapid review and meta-analysis. *Clin. Microbiol. Infect.* **2020**, *26*, 1622–1629. [CrossRef]
23. Lansbury, L.; Lim, B.; Baskaran, V.; Lim, W.S. Co-infections in people with COVID-19: A systematic review and meta-analysis. *J. Infect.* **2020**, *81*, 266–275. [CrossRef] [PubMed]
24. Czeisler, M.É.; Garcia-Williams, A.G.; Molinari, N.-A.; Gharpure, R.; Li, Y.; Barrett, C.E.; Robbins, R.; Facer-Childs, E.R.; Barger, L.K.; Czeisler, C.A.; et al. Demographic Characteristics, Experiences, and Beliefs Associated with Hand Hygiene Among Adults during the COVID-19 Pandemic—United States, June 24–30, 2020. *MMWR Morb. Mortal. Wkly. Rep.* **2020**, *69*, 1485–1491. [CrossRef]

25. Guzek, D.; Skolmowska, D.; Głąbska, D. Analysis of Gender-Dependent Personal Protective Behaviors in a National Sample: Polish Adolescents' COVID-19 Experience (PLACE-19) Study. *Int. J. Environ. Res. Public Health* **2020**, *17*, 5770. [CrossRef] [PubMed]
26. Sax, H.; Uçkay, I.; Richet, H.; Allegranzi, B.; Pittet, D. Determinants of Good Adherence to Hand Hygiene among Healthcare Workers Who Have Extensive Exposure to Hand Hygiene Campaigns. *Infect. Control Hosp. Epidemiol.* **2007**, *28*, 1267–1274. [CrossRef]
27. Nørgaard, S.K.; Vestergaard, L.S.; Nielsen, J.; Richter, L.; Schmid, D.; Bustos, N.; Braye, T.; Athanasiadou, M.; Lytras, T.; Denissov, G.; et al. Real-time monitoring shows substantial excess all-cause mortality during second wave of COVID-19 in Europe, October to December 2020. *Eurosurveillance* **2021**, *26*, 2002023. [CrossRef] [PubMed]
28. Siettos, C.; Anastassopoulou, C.; Tsiamis, C.; Vrioni, G.; Tsakris, A. A bulletin from Greece: A health system under the pressure of the second COVID-19 wave. *Pathog. Glob. Health* **2021**, *115*, 133–134. [CrossRef] [PubMed]
29. Post, L.; Culler, K.; Moss, C.B.; Murphy, R.L.; Achenbach, C.J.; Ison, M.G.; Resnick, D.; Singh, L.N.; White, J.; Boctor, M.J.; et al. Surveillance of the Second Wave of COVID-19 in Europe: Longitudinal Trend Analyses. *JMIR Public Health Surveill.* **2021**, *7*, e25695. [CrossRef] [PubMed]
30. Lang, R.; Benham, J.L.; Atabati, O.; Hollis, A.; Tombe, T.; Shaffer, B.; Burns, K.K.; MacKean, G.; Léveillé, T.; McCormack, B.; et al. Attitudes, behaviours and barriers to public health measures for COVID-19: A survey to inform public health messaging. *BMC Public Health* **2021**, *21*, 1–15. [CrossRef]
31. McKee, M.; Rajan, S. What can we learn from Israel's rapid roll out of COVID 19 vaccination? *Isr. J. Health Policy Res.* **2021**, *10*, 1–4. [CrossRef]
32. Wake, A.D. The Willingness to Receive COVID-19 Vaccine and Its Associated Factors: "Vaccination Refusal Could Prolong the War of This Pandemic"—A Systematic Review. *Risk Manag. Healthc. Policy* **2021**, *14*, 2609–2623. [CrossRef] [PubMed]
33. Spernovasilis, N.; Ierodiakonou, D.; Spanias, C.; Mathioudaki, A.; Ioannou, P.; Petrakis, E.; Kofteridis, D. Doctors' Perceptions, Attitudes and Practices towards the Management of Multidrug-Resistant Organism Infections after the Implementation of an Antimicrobial Stewardship Programme during the COVID-19 Pandemic. *Trop. Med. Infect. Dis.* **2021**, *6*, 20. [CrossRef] [PubMed]
34. Perozziello, A.; Lescure, F.X.; Truel, A.; Routelous, C.; Vaillant, L.; Yazdanpanah, Y.; Lucet, J.C.; CEFECA Study Group; Liem-Binh, L.N.; Bruno, M.; et al. Prescribers' experience and opinions on antimicrobial stewardship programmes in hospitals: A French nationwide survey. *J. Antimicrob. Chemother.* **2019**, *74*, 2451–2458. [CrossRef] [PubMed]

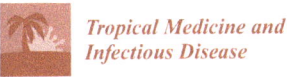

Communication

High Effectiveness of SARS-CoV-2 Vaccines in Reducing COVID-19-Related Deaths in over 75-Year-Olds, Ceará State, Brazil

Carlos Henrique Alencar [1,2,*], Luciano Pamplona de Góes Cavalcanti [1,2,3], Magda Moura de Almeida [1,4], Patrícia Pereira Lima Barbosa [1], Kellyn Kessiene de Sousa Cavalcante [1,4], Déborah Nunes de Melo [1], Bruno Cavalcante Fales de Brito Alves [3] and Jorg Heukelbach [1]

1. School of Medicine, Post Graduate Program in Public Health, Federal University of Ceará, Fortaleza 60430-140, Brazil; pamplona.luciano@gmail.com (L.P.G.C.); magda.almeida.mfc@gmail.com (M.M.A.); patricialima18@yahoo.com.br (P.P.L.B.); kellynveterinaria@hotmail.com (K.K.S.C.); deborahnmb@gmail.com (D.N.M.); heukelbach@web.de (J.H.)
2. School of Medicine, Post Graduate Program in Pathology, Federal University of Ceará, Fortaleza 60411-750, Brazil
3. Christus University Center, Fortaleza 60190-180, Brazil; brunocafa@gmail.com
4. Health Secretariat of Ceará State, Fortaleza 60060-440, Brazil
* Correspondence: carllosalencar@ufc.br; Tel.: +55-85-3366-8045

Abstract: In Brazil, the SARS-CoV-2 vaccination program has so far prioritized people over 75 years of age. By the end of March 2021, in Ceará State, a total of 313,328 elderly people had received at least one dose of vaccine (45% Oxford-AstraZeneca/Fiocruz and 55% CoronaVac-Sinovac/Butantan), and 159,970 had received two doses (83% CoronaVac-Sinovac/Butantan and 17% Oxford-AstraZeneca/Fiocruz). After a single dose, there was already a significant reduction in COVID 19-related deaths (protection ratio: 19.31 (95% CI: 18.20–20.48), attributable protection ratio: 94.8%); higher protection ratios were observed after the application of two doses of the vaccine (132.67; 95% CI: 109.88–160.18), with an attributable protection ratio of 99.2%. SARS-CoV-2 vaccines are highly effective in reducing the number of COVID-19-related deaths in over 75-year-olds in Brazil, one of the hardest hit countries by the current pandemic.

Keywords: COVID-19; SARS-CoV-2; COVID-19 vaccines; mortality; epidemiology; public health

1. Introduction

SARS-CoV-2 vaccines can reduce disease occurrence and transmission in a population. This is essential to reduce both morbidity and mortality from SARS-CoV-2 [1]. Consequently, there is a need for evidence on the effectiveness of vaccines to protect not only against SARS-CoV-2 symptoms but also to reduce COVID-19-related case fatality rates [2]. However, the reduction in the occurrence of severe disease and death is difficult to evaluate in phase 3 clinical trials, mainly due to the high number of participants required [1]. Thus, the effectiveness of SARS-CoV-2 vaccines in relation to case fatality has to be inferred from other sources of data, such as mortality statistics [3].

In Brazil, by the end of June 2021, more than 18.5 million cases and more than 500,000 deaths were confirmed, with a case fatality rate of 2.8% [4]. The state of Ceará, with a population of 8.8 million, was one of the first Brazilian states to confirm sustained transmission of COVID-19 in 2020 [5]. Despite the rapid implementation of control measures, Ceará stands out with more than 880,000 cases and almost 22,500 deaths by the end of June 2021 [4]. The case fatality rate was 2.5%, and there was a high rate of hospital bed occupancy (>90%), while different strains of SARS-CoV-2 were circulating [5].

A recent case-control study in England, including almost 160,000 adults aged over 70 years, evidenced a significant reduction in symptomatic COVID-19 cases and severe symptoms after a single dose of the Oxford-AstraZeneca vaccine [6]. A recent study with Brazilian data showed an association between the rapid increase in vaccination coverage of the older population and relative mortality, as compared to younger individuals, in a setting where the gamma variant was predominant, and the most widely used vaccine was CoronaVac-Sinovac/Butantan [7]. The Brazilian Ministry of Health has made available both vaccines from Oxford-AstraZeneca/Fiocruz and CoronaVac-Sinovac/Butantan. In Ceará, by May 2021, more than 1.7 million people had taken at least one dose of a vaccine, with more than 500 thousand people having received two doses [8]. In this study, we evaluated the hypothesis that COVID-19 vaccinations had a considerable impact on reducing the number of deaths due to COVID-19 in the state of Ceará, Northeast Brazil, in the year 2021.

2. Materials and Methods

People aged 75 years or older were included since this age group was prioritized by the Brazilian Immunization Program and, thus, had a higher proportion of vaccination coverage at the beginning of the campaign. For the year 2021, the estimated population in this age group was 354,269 people (IBGE—Brazilian Institute of Geography and Statistics/*Instituto Brasileiro de Geografia e Estatística*).

We used data from the National Mortality System (SIM) and from the Immunization Program (SIPNI), between 17 January and 11 May 2021. The SIM database records all deaths that occur in Brazil. We selected death records with COVID-19 as the underlying cause of death. The SIPNI aims to coordinate immunization actions throughout Brazil, and records the immunobiological doses applied. The number of unvaccinated people was calculated as the difference between the estimated population and the number of vaccinated individuals. We included only individuals who had received at least one COVID-19 vaccine application. After removing duplicates, the databases were probabilistically related by means of people's names (*soundex*) and respective dates of birth, using Stata 15.1 software. The outcome was defined as people who died 21 days or later after the first dose of vaccine. We stratified the vaccinated population by number of doses, vaccine type and age group, and calculated the proportion of deaths as well as the protection ratio for deaths and percentage attributable protection ratio for deaths, and their respective 95% confidence intervals. All data in this study were extracted from secondary databases. The use of data was authorized by the Secretary of Health of the State of Ceará. As the study consisted of an analysis of secondary data, no informed consent was sought.

3. Results

A total of 313,328 elderly people (88.4% of the total population > 75 years) had received at least one dose of a vaccine, 44.5% from Oxford-AstraZeneca/Fiocruz and 55.5% from CoronaVac. A total of 159,970 had received two doses, 83.0% from CoronaVac-Sinovac/Butantan and 17.0% from Oxford-AstraZeneca/Fiocruz. The occurrence of deaths among the unvaccinated elderly was more than 132 times higher, as compared to those who had received two doses of a vaccine, with a protection ratio for deaths of 99.2%. After a single dose of a vaccine, the protection ratio was 19.3 (Table 1). The effect was more pronounced with increasing age.

Table 1. Protection ratios for death and percentage attributable protection ratios for deaths by COVID-19, stratified by number of doses applied, vaccine type and age group over 75 year-olds in the state of Ceará, Brazil, 2021.

Variables	N	Deaths	% Deaths	Protection Ratio (95% CI)	Attributable Protection Ratio (%) (95%CI)
Number of doses and type of vaccine:					
Oxford-AstraZeneca/Fiocruz 1st dose	139,322	716	0.51	17.91 (16.55–19.39)	94.4 (93.9–94.8)
CoronaVac-Sinovac/Butantan 1st dose	174,006	778	0.45	20.59 (19.07–22.22)	95.1 (94.7–95.5)
Vaccinated 1st dose	313,328	1494	0.48	19.31 (18.20–20.48)	94.8 (94.5–95.1)
Oxford-AstraZeneca/Fiocruz 1st and 2nd dose	27,193	3	0.01	834.45 (269.03–2588.18)	99.8 (99.6–99.9)
CoronaVac-Sinovac/Butantan 1st and 2nd dose	132,777	108	0.08	113.17 (93.50–136.99)	99.1 (98.9–99.3)
Vaccinated 1st and 2nd dose	159,970	111	0.07	132.67 (109.88–160.18)	99.2 (99.1–99.4)
Not vaccinated	40,941	3769	9.21	1	-
Age Group–1st dose only:					
75 to 79 years					
Oxford-AstraZeneca/Fiocruz	32,749	141	0.43	8.39 (7.03–10.00)	88.0 (85.8–90.0)
CoronaVac-Sinovac/Butantan	97,072	481	0.50	7.29 (6.54–8.12)	86.3 (84.7–87.7)
Vaccinated	129,821	622	0.48	7.53 (6.82–8.33)	86.7 (85.3–88.0)
Not vaccinated	26,857	1010	3.76	1	-
80 to 89 years					
Oxford-AstraZeneca/Fiocruz	78,474	371	0.47	31.89 (28.59–35.58)	96.8 (96.5–97.2)
CoronaVac-Sinovac/Butantan	70,327	256	0.36	41.42 (36.42–47.12)	97.6 (97.2–97.9)
Vaccinated	148,801	627	0.42	35.78 (32.77–39.07)	97.2 (96.9–97.4)
Not vaccinated	13,336	2011	15.08	1	-
90 years or more					
Oxford-AstraZeneca/Fiocruz	28,099	204	0.73	137.74 (120.13–157.92)	99.2 (99.1–99.4)
CoronaVac-Sinovac/Butantan	6,607	41	0.62	161.14 (118.76–218.64)	99.3 (99.1–99.5)
Vaccinated	34,706	245	0.71	141.65 (125.04–160.48)	99.3 (99.2–99.4)
Not vaccinated	748	748	100.00	1	-

4. Discussion

Our data showed an impressive reduction in COVID-19-related deaths in older age groups in Ceará State, which is the population strata at highest risk for severe disease and death. Previous studies have shown that, by May 2021, more than 40,000 deaths had been prevented due to vaccination of the elderly population in Brazil with the Oxford-AstraZeneca and CoronaVac-Sinovac/Butantan vaccines [7]. Similar findings were found in the US after use of the first dose of Pfizer-BioNTech, particularly in older adults [9]. A study in Tennessee/USA showed a reduction of more than 95% in mortality in the vaccinated elderly population between December 2020 and March 2021 [10].

Considering the difficulties in the vaccine supply chain and their availability, it is important that the vaccines from both major producers showed a high effectiveness in reducing COVID-19-related deaths, even after a single dose. Furthermore, as predicted by Bolcato et al. in 2020, there may be problems that occur, such as insufficient production of vaccine doses for the entire population, or with different vaccination strategies and different times between doses, generating the need for difficult prioritization decisions [11]. In this context, the ability of a vaccine to protect against serious illness and death should be considered the most important outcome, since hospital admissions, especially in intensive care units, represent the greatest burden on health systems and has led several countries to face a collapse in their health systems. The global crisis generated by the coronavirus pandemic highlighted, once again, the importance of vaccination programs as effective public health measures, and brought about new mechanisms that may become models for future responses to regional epidemics and pandemics, with a greater variety of platforms and joint work to overcome challenges and accelerate vaccine development, manufacturing and delivery [12]. It is worth noting that the duration of protection after recovery from COVID-19 corresponds somewhat to the duration of protection provided by the vaccine [13].

For Hodgson et al. (2021), the beneficial effects of a vaccine can be assessed if the vaccine is effective in older adults and if there is a wide distribution of the vaccine [1]. The evaluation of asymptomatic SARS-CoV-2 infection is an important clinical outcome in the evaluation of vaccines, but is certainly of less public health importance than its effectiveness against death. In Italy, for example, the number of infections in nursing homes was particularly high, with a high mortality rate. Yet it must be recognized that the current situation of social disparity does not facilitate equal opportunities for all. As a result, the elderly will continue to experience moments of loneliness, despite efforts to reduce them [14].

Equal access to COVID-19 vaccines in all countries will continue to be a goal to be pursued. But the experience of previous pandemics suggests that access will be limited in low and middle income countries, despite the rapid development of some new candidate vaccines. Thus, the WHO proposal, with the COVAX Facility program, represents an attempt to facilitate multilateral cooperation to procure and distribute two billion doses of COVID-19 vaccines equitably in all countries of the world by the end of 2021 [15].

Our study is subject to some limitations, such as the use of secondary mortality data that may be subject to some errors. The smaller number of second doses by AstraZeneca in our study is basically due to the longer period between the two doses and, therefore, the population had not yet received the second dose during the study period. We also observed that the population of people vaccinated in the age group over 90 years was higher than the estimated population for this age group, this fact is due to the last census being conducted in 2010. We used the population projection for the year 2021, but there was still a difference of 1900 more people vaccinated in the population over 90 years of age. The estimated population was adjusted to the vaccinated population and, thus, data should be interpreted with care. Data on the antibody response of vaccinated individuals were not available, which may limit interpretation of results. However, we obtained population-based data from a population with a high vaccination coverage, and the study results can, thus, be considered as robust and valid.

5. Conclusions

SARS-CoV-2 vaccines are highly effective in reducing the number of COVID-19-related deaths in over 75 year-olds in Brazil, one of the hardest hit countries by the current pandemic.

Author Contributions: Conceptualization, C.H.A., L.P.G.C. and J.H.; methodology, C.H.A. and J.H.; formal analysis, C.H.A.; writing—original draft preparation, C.H.A., L.P.G.C. and J.H.; writing—review and editing, C.H.A., L.P.G.C., M.M.A., P.P.L.B., K.K.S.C., D.N.M., B.C.F.B.A. and J.H. All authors have read and agreed to the published version of the manuscript. C.H.A., L.P.G.C. and J.H. contributed equally.

Funding: This research did not receive external funding.

Informed Consent Statement: Patient consent was waived due to the research being conducted with secondary data from the immunization and mortality information systems. We obtained a declaration from the Ethical Review Board of the Federal University of Ceará (Fortaleza, Brazil) exempting us from the need for ethical clearance for this study. This exemption from ethical clearance is based on Brazilian laws: Law No. 12,527 of 18 November 2011 and National Health Council (CNS) Resolution No. 510 of 7 April 2016.

Data Availability Statement: The data presented in this study are publicly available in: https://integrasus.saude.ce.gov.br/#/indicadores/indicadores-coronavirus/indice-transparencia (accessed on 13 July 2021).

Acknowledgments: L.P.G.C. and J.H. are research fellows at the Conselho Nacional de Desenvolvimento Científico e Tecnológico (CNPq/Brazil).

Conflicts of Interest: The authors declare no conflict of interest.

References

1. Hodgson, S.H.; Mansatta, K.; Mallett, G.; Harris, V.; Emary, K.R.; Pollard, A.J. What defines an efficacious COVID-19 vaccine? A review of the challenges assessing the clinical efficacy of vaccines against SARS-CoV-2. *Lancet Infect. Dis.* **2021**, *21*, e26–e35. [CrossRef]
2. Cook, T.; Roberts, J. Impact of vaccination by priority group on UK deaths, hospital admissions and intensive care admissions from COVID-19. *Anaesthesia* **2021**, *76*, 608–616. [CrossRef] [PubMed]
3. Gee, J. First month of COVID-19 vaccine safety monitoring—United States, 14 December 2020–13 January 2021. *MMWR Morb. Mortal. Wkly. Rep.* **2021**, *70*. [CrossRef] [PubMed]
4. Brasil. COVID19—Painel Coronavírus 2021. Available online: https://covid.saude.gov.br (accessed on 29 June 2021).
5. Lemos, D.R.Q.; D'angelo, S.M.; Farias, L.A.B.G.; Almeida, M.M.; Gomes, R.G.; Pinto, G.P.; Cavalcante Filho, J.N.; Feijão, L.X.; Cardoso, A.R.P.; Lima, T.B.R. Health system collapse 45 days after the detection of COVID-19 in Ceará, Northeast Brazil: A preliminary analysis. *Rev. Soc. Bras. Med. Trop.* **2020**, *53*, e20200354. [CrossRef] [PubMed]
6. Lopez Bernal, J.; Andrews, N.; Gower, C.; Robertson, C.; Stowe, J.; Tessier, E.; Simmons, R.; Cottrell, S.; Roberts, R.; O'Doherty, M.; et al. Effectiveness of the Pfizer-BioNTech and Oxford-AstraZeneca vaccines on covid-19 related symptoms, hospital admissions, and mortality in older adults in England: Test negative case-control study. *BMJ* **2021**, *373*, n1088. [CrossRef] [PubMed]
7. Victora, C.; Castro, M.C.; Gurzenda, S.; de Medeiros, A.C.; França, G.; Barros, A.J.D. Estimating the early impact of vaccination against COVID-19 on deaths among elderly people in Brazil: Analyses of routinely-collected data on vaccine coverage and mortality. *medRxiv* **2021**, *2021*. [CrossRef]
8. Ceará. Painel de Transparência—Vacinômetro Covid Ceará: Secretaria de Saúde do Estado do Ceará. 2021. Available online: https://integrasus.saude.ce.gov.br/#/indicadores/indicadores-coronavirus/vacinometro-covid (accessed on 25 June 2021).
9. Christie, A.; Henley, S.J.; Mattocks, L.; Fernando, R.; Lansky, A.; Ahmad, F.B.; Adjemian, J.; Anderson, R.N.; Binder, A.M.; Carey, K.; et al. Decreases in COVID-19 Cases, Emergency Department Visits, Hospital Admissions, and Deaths Among Older Adults Following the Introduction of COVID-19 Vaccine—United States, 6 September 2020–1 May 2021. *MMWR Morb. Mortal. Wkly. Rep.* **2021**, *70*, 858–864. [CrossRef] [PubMed]
10. Roghani, A. The Influence of Covid-19 Vaccine on Daily Cases, Hospitalization, and Death Rate in Tennessee: A Case Study in the United States. *medRxiv* **2021**, *2021*. [CrossRef]
11. Bolcato, M.; Aurilio, M.T.; Aprile, A.; Di Mizio, G.; Della Pietra, B.; Feola, A. Take-Home Messages from the COVID-19 Pandemic: Strengths and Pitfalls of the Italian National Health Service from a Medico-Legal Point of View. *Healthcare* **2021**, *9*, 17. [CrossRef] [PubMed]
12. Pagliusi, S.; Hayman, B.; Jarrett, S. Vaccines for a healthy future: 21st DCVMN Annual General Meeting 2020 report. *Vaccine* **2021**, *39*, 2479–2488. [CrossRef] [PubMed]

13. Voysey, M.; Clemens, S.A.C.; Madhi, S.A.; Weckx, L.Y.; Folegatti, P.M.; Aley, P.K.; Angus, B.; Baillie, V.L.; Barnabas, S.L.; Bhorat, Q.E. Safety and efficacy of the ChAdOx1 nCoV-19 vaccine (AZD1222) against SARS-CoV-2: An interim analysis of four randomised controlled trials in Brazil, South Africa, and the UK. *Lancet* **2021**, *397*, 99–111. [CrossRef]
14. Bolcato, M.; Trabucco Aurilio, M.; Di Mizio, G.; Piccioni, A.; Feola, A.; Bonsignore, A.; Tettamanti, C.; Ciliberti, R.; Rodriguez, D.; Aprile, A. The Difficult Balance between Ensuring the Right of Nursing Home Residents to Communication and Their Safety. *Int. J. Environ. Res. Public Health* **2021**, *18*, 2484. [CrossRef] [PubMed]
15. Eccleston-Turner, M.; Upton, H. International Collaboration to Ensure Equitable Access to Vaccines for COVID-19: The ACT-Accelerator and the COVAX Facility. *Milbank Q.* **2021**. [CrossRef] [PubMed]

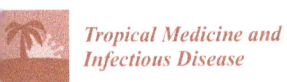

Article

Persistent Symptoms in Post-COVID-19 Patients Attending Follow-Up OPD at Sukraraj Tropical and Infectious Disease Hospital (STIDH), Kathmandu, Nepal

Anup Bastola [1], Richa Nepal [2,*], Bikesh Shrestha [2], Kijan Maharjan [2], Sanjay Shrestha [2], Bimal Sharma Chalise [2] and Jenish Neupane [2]

1 Department of Tropical Medicine, Sukraraj Tropical and Infectious Disease Hospital, Teku, Kathmandu 44600, Nepal; docanup11@gmail.com
2 Department of Internal Medicine, Sukraraj Tropical and Infectious Disease Hospital, Teku, Kathmandu 44600, Nepal; Bkeshshrestha4@gmail.com (B.S.); Kijan1069@gmail.com (K.M.); Shrestha834@gmail.com (S.S.); bschalise@gmail.com (B.S.C.); drneupanejenish@gmail.com (J.N.)
* Correspondence: nepaldeepika123@gmail.com; Tel.: +977-9860236283

Abstract: The long-term effects of COVID-19 among survivors is a matter of concern. This research aimed to study persistent symptoms in post-COVID-19 patients attending a follow-up clinic at a tertiary care hospital in Nepal. All patients, presenting to the outpatient clinic during the study duration of six weeks, with history of positive reverse transcriptase- polymerase chain reaction for severe acute respiratory syndrome-coronavirus-2 (SARS-CoV-2) at least two weeks prior to presentation, were included. The duration of follow-up ranged from 15 till 150 days with the mean duration of 28 days after diagnosis of COVID-19. Of 118 patients, 43 (36.4%) had a history of mild COVID-19, 15 (12.8%) had moderate, and 60 (50.8%) had severe. At the time of presentation, 97 (82.2%) patients reported that they had at least one persistent/new symptom beyond two weeks from the diagnosis of COVID-19. Dyspnea, fatigue, chest heaviness, and cough were the commonest persistent complaints in 48 (40.7%), 39 (33.1%), 33 (28%), and 32 (27.1%) patients, respectively. The findings in our study highlight the need for extended monitoring of post-COVID-19 patients following discharge, in order to understand and mitigate long-term implications of the disease.

Keywords: COVID-19; Nepal; post-acute COVID-19 syndrome

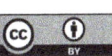

1. Introduction

More than a year after reporting Coronavirus Disease-2019 (COVID-19) for the first time in China, the disease is unrelenting, with more than 147 million cases and 3.1 million deaths worldwide, as of 28 April 2021 [1]. Persistent/new symptoms following convalescence of the clinical disease and/or microbiological recovery have been observed in a large fraction of COVID-19 patients [2]. To date, there is no clear consensus on the definition of such a group of patients. Long COVID, long haul COVID, chronic COVID syndrome, post-COVID-19 syndrome, and post-acute COVID-19 are the different terminologies currently in use for the condition characterized by the persistence of symptoms beyond the acute phase of COVID-19 [3].

Post-COVID-19 patients continue to have persistent symptoms or may have new symptoms following apparent clinical recovery as a result of the consequences of organ damage during acute COVID-19 infection, neurobehavioral abnormalities due to the disease process or hospital admission and intensive care strategies. A perplexing finding noted by physicians in several parts of the world was the prevalence of long COVID unrelated to severity of illness of COVID-19, unlike other diseases, where rigorous intensive care strategies in severely ill patients were associated with long-term health implications in survivors [4].

There have been unprecedented efforts from the scientific community worldwide for the diagnosis, treatment, and prevention of COVID-19; however, little has been done to address the potential long-term health implications for more than 95% COVID-19 patients who have recovered from this novel disease worldwide. Signs and symptoms that fail to return to a healthy baseline status beyond two weeks from the disease onset could be considered to a long-term effect of COVID-19 in apparently recovered post-COVID-19 patients [5]. This research aims to study persistent or new symptoms in post-COVID-19 patients presenting to a tertiary level infectious disease hospital in central Nepal.

2. Materials and Methods

2.1. Study Design and Settings

This was a descriptive, cross-sectional study conducted among post-COVID-19 patients who had presented to the follow-up outpatient department of a central level infectious disease government hospital, Sukraraj Tropical and Infectious Disease Hospital (STIDH) in Kathmandu, the capital city of Nepal. All patients diagnosed with COVID-19 by positive real time polymerase chain reaction (RT-PCR) for SARS-CoV-2, at least two weeks prior to presentation, were included in our study. Data collection was done over the period of six weeks from 1 March 2021 to 14 April 2021. All patients who had been in home isolation or were discharged following hospital admission from STIDH or from any other hospital during their acute COVID-19 illness were included in this study.

2.2. Data Collection

Data collection was done through a face-to-face interview by using a standardized structured questionnaire after consent for voluntary participation was obtained. History taking and relevant clinical examination were done by two experienced attending physicians. Patients were asked to answer Yes/No questions for the symptoms related to post-COVID pathology. Data related to course of COVID-19 illness and index admission were collected retrospectively from the patients, and by reviewing past medical records/discharge sheets brought by patients in the follow-up OPD. Cronbach's alpha was computed for reliability analysis of the questionnaire using responses from the first fifty consecutive participants. The value was calculated as 0.84 and found to be acceptable.

Patients were asked to report newly occurring or persistent symptoms, or any other symptom worse than before COVID-19 development. The symptoms that did not return to baseline and lasted for more than two weeks following diagnosis of COVID-19 were labeled as persistent symptoms and those symptoms that appeared after two weeks of diagnosis of COVID-19, and were not attributed to other diseases, were labeled as new symptoms in post-COVID-19 patients. Dyspnea/shortness of breath, fatigue, chest heaviness, cough, chest pain, palpitations, anosmia/hyposmia, ageusia/hypogeusia, decreased appetite, headache, and throat discomfort were the persistent symptoms reported by post-COVID-19 patients in our study. Likewise, insomnia, anxiety, hot flushes, parosmia, burning sensation along limbs, impaired concentration, and burning sensation in the perinostrillar area were the new symptoms reported by post-COVID-19 patients in our study. Level of dyspnea/shortness of breath were defined in terms of the Modified Medical Research Council (MMRC) dyspnea scale, where higher scores corresponded to increased level of dyspnea.

2.3. Data Analysis

Data was entered in Microsoft Excel and then analyzed with a statistical package for social sciences (SPSS) version 25. Descriptive analyses were done using frequencies and percentages for categorical variables, and means and standard deviation for continuous variables. Bivariate analysis was done using Chi square and Fisher's exact test, where appropriate. p value < 0.05 was considered to be significant.

3. Results

Out of 118 patients enrolled in our study, 81 (68.6%) were males and 37 (31.4%) were females with the male: female ratio of approximately 2.2:1. The mean age of presentation was 49.7 ± 15.01 years with minimum age of 25 years and maximum age of 87 years. Thirty-four (28.8%) patients were aged 60 and above, whereas the majority of patients in our study were in the age group 30 to 59 years (64.4%). The most common comorbidity among post-COVID-19 patients who had presented to the follow-up OPD in our study was hypertension (24.6%), followed by diabetes mellitus (14.4%), and chronic respiratory diseases (7.6%). Sixty-three (53.4%) patients did not have any comorbidities in our study. The duration of follow-up of post-COVID-19 patients ranged from 15 to 150 days with mean duration of 28 days (S.D—17.5 days) after diagnosis. More than two-third of the total patients (66.9%) had their first follow-up within three to four weeks of diagnosis of COVID-19, 25 (21.2%) patients presented within five to six weeks, nine (7.6%) patients presented within seven to eight weeks, three (2.5%) patients presented within nine to twelve weeks, and two (1.7%) patients presented after three months of diagnosis of COVID-19 (Table 1).

Table 1. Baseline characteristics of post-COVID-19 patients presenting to follow-up OPD at STIDH (N-118).

Baseline Characteristics		Frequency n (%)
Gender	Male	81 (68.6)
	Female	37 (31.4)
Age group	less than 30 years	8 (6.8)
	30 to 59 years	76 (64.4)
	60 to 74 years	26 (22)
	75 years and above	8 (6.8)
Comorbidities	Hypertension	29 (24.6)
	Diabetes mellitus	17 (14.4)
	Chronic respiratory diseases	9 (7.6)
	Heart disease	6 (5.1)
	Hypothyroidism	8 (6.8)
	Psychiatric illness	5 (4.2)
	Cerebrovascular disease	1 (0.8)
	Seizure disorder	1 (0.8)
	Rheumatoid arthritis	1 (0.8)
	None	63 (53.4)
Time since diagnosis of COVID-19 at first-follow up	3 to 4 weeks	79 (66.9)
	5 to 6 weeks	25 (21.2)
	7 to 8 weeks	9 (7.6)
	9 to 12 weeks	3 (2.5)
	More than 12 weeks	2 (1.7)

Table 2 enlists the symptoms during the acute phase of COVID-19 illness, as reported by the study participants in the follow-up OPD of STIDH. The most common symptoms were fever (74.6%), myalgia (74.6%), cough (73.7%), and dyspnea (60.2%). Anosmia/hyposmia and ageusia/dysgeusia were reported by 49.2% and 45.8% patients, respectively. forty-three (36.4%) patients had mild COVID-19, 15 (12.8%) had moderate COVID-19, and 60 (50.8%) had severe COVID-19 in our study. Out of the total number of patients, 34 (28.8%) were admitted to the ward and 38 (32.2%) to intensive care units during the acute phase of COVID-19 infection (Table 3). The mean duration of hospital admission for patients who got admitted was 9.43 ± 5.76 days with minimum duration of one day and maximum duration of 33 days.

Table 2. Symptomatology during COVID-19 illness of post-COVID patients presenting to follow-up OPD at STIDH (N-118).

Symptoms	Frequency n (%)
Fever	88 (74.6)
Myalgia/Body ache	88 (74.6)
Cough	87 (73.7)
Shortness of breath	71 (60.2)
Anosmia/Hyposmia	58 (49.2)
Ageusia/Dysgeusia	54 (45.8)
Headache	50 (42.4)
Chest pain	38 (32.2)
Decreased appetite	37 (31.4)
Diarrhoea	34 (28.8)
Sore throat	30 (25.4)
Runny nose	24 (20.3)
Nausea/Vomiting	17 (14.4)
Dizziness	14 (11.9)
Abdominal pain	7 (5.9)
Hemoptysis	3 (2.5)

At the time of presentation of the first follow-up at STIDH OPD, 97 (82.2%) patients had reported that they had at least one persistent/new symptom beyond two weeks from diagnosis of COVID-19 infection (Figure 1). Twenty-three (19.5%) patients had one symptom, 52 (44.1%) had two to four symptoms, and 22 (18.6%) had five or more symptoms at their first follow-up visit. Twenty-one (17.8%) patients did not have any complaint during their follow-up visit at STIDH (Figure 2). Table 4 enlists the symptoms that were persistent/had newly emerged following acute disease in the post-COVID-19 patients in our study. Dyspnea, fatigue, chest heaviness, and cough were the commonest complaints present in 48 (40.7%), 39 (33.1%), 33 (28%), and 32 (27.1%) patients, respectively. Insomnia and anxiety was present in 19 (16.1%) and 16 (13.6%) post-COVID patients. Anosmia/hyposmia was persistent in 11 (9.3%) and ageusia/hypogeusia was persistent in 8 (6.8%) patients during their first follow-up visit (Table 4).

Out of 48 patients in our study who reported dyspnea to be persistent at their first follow-up visit, 29 (24.6%) had MMRC 1 symptoms, 14 (11.9%) had MMRC 2 symptoms, 5 (4.2%) had MMRC 3 symptoms, and none had MMRC 4 symptoms. Resting hypoxia (room air oxygen saturation less than 94%) was recorded in 24 (20.33%) patients, out of which 15 (12.7%) had mild hypoxia (oxygen saturation 90 to 93%), 3 (2.5%) had moderate hypoxia (oxygen saturation 85 to 89%), and 6 (5.1%) had severe hypoxia (oxygen saturation less than 85%). Sixteen (13.6%) patients who had resting hypoxia were using domiciliary oxygen therapy at home, though intermittently (Table 5).

Table 3. Course of COVID-19 illness in post-COVID patients presenting to follow-up OPD at STIDH (N-118).

Course of COVID-19 Illness		Frequency n (%)
Severity of COVID-19	Mild	43 (36.4)
	Moderate	15 (12.8)
	Severe	60 (50.8)
Mode of isolation during COVID-19	Home	46 (39)
	Ward admission	34 (28.8)
	ICU admission	38 (32.2)
Duration of hospital admission	None	46 (39)
	less than one week	20 (16.9)
	one to two weeks	43 (36.4)
	three to four weeks	6 (5.1)
	more than four weeks	3 (2.5)
Highest oxygen delivery device used during hospital stay	None	58 (49.2)
	Nasal cannula	44 (37.3)
	Face mask	9 (7.6)
	Non- invasive ventilation	7 (5.9)
	Invasive ventilation	0 (0)
Use of COVID-19 specific medications during hospital stay	Oral or intravenous steroids	65 (55.5)
	Remdesivir	68 (57.6)
	Convalescent plasma therapy	14 (11.9)

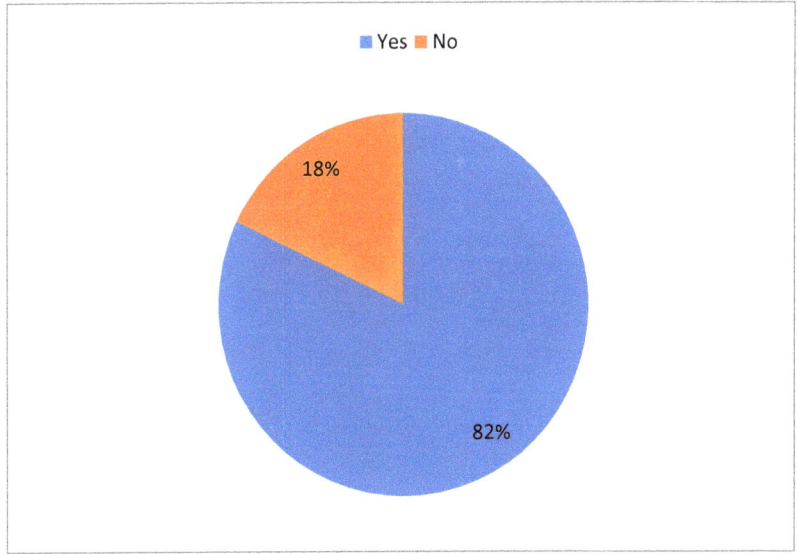

Figure 1. Distribution of post-COVID patients with at least one persistent/new symptom over two weeks after acute COVID-19 infection (N-118).

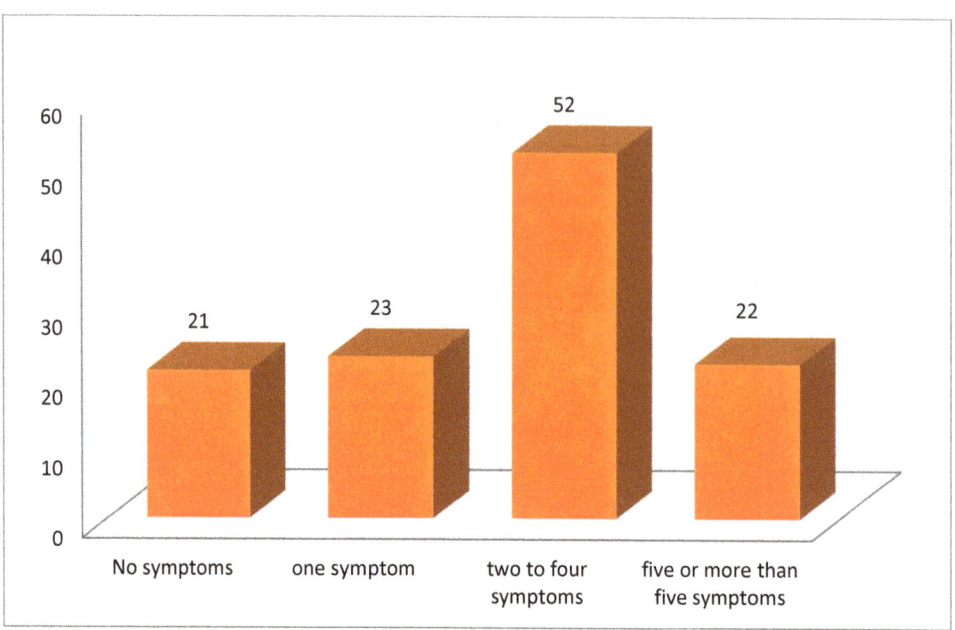

Figure 2. Distribution of post-COVID patients with the number of persistent/new symptoms during their first follow-up visit (N-118).

Table 4. Persistent/new symptoms in post-COVID-19 patients presenting to follow-up OPD at STIDH (N-118).

Symptoms	Frequency n (%)
Shortness of breath	48 (40.7)
Fatigue	39 (33.1)
Chest heaviness	33 (28.0)
Cough	32 (27.1)
Chest pain	23 (19.4)
Insomnia	19 (16.1)
Anxiety	16 (13.6)
Anosmia/Hyposmia	11 (9.3)
Palpitations	11 (9.3)
Ageusia/Hypogeusia	8 (6.8)
Decreased appetite	7 (5.9)
Headache	4 (3.3)
Throat discomfort	3 (2.5)
Burning sensation along limbs	3 (2.5)
Impaired concentration	2 (1.7)
Hot flushes	1 (0.8)
Parosmia	1 (0.8)
Burning sensation in the perinostrillar area	1 (0.8)

Table 5. Oxygenation status of post-COVID-19 patients presenting to follow-up OPD at STIDH (N-118).

Oxygenation Related Parameters		Frequency n (%)
Grade of dyspnea during first follow-up	MMRC 0	70 (59.3)
	MMRC 1	29 (24.6)
	MMRC 2	14 (11.9)
	MMRC 3	5 (4.2)
	MMRC 4	0 (0)
Use of domiciliary oxygen during the first follow-up visit	Yes	16 (13.6)
	No	102 (86.4)
Oxygen saturation at rest during the first follow-up visit	≥94%	94 (79.7)
	90 to 93%	15 (12.7)
	85 to 89%	3 (2.5)
	80 to 84%	4 (3.4)
	75 to 79%	2 (1.7)

On bivariate analysis of the presence of at least one persistent/new symptom in post-COVID-19 patients to some pertinent baseline characteristics, no significant association was demonstrated with age groups, gender, presence of any comorbidity, or severity of acute COVID-19 illness (p value- 0.177, 0.463, 0.919, and 0.056, respectively). However, the presence of at least one persistent/new symptom in post-COVID-19 patients was significantly associated to mode of isolation during their acute COVID-19 illness (p value 0.040) (Table 6).

Table 6. Association of the presence of at least one persistent/new symptom in post-COVID-19 patients with baseline characteristics (N-118).

		Presence of at Least One Persistent/New Symptom in Post-COVID Patients		p Value
		Yes	No	
Gender	Male	68	13	0.463
	Female	29	8	
Age groups	Less than 30 years	7	2	0.177
	30 to 59 years	58	17	
	60 to 74 years	23	2	
	More than 75 years	9	0	
At least one comorbidity	Yes	45	10	0.919
	No	52	11	
Severity of COVID-19	Mild	31	12	0.056
	Moderate	12	3	
	Severe	54	6	
Mode of isolation	Home	34	12	0.040 *
	Ward	27	7	
	ICU	36	2	

* p value < 0.05.

4. Discussion

As the COVID-19 pandemic continues unabated, a vast majority of survivors have presented to healthcare providers with a multitude of signs and symptoms representing possible long-term effects following acute COVID-19 infection [6]. With the persistence of debilitating complaints by the survivors of previous coronavirus infections like Severe Acute Respiratory Syndrome (SARS) in 2003 and Middle East Respiratory Syndrome (MERS) in 2012, the current concern regarding long haulers of COVID-19 seems justified [7]. In a systematic review on the long-term effects of COVID-19 by Leon et al., 80% post-COVID-19 patients (95% confidence interval 65–92%) continue to have one or more symptoms following two weeks of acute COVID-19 infection [5]. Another study by Morin et al. reported that 51% patients had at least one symptom after four months of diagnosis of COVID-19 in a cohort of 478 hospitalized patients [8]. Similarly, in a review by Pavli et al., the incidence of post-COVID syndrome was estimated to be 10 to 35% among patients who were treated on an outpatient basis, and reached 85% among patients who were hospitalized [9]. In our study, around 82.2% patients, with a recent history of confirmed COVID-19 infection, continue to have at least one persistent/new symptom beyond two weeks of diagnosis.

Shortness of breath was the commonest complaint reported by 40.7% patients at mean follow-up duration of 28 days in our study. In a study done in Italy by Carfi et al., fatigue (53.1%) and dyspnea (43.4%) were the commonest complaints of post-COVID-19 patients at mean follow-up duration of 60 days [10]. Persistent dyspnea could result due to the underlying pathology of impaired diffusion capacity, impaired respiratory muscle strength, and fibrotic abnormalities in post-COVID lungs, which were more frequently encountered in severe forms of COVID-19 following convalescence [11]. Another study from China reported fatigue (63%) and sleep disturbances (26%) to be persistent among post-COVID-19 patients at the median duration of six months from the disease onset [12]. Our study reported fatigue in 33.1% patients, whereas insomnia and anxiety were persistent in 16.1% and 13.6% patients during their first follow-up visit following COVID-19. Post viral fatigue has been postulated to result from immune dysregulation and autonomic alterations following COVID-19 infection [13]. Psychological effects following recovery from acute COVID-19 illness could result due to direct viral effects on cognition or may result from the social circumstances related to disease like loss of loved ones, spanning fears about future, job loss, anticipation anxiety, lockdown, and intensive care strategies following which the patient survived [14].

Neurological symptoms like anosmia/hyposmia and ageusia/dysgeusia were found to be persistent in 9.3% and 6.8% patients at their first follow-up visit. One patient reported perception of foul smell and altered smell pattern suggestive of parosmia even after three months of mild COVID-19 infection. Post-infectious olfactory dysfunction in form of misperception of existing odors has been previously reported as a delayed complication following COVID-19 [15]. Similarly, another patient reported a new onset of burning sensation and lancating pain at the left perinostrillar and maxillary area eight weeks following recovery from mild COVID-19 infection, suggestive of left-sided trigeminal neuralgia. The existence of trigeminal neuralgia in relation to SARS-CoV-2 has been recently described in the literature as one of the uncommon manifestations of COVID-19 [16]. Two (1.7%) patients complained of impaired concentration following COVID-19, of which one was below 30 years of age who did not require hospital admission and the other was above 75 years of age, treated in an intensive care unit. 'Brain fog' is a colloquial term being used to describe the cognitive difficulties faced by a large group of patients following COVID-19. Neuroinflammation, resulting from the pathogenic and stress stimuli, is the proposed mechanism for this condition, though concrete evidence is yet to be seen [17].

Around two-third (65.3%) of total patients said that they did not feel as normal as before the diagnosis at mean duration of 28 days following COVID-19 infection. Eighteen percent of the total patients reported more than four persistent symptoms during their follow-up visit at STIDH. An important finding in our study was that the presence of at least one persistent/new symptom in post-COVID-19 patients did not correlate with age groups, gender, comorbidities, or severity of COVID-19. Similar findings were also mentioned by Rio et al., who stated that long COVID symptoms did not correlate with chronic comorbidities or severity of acute COVID-19 illness. [18]. Likewise, Terfonde et al. stressed on the persistence of symptoms in younger group of patients without any comorbid conditions, such that could result in a prolonged road to recovery to usual state of health, leading to absenteeism from work and poor quality of life [19]. Significant association was demonstrated between the presence of at least one persistent/new symptom in post-COVID-19 patients to mode of isolation (Table 6), whereby patients who were treated in an intensive care unit had higher chances of getting at least one prolonged symptom beyond two weeks from diagnosis of COVID-19. Post intensive care syndrome is a well-defined morbid entity, which has been described in patients after discharge from an intensive care unit following severe illnesses. However, post-COVID syndrome has been described not only in patients who were discharged from intensive care but also in those that did not seek medical help and recovered at home [18]. Thus, our finding regarding the association of mode of isolation to persistence of post-COVID symptoms needs further evaluation.

The emergence of multiple variants of SARS-CoV-2 in recent times is a matter of grave concern that raises the question of a possible escape from vaccine-induced immunity and could be a major driving force for perpetuality of the current pandemic. Healthcare workers need to be aware of the persistence of multitude of symptoms in COVID-19 patients post discharge, and ways to mitigate it. The physical and psychological burden on survivors of this novel disease is yet to be addressed in a holistic way. Despite the fact that the scientific community is still in search for a breakthrough to save lives during the acute phase of the disease, the post-COVID morbidity of millions cannot be ignored. This study addresses the post-COVID symptomatology in one of the tertiary care centers in Nepal and represents data from low- and middle-income countries in South Asia. With a third wave of COVID-19 looming round the corner in South Asia, more studies need to be planned to investigate the long-term consequences of COVID-19.

This was a single-centered study and had a small sample size. Larger studies need to be conducted to know the actual burden of persistent symptoms in post-COVID-19 patients. An important point of consideration is that this was a hospital-based study; thus, the actual prevalence of post-COVID-19 symptoms might have been overestimated. A single follow-up visit was only considered in this study. Longer duration of follow-up is warranted to study the evolution of persistent symptoms in post-COVID-19 patients.

5. Conclusions

This study concluded that there was a high prevalence of persistent symptoms in post-COVID-19 patients. Post-COVID-19 symptoms had no association with age group, gender, presence of any comorbidity, or severity of disease. Healthcare workers need to acknowledge this fact and be aware of the long haulers of COVID-19 so that necessary therapeutic and rehabilitative services can be offered to such groups of patients. Our findings highlight the need for long-term monitoring of COVID-19 patients post convalescence, to understand the implications and consequences of persistent symptoms in the well-being of these apparently recovered COVID-19 patients.

Author Contributions: Conceptualization, A.B.; methodology, R.N.; software, B.S.; validation, A.B., R.N.; formal analysis, K.M; investigation, S.S.; resources, R.N. and J.N.; data curation, B.S. and K.M.; writing—original draft preparation, R.N.; writing—review and editing, A.B.; visualization, J.N. and S.S.; supervision, B.S.C. All authors have read and agreed to the published version of the manuscript.

Funding: This research received no external funding.

Institutional Review Board Statement: The study was conducted according to the guidelines of the Declaration of Helsinki, and approved by the Ethical Review Board of Nepal Health Research Council (Reference number: 2235/date of approval 23-02-2021).

Informed Consent Statement: Written informed consent has been obtained from the patients to publish this paper.

Data Availability Statement: The datasets supporting the conclusions have been included in this article. Source data can be made available on request by the corresponding author.

Conflicts of Interest: The authors declare no conflict of interest.

References

1. World Health Organization. WHO Coronavirus (COVID-19) Dashboard [Internet]. 2021. Available online: https://covid19.who.int/ (accessed on 28 April 2021).
2. Higgins, V.; Sohaei, D.; Diamandis, E.P.; Prassas, I. COVID-19: From3 an acute to chronic disease? Potential long-term health consequences. *Crit. Rev. Clin. Lab. Sci.* **2020**, 1–23. [CrossRef] [PubMed]
3. Baig, A.M. Chronic COVID Syndrome: Need for an appropriate medical terminology for Long-COVID and COVID Long-Haulers. *J. Med. Virol.* **2020**. [CrossRef] [PubMed]
4. Rubin, R. As their numbers grow, COVID-19 "long haulers" stump experts. *JAMA* **2020**, *324*, 1381–1383. [CrossRef] [PubMed]
5. Lopez-Leon, S.; Wegman-Ostrosky, T.; Perelman, C.; Sepulveda, R.; Rebolledo, P.A.; Cuapio, A.; Villapol, S. More than 50 Long-Term Effects of COVID-19: A Systematic Review and Meta-Analysis. Available at SSRN 3769978. 1 January 2021. Available online: https://dx.doi.org/10.2139/ssrn.3769978 (accessed on 29 April 2021).
6. Meagher, T. Long COVID-An Early Perspective. *J. Insur. Med.* **2021**, *49*, 19–23. [CrossRef] [PubMed]
7. Ahmed, H.; Patel, K.; Greenwood, D.C.; Halpin, S.; Lewthwaite, P.; Salawu, A.; Eyre, L.; Breen, A.; O'Connor, R.; Jones, A.; et al. Long-term clinical outcomes in survivors of severe acute respiratory syndrome (SARS) and Middle East respiratory syndrome (MERS) coronavirus outbreaks after hospitalisation or ICU admission: A systematic review and meta-analysis. *J. Rehabil. Med.* **2020**, *52*, 1–11. [CrossRef]
8. Morin, L.; Savale, L.; Pham, T.; Colle, R.; Figueiredo, S.; Harrois, A.; Gasnier, M.; Lecoq, A.L.; Meyrignac, O.; Noel, N.; et al. Four-month clinical status of a cohort of patients after hospitalization for COVID-19. *JAMA* **2021**, *325*, 1525–1534. [CrossRef] [PubMed]
9. Pavli, A.; Theodoridou, M.; Maltezou, H.C. Post-COVID syndrome: Incidence, clinical spectrum, and challenges for primary healthcare professionals. *Arch. Med. Res.* **2021**. [CrossRef] [PubMed]
10. Carfì, A.; Bernabei, R.; Landi, F. Persistent symptoms in patients after acute COVID-19. *JAMA* **2020**, *324*, 603–605. [CrossRef] [PubMed]
11. Huang, Y.; Tan, C.; Wu, J.; Chen, M.; Wang, Z.; Luo, L.; Zhou, X.; Liu, X.; Huang, X.; Yuan, S.; et al. Impact of coronavirus disease 2019 on pulmonary function in early convalescence phase. *Respir. Res.* **2020**, *21*, 1–10. [CrossRef] [PubMed]
12. Huang, C.; Huang, L.; Wang, Y.; Li, X.; Ren, L.; Gu, X.; Kang, L.; Guo, L.; Liu, M.; Zhou, X.; et al. 6-month consequences of COVID-19 in patients discharged from hospital: A cohort study. *Lancet* **2021**. [CrossRef]
13. Simani, L.; Ramezani, M.; Darazam, I.A.; Sagharichi, M.; Aalipour, M.A.; Ghorbani, F.; Pakdaman, H. Prevalence and correlates of chronic fatigue syndrome and post-traumatic stress disorder after the outbreak of the COVID-19. *J. Neurovirology* **2021**, *27*, 154–159. [CrossRef]
14. Mendelson, M.; Nel, J.; Blumberg, L.; Madhi, S.A.; Dryden, M.; Stevens, W.; Venter, F.W. Long-COVID: An evolving problem with an extensive impact. *SAMJ S. Afr. Med. J.* **2021**, *111*, 10–12. [CrossRef]
15. Duyan, M.; Ozturan, I.U.; Altas, M. Delayed Parosmia Following SARS-CoV-2 Infection: A Rare Late Complication of COVID-19. *SN Compr. Clin. Med.* **2021**, *3*, 1200–1202. [CrossRef] [PubMed]
16. Molina-Gil, J.; González-Fernández, L.; García-Cabo, C. Trigeminal neuralgia as the sole neurological manifestation of COVID-19: A case report. *Headache J. Head Face Pain* **2021**, *61*, 560–562. [CrossRef] [PubMed]
17. Theoharides, T.C.; Cholevas, C.; Polyzoidis, K.; Politis, A. Long-COVID syndrome-associated brain fog and chemofog: Luteolin to the rescue. *BioFactors* **2021**, *47*, 232–241. [CrossRef] [PubMed]
18. Del Rio, C.; Collins, L.F.; Malani, P. Long-term health consequences of COVID-19. *JAMA* **2020**, *324*, 1723–1724. [CrossRef] [PubMed]
19. Tenforde, M.W.; Kim, S.S.; Lindsell, C.J.; Rose, E.B.; Shapiro, N.I.; Files, D.C.; Gibbs, K.W.; Erickson, H.L.; Steingrub, J.S.; Smithline, H.A.; et al. Symptom duration and risk factors for delayed return to usual health among outpatients with COVID-19 in a multistate health care systems network—United States, March–June 2020. *Morb. Mortal. Wkly. Rep.* **2020**, *69*, 993. [CrossRef] [PubMed]

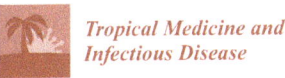

Perspective

Real-Time Operational Research: Case Studies from the Field of Tuberculosis and Lessons Learnt

Anthony D. Harries [1,2,*], Pruthu Thekkur [1,3], Irene Mbithi [4], Jeremiah Muhwa Chakaya [4,5,6], Hannock Tweya [7], Kudakwashe C. Takarinda [8], Ajay M. V. Kumar [1,3,9], Srinath Satyanarayana [1,3], Selma Dar Berger [1], I. D. Rusen [10], Mohammed Khogali [11] and Rony Zachariah [11]

1. International Union against Tuberculosis and Lung Disease (The Union), 75006 Paris, France; Pruthu.TK@theunion.org (P.T.); akumar@theunion.org (A.M.V.K.); SSrinath@theunion.org (S.S.); sberger@theunion.org (S.D.B.)
2. Department of Clinical Research, Faculty of Infectious and Tropical Diseases, London School of Hygiene and Tropical Medicine, London WC1E 7HT, UK
3. The Union South-East Asia Office, C-6 Qutub Institutional Area, New Delhi 110016, India
4. Respiratory Society of Kenya, Regent Court, Nairobi P.O. Box 27789-00506, Kenya; imbithi@resok.org (I.M.); Jeremiah.Muhwa@lstmed.uk (J.M.C.)
5. Department of Medicine, Therapeutics and Dermatology, Kenyatta University, Nairobi P.O. Box 43844-00100, Kenya
6. Department of Clinical Sciences, Liverpool School of Tropical Medicine, Liverpool L3 5QA, UK
7. The Lighthouse, Kamuzu Central Hospital, Lilongwe P.O. Box 106, Malawi; htweya@lighthouse.org.mw
8. AIDS and TB Department, Ministry of Health and Child Care, Causeway, Harare P.O. Box CY 1122, Zimbabwe; kctakarinda@gmail.com
9. Yenepoya Medical College, Yenepoya (Deemed to be University), Mangalore 575018, India
10. Vital Strategies, New York, NY 10005, USA; irusen@vitalstrategies.org
11. Special Programme for Research and Training in Tropical Disease (TDR), World Health Organization, 1211 Geneva 27, Switzerland; khogalim@who.int (M.K.); zachariahr@who.int (R.Z.)
* Correspondence: adharries@theunion.org; Tel.: +44-(0)-1962-714-297

Abstract: Real-time operational research can be defined as research on strategies or interventions to assess if they are feasible, working as planned, scalable and effective. The research involves primary data collection, periodic analysis during the conduct of the study and dissemination of the findings to policy makers for timely action. This paper aims to illustrate the use of real-time operational research and discuss how to make it happen. Four case studies are presented from the field of tuberculosis. These include (i) mis-registration of recurrent tuberculosis in Malawi; (ii) HIV testing and adjunctive cotrimoxazole to reduce mortality in TB patients in Malawi; (iii) screening TB patients for diabetes mellitus in India; and (iv) mitigating the impact of COVID-19 on TB case detection in capital cities in Kenya, Malawi and Zimbabwe. The important ingredients of real-time operational research are sound ethics; relevant research; adherence to international standards of conducting and reporting on research; consideration of comparison groups; timely data collection; dissemination to key stakeholders; capacity building; and funding. Operational research can improve the delivery of established health interventions and ensure the deployment of new interventions as they become available, irrespective of diseases. This is particularly important when public health emergencies, including pandemics, threaten health services.

Keywords: operational research; real-time operational research; tuberculosis; COVID-19; ethics; research capacity building; Malawi; Kenya; Zimbabwe; India

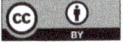

1. Introduction

Over the years, the terms "operational research", "operations research", "implementation research", "health systems research" and "health services research" have been used interchangeably to describe research conducted in health programmes using routinely collected data to try and effect change in policy and/or practice. Ask 20 operational research scientists to define what is meant by these types of research, and the likelihood is that you will get 20 different answers.

As a group working both independently and together over 30 years in health programmes in low- and middle-income countries, we have proposed a pragmatic definition of operational research: "the search for knowledge on interventions, strategies or tools that can enhance the quality, effectiveness, or coverage of programmes in which the research is being conducted" [1].

The premise that underpins this type of research is that we routinely collect mounds of data from all levels of the health system. These data can include daily out-patient attendances, daily in-patient admissions and discharges, data about patient screening, diagnostic services, enrolment to care, treatment outcomes and so on. The data are usually collected and collated as aggregate numbers in paper-based reports or electronic data sets and, more often than not, are stored away as reports in shelves or databases and rarely used after that. Operational research seeks to utilise these data, transform the data into useful information about how the health system works and use that evidence for decision making to improve public health, be it at the local, national or international level [2,3].

The operational research that we most frequently see being done uses secondary data that have been routinely collected over months or years and are used to produce information and evidence about disease control programmes, health services or health systems. However, operational research can be carried out using primary data. We would regard this as real-time operational research and define it more comprehensively as "any operational research involving primary data collection, periodic analysis and interpretation at regular intervals during the conduct of the study and dissemination of findings to policy makers for timely action." This type of research is more labour intensive and demanding than research using previously available records. However, it is key to the effective implementation of proven interventions and to show how new products (for example, vaccines, diagnostics and treatments) can be introduced and deployed, ensuring they are available to everyone who needs them. Real-time operational research is not an academic exercise, but rather a formal evaluation of public health practice that needs to be firmly integrated and embedded within health service delivery.

This paper aims to illustrate the use and effectiveness of real-time operational research. Specific objectives are to: (i) focus on tuberculosis (TB) and show how four real-time operational research studies were conducted in Africa and Asia, with the findings leading to important changes in policy and practice; and (ii) consider and discuss how to make real-time operational research happen on the ground and be effective.

2. Four Case Studies of Real-Time Operational Research on TB

2.1. Incorrect Registration of New and Recurrent TB in Malawi

In 1999, the National TB Programme (NTP) in Malawi became concerned about the declining numbers of patients registered nationally as 'recurrent TB'. The country was in the midst of amid a catastrophic human immunodeficiency virus (HIV) epidemic, and previous clinical studies done throughout sub-Saharan Africa had shown that HIV was strongly associated with recurrent TB [4–7]. The declining numbers of patients with recurrent TB in Malawi did not make sense, and the NTP was concerned that patients with recurrent TB were being misregistered as having new TB. A real-time operational research project was started after receiving ethics approval from the Malawi National Health Science Research Committee.

All 43 hospitals in the country that registered and treated TB patients were visited in each of the three regions over a few months during the NTP routine supervision schedules. All patients in the hospital registered with new TB were interviewed using a structured questionnaire, and they were asked whether they had ever had previous TB and treatment: if this was the case, the patient was recorded as having recurrent TB. Wherever possible, affirmative patient responses were verified using out-patient identity cards of previous TB treatment. At the end of each regional supervision, the data were analysed and discussed before moving to the next region to see if the simple protocol should be continued to be used or changed—in the event, no changes were made. The key findings at the end of the study are shown in Table 1 [8].

Table 1. Recurrent tuberculosis in patients registered in Malawi as having "new" tuberculosis.

Characteristics	Registered as New TB	Found to Have Had Previous (Recurrent) TB		OR (95% CI)	p-Value
	N	n	(%)		
All types of TB	1254	94	(7.5)		
Smear-Positive PTB	746	34	(4.6)	Ref	
Smear-Negative PTB	282	40	(14.2)	3.5 (2.1–5.7)	<0.001
Extrapulmonary TB	226	20	(8.8)	2.0 (1.1–3.7)	<0.05

TB = tuberculosis; PTB = pulmonary tuberculosis; OR = odds ratio; CI = confidence interval. Adapted from [8].

The study confirmed the NTP hypothesis that a substantial number of patients with recurrent TB were misregistered as having new TB. The mistake was significantly more common in patients with smear-negative pulmonary TB (PTB) and extrapulmonary TB than those with smear-positive PTB. This had important programmatic implications. First, not only were patients being misregistered in the country, but this incorrect information was being transmitted to the World Health Organization (WHO) and published in the annual WHO Global TB Reports. Second, anti-TB treatment at that time was different for new and recurrent TB patients, so some patients were incorrectly treated.

The NTP acted swiftly and decisively. Within three months, all NTP staff were briefed about the findings and were retrained, and new guidelines on how to properly register and treat TB patients were developed [9]. These guidelines were disseminated in-country, and the National TB Manual (which was the blueprint for TB control activities in the country) was updated.

The following year, the study was repeated using the same methodology to see if these interventions had worked. A considerable improvement was noted with large reductions in numbers and proportions of patients being misregistered [10]. The mis-registration of smear-negative PTB and extrapulmonary TB declined from 14.2% to 4.7% and from 8.8% to 0.9%, respectively. Over the next few years, recurrent TB as a proportion of all nationally registered TB patients rose from 3% in 1999 to 12% five or six years later, and this was probably a true reflection of the pattern of TB in the country at those times (source: Malawi NTP). The research led to a more accurate reporting of recurrent TB and patients receiving the correct treatment for that time.

2.2. HIV Testing and Adjunctive Cotrimoxazole to Reduce Mortality in TB Patients in Malawi

The advent of HIV in Malawi severely affected the NTP. Case numbers rose dramatically and treatment success, having been excellent at 90% or higher in the pre-HIV era, declined dramatically. A study of over 800 TB patients consecutively registered and treated in 1995 at a large district hospital found that 31% had died by the end of treatment [11]. In this study, HIV-positive patients had a 2.3 times higher hazard of death than HIV-negative patients.

During the whole of the 1990s, antiretroviral therapy (ART) was not available in sub-Saharan Africa. However, a randomised controlled trial in Cote d'Ivoire, West Africa, conducted between 1995 and 1998, showed that adjunctive cotrimoxazole administered to HIV-positive TB patients reduced their mortality by 48% [12]. Based on this evidence, the Ministry of Health in Malawi asked the NTP to assess whether a package of voluntary counselling, HIV testing and adjunctive cotrimoxazole (for those found HIV-positive) might reduce the high mortality in TB patients routinely registered for treatment.

After receiving ethical approval from the Malawi National Health Science Research Committee, a real-time operational research project was started in Thyolo District, Southern Malawi, conducted jointly by Medecins Sans Frontieres and the NTP [13]. Between July

1999 and June 2020, all TB patients who started on anti-TB treatment were offered voluntary counselling and HIV testing. Those found to be HIV-positive were offered adjunctive cotrimoxazole provided there were no contraindications. Side effects were monitored clinically. Patients were followed up in the usual way on a regular monthly and quarterly basis with close supervision. There was periodic analysis of the data and regular meetings held with various stakeholders including the NTP director. The end-of treatment outcomes in this cohort (the intervention group) were compared with end-of-treatment outcomes in the cohort of TB patients registered the previous year between July 1998 and June 1999, in whom counselling, HIV testing and cotrimoxazole were not offered (the historical control group). Case fatality was the primary endpoint, and additional efforts were made to determine whether patients in each cohort who were lost to follow-up or transferred out of the district during treatment had died during the treatment period.

Of the 1061 TB patients in the intervention cohort, 91% were HIV tested, of whom 77% were HIV-positive, of whom 94% were given adjunctive cotrimoxazole. Of those receiving cotrimoxazole, 2% had reversible, non-serious, dermatological reactions. The numbers and proportions of patients in the intervention and control cohorts who died by the end of anti-TB treatment are shown in Table 2 [13]. There was a significant decrease in death for the whole intervention cohort compared with the control cohort, and this was particularly noted in those with smear negative PTB and in those registered with new TB. The number of TB patients needed to treat with counselling, HIV testing and adjunctive cotrimoxazole to prevent one death during anti-TB treatment was 12.5.

Table 2. Death in TB patients in the intervention (HIV testing and cotrimoxazole) and control groups, Thyolo District, Malawi.

Characteristics	Death [Total Enrolled on Treatment / Died / (%)]						p-Value
	HIV Testing and Cotrimoxazole Cohort			Control Cohort			
	Total N	Died N	Died (%)	Total n	Died n	Died (%)	
All TB patients	1061	299	(28)	925	333	(36)	<0.001
TB Type:							
Smear-Positive PTB	464	91	(20)	340	74	(22)	0.5
Smear-Negative PTB	282	105	(37)	288	140	(49)	<0.01
Extrapulmonary TB	315	103	(33)	297	119	(40)	0.05
TB Category:							
New	967	267	(28)	897	326	(36)	<0.001
Previously Treated	94	32	(34)	28	7	(25)	0.4

TB = tuberculosis; PTB = pulmonary tuberculosis; chi square tests used to calculate the *p* value. Adapted from [13].

The study showed that it was feasible and safe for the NTP at the district level to implement the package of interventions, and it was effective at reducing mortality. Another real-time implementation research study with a slightly different methodology, conducted in the North of Malawi, produced almost identical results [14].

Once the studies had been completed, a Ministry of Health meeting was arranged with many stakeholders to discuss the results and the implications, which resulted in a policy of HIV testing and adjunctive cotrimoxazole being recommended for all TB patients in the country [15]. This policy was implemented and scaled up over several years and provided the framework for treating HIV-positive TB patients with ART once this treatment became available from 2004. The impact was huge. Death during anti-TB treatment in patients with smear-positive PTB decreased from 19% in 2002 to 7.5% in 2008, and this was associated with a striking increase in treatment success, which rose from 72% to 86% [15].

2.3. Screening TB Patients for Diabetes Mellitus in India

In 2007 and 2008, two systematic reviews showed that people with diabetes mellitus (DM) had a 2–3 times increased risk of developing TB than the general population [16,17].

Stakeholder meetings and further reviews of the literature led to the WHO and the International Union Against Tuberculosis and Lung Disease (The Union) launching a Framework for Collaborative Activities to Reduce the Dual Burden of TB and DM [18]. Integral to this framework was the recommendation to undertake bi-directional screening for the two diseases. At that time, how this was best done and monitored in routine health care settings was unknown. Several real-time operational research studies were therefore set up in China and India [19–22]. Overall ethical approval was obtained from The Union Ethics Advisory Group. Formal national ethics approval was deemed to not be necessary in the two countries, as these were judged to be programmatic feasibility studies, although in some cases, local ethics approval at health facility sites was obtained.

One of these studies focused on screening TB patients for DM in eight tertiary care hospitals and 67 peripheral health institutions in India [21]. After a two-day consultative meeting between the national programme managers, national experts, and representatives from the Union, WHO and the World Diabetes Foundation, the screening methodology, the recording and reporting registers and the necessary training of front-line staff were agreed upon. The human resources and costs needed for screening and supervision were found within the routine health service budget. The screening was as follows: all registered TB patients were asked whether they had DM or were on anti-DM medication. Those saying they had no DM were offered random blood glucose (RBG) testing. If RBG $\geq$ 110 mg/dl, patients were asked to return a few days later for a fasting blood glucose (FBG). If FBG $\geq$ 126 mg/dl, the patient was diagnosed as having presumptive DM and referred to diabetes services for a definitive diagnosis and enrolment to care.

Implementation started in January 2012. During the conduct of the study, there was periodic analysis of the data, and a presentation of interim results was made to the India NTP director. Nine months after starting, in September 2012, the final results were collated and analysed. The key findings are shown in Table 3.

Table 3. Screening of TB patients for Diabetes Mellitus in selected health facilities in India.

Screening Process for TB Patients	Number	(%)
Patients registered with TB	8269	
Known diagnosis of DM	682	(8)
Needing to be screened with RBG	7587	
Screened with RBG	7467	(98)
RBG$\geq$110 mg/dl and needing to be screened with FBG	2838	
Screened with FBG	2703	(95)
FBG$\geq$126 mg/dl and newly diagnosed with DM	402	(5)
Known and newly diagnosed with DM	1084	(13)
Known and newly diagnosed with DM and referred to DM care	1033	(95)
Known and newly diagnosed with DM and reaching DM care	1020	

TB = tuberculosis; DM = diabetes mellitus; RBG = random blood glucose; FBG = fasting blood glucose; adapted from [21].

Of those registered for TB, 8% had a known diagnosis of DM. The screening procedures for those with no known diagnosis of DM worked well, with 95% or more of patients needing the RBG and FBG tests receiving them. Altogether, 13% of the cohort had presumptive DM (8% with a known diagnosis of DM and 5% with a new diagnosis of DM), and most of those were referred to and reached DM care services for further evaluation.

Within a few weeks of the study completion, the findings were discussed at a large national meeting with all the stakeholders present. Following the meeting, there was a rapid national policy decision to screen all TB patients in India for DM routinely. This decision was made about eight months ahead of the scientific publication of the research findings [23]. The policy has since been translated into practice in various states in India.

The same process of a national stakeholder's meeting, followed by implementation, and a second national stakeholder's meeting took place in China [19]. Six sites (five hospitals and one TB clinic) were selected. The study was regarded as a pilot project to assess the feasibility of the DM screening approach with a view to learning lessons for national scale-up. As such, upon completion of the project, the national authorities in China recommended further evaluations rather than a policy decision to change practice.

2.4. Mitigating the Impact of COVID-19 on TB Services in Three African Countries

In early January 2020, a new coronavirus, named severe acute respiratory syndrome coronavirus 2 (SARS-CoV-2), was linked to several atypical pneumonia cases in China. The disease caused by this new virus was subsequently named coronavirus disease 2019 (COVID-19). Spread occurred rapidly worldwide, and on 11 March 2020, the WHO declared COVID-19 to be a global pandemic. Most countries affected by COVID-19 authorised national lockdowns with restricted movements of the population to curb transmission of infection.

In high TB-burden countries, there was concern that the national lockdowns, combined with community fear of health facilities as places to contract COVID-19, would severely affect TB and HIV programme services. In the capital cities of three African countries (Kenya, Zimbabwe and Malawi), an operational research project was approved in April 2020 to assess whether a real-time monthly surveillance of TB and HIV activities instead of the usual quarterly surveillance might help to counteract the anticipated negative impact on TB and HIV services. It was hypothesised that if there were declines in case numbers or treatment outcomes, then the TB and HIV programmes could act more quickly on monthly information rather than waiting for quarterly information to reverse these trends. It was agreed that data would be collected and collated monthly using an EpiCollect5 application and reports sent monthly to the TB and HIV programme directors and all the other stakeholders included in the project.

The key objectives in each country were to collect, collate and report on specific TB and HIV-related data during the COVID-19 period (March 2020 to February 2021) and compare these data with those collected in the pre-COVID-19 period (March 2019 to February 2020) in which data were collected and collated retrospectively. Overall ethics approval was obtained from the Union Ethics Advisory Group, the Kenya Medical Research Institute, and Zimbabwe's Medical Research Council. The Malawi National Health Science Research Committee waived the need for formal ethics approval on the grounds that this was programmatic work [24–26].

With respect to TB case detection, the key findings are shown in Table 4. In all three countries, the overall numbers of people presenting with presumptive PTB for investigation decreased, as did the numbers diagnosed with TB and registered for treatment.

Table 4. Numbers with presumptive PTB and registered TB in the pre-COVID-19 and COVID-19 periods in Kenya, Malawi and Zimbabwe.

Numbers Recorded with Presumptive PTB	Pre-COVID-19 March 2019–February 2020	COVID-19 March 2020–February 2021	Difference % between Pre-COVID-19 and COVID-19
Kenya	28,038	19,295	31.2% decrease
Malawi	11,271	6137	45.6% decrease
Zimbabwe	3270	1941	40.6% decrease
Numbers Diagnosed and Registered with TB	Pre-COVID-19 March 2019–February 2020	COVID-19 March 20–February 2021	Difference % between pre-COVID-19 and COVID-19
Kenya	3716	2676	28.0% decrease
Malawi	1822	1474	19.1% decrease
Zimbabwe	1078	715	33.7% decrease

PTB = pulmonary tuberculosis; TB = tuberculosis; adapted from [24–26].

After the initial lockdown period, which lasted several months in the three countries, measures to improve TB case detection were put in place. Using monthly comparative data with the pre-COVID-19 period, the differences in numbers of patients with presumptive and registered TB in the first 6-months of the COVID-19 period compared with the second 6-months of the COVID-19 period are shown in Table 5.

Table 5. Numbers with presumptive PTB and registered TB between first 6-months and second 6-months of COVID-19 in Kenya, Malawi and Zimbabwe.

Numbers Recorded with Presumptive TB	Percentage Difference Compared with Equivalent Pre-COVID-19 Period	
	COVID-19: First 6-Months March 2020–August 2020	COVID-19: Second 6-Months September 2020–February 2021
Kenya	−53%	+5%
Malawi	−50%	−40%
Zimbabwe	−36%	−45%
Numbers Diagnosed and Registered with TB	COVID-19: first 6-months March 2020–August 2020	COVID-19: second 6-months September 2020–February 2021
Kenya	−35%	−20%
Malawi	−23%	−15%
Zimbabwe	−30%	−37%

PTB = pulmonary tuberculosis; TB = tuberculosis; adapted from [24–26].

In Kenya, there were considerable improvements, despite industrial strike action in the health sector, which negatively affected the health services between November 2020 and January 2021. The interventions to improve TB case finding included: (i) integrated screening and fast-tracking of investigations for TB and COVID-19 in patients presenting with respiratory symptoms; (ii) active TB case finding in hot spots in the city; (iii) enhanced TB case finding that included screening of TB through mobile phones using a dedicated Unstructured Supplementary Service Data (USSD) dialling code, asking patients to dial into a toll-free TB screening call centre operated by health care workers and use of automated TB screening machines positioned at strategic spots in the community; (iv) active tracing of close contacts of index patients and (v) improved TB screening amongst people living with HIV [24].

In Malawi, there were modest improvements. The programme aimed to keep services running; healthcare workers were asked to inquire about TB symptoms in those attending out-patient departments proactively, and there was an active tracing of patients needing to be registered [25].

In Zimbabwe, there was a deterioration in TB case finding services. The interventions put in place included: (i) integrated screening and fast-tracking of investigations for TB and COVID-19 in patients presenting with respiratory symptoms; (ii) improved contact tracing in selected facilities; and (iii) the promotion of strict infection control practices at health facilities to encourage symptomatic patients to attend. Unfortunately, the country had widespread industrial strike action in the health sector between July and September 2020, and between December 2020 and January 2021, there were stock-outs of TB diagnostic reagents, which greatly reduced the ability to diagnose TB [26].

In all three countries, the data collection was led and monitored by country coordinators engaged explicitly for the study. They worked with a central monitoring and evaluation coordinator at The Union to put together the monthly reports for each country. In brief, two weeks after the end of each month, the TB and HIV data were collated, validated and presented in a monthly report as a series of figures, tables and narrative. These were sent to the TB and HIV programme directors, usually within a week of putting the data together, and shared with the study sites as well as all the other stakeholders involved in the project. The TB programme directors reviewed the monthly surveillance reports, which they received within four weeks of the end of the month and used the data for decision making. Cause and effect are difficult to disentangle from a study like this. Still, it is likely that timely access to data helped the programmes' efforts to maintain services during this challenging time.

The three studies have helped shed light on additional ways to improve TB case finding. Further innovative approaches that would benefit from real-time implementation research during the COVID-19 pandemic might include: (i) the strengthening of sputum specimen transportation to and from laboratories; (ii) the use of saliva as an alternative to sputum for diagnosing TB and COVID-19; (iii) the use of adequately equipped mobile vans with on-site Xpert MTB/RIF assays and ultraportable chest x-rays to provide diagnostic outreach; (iv) the application of digital platforms and connectivity solutions to maintain contact with patients during the lockdown periods and to ensure rapid delivery of test results for those being investigated; and iv) mobilization of TB survivors to facilitate contact tracing and active screening for TB in high-risk groups [27,28].

3. Making Real-Time Operational Research Happen and Ensuring It Is Effective

Real-time operational research, as discussed earlier, is more labour intensive than research based around the collection of secondary data. There are a number of issues that must be considered, discussed and agreed upon when planning and implementing such studies.

3.1. Ethics

A sound ethics framework must underpin the research studies, with an understanding that informed consent may be required from patients (this was deemed not to be needed in any of the four TB case studies) and the benefits and risks of any intervention may need careful assessment from a human rights perspective and the disease control programme itself [29]. In the four case studies, ethics approval was always sought, although in some cases, the National Scientific and Research Ethics Committee waived the need for a formal ethics review.

3.2. Research Relevance and Prioritization at the Country Level

The research must be relevant and a priority for the country and the disease control programme. The operational research studies in the four examples were all priorities for the national TB programmes. Programme directors were kept closely in touch with the data collection and analysis that occurred during the study and were all involved in the stakeholder meetings at the conclusion of the study. As such, the results were influential in shaping policy and practice on the ground and making a difference for the better.

Real-time operational research is beneficial in pandemic and epidemic situations where countries are desperate to maintain routine health services despite numerous challenges. The anticipated negative impact of COVID-19 on TB and HIV services in Kenya, Malawi and Zimbabwe was a case in point, where monthly instead of quarterly surveillance was welcomed and instituted by the disease control programmes to try and counteract the dramatic decreases in TB case detection and HIV testing. The data were also used to assess new strategies implemented to counteract the adverse effects of COVID-19 [24–26].

Another example is the Ebola Virus Disease (EVD) outbreak in Sierra Leone and Liberia in 2014. Operational research carried out after the EVD outbreak showed the adverse effects of EVD on the ability of the programmes to diagnose TB and provide HIV testing [30,31]. While this research provided useful information about what to do in the event of further EVD outbreaks, real-time operational research at the time of the 2014 EVD outbreak might have helped the programmes better weather the storm, as was shown for example with TB services in neighbouring Guinea [32].

3.3. Research That Adheres to International Standards of the Conduct and Reporting of Research

The research, whether this is designed as a cross-sectional study, a cohort study or a case-control study, must be conducted and reported according to international standard guidelines [33]. The majority of the operational research studies that focus on quantitative data are observational designs and should follow the Strengthening the Reporting of Observational Studies in Epidemiology (STROBE) guidelines [34]. Qualitative research studies should follow the Standards for Reporting Qualitative Research (SRQR) [35] or the consolidated criteria for reporting qualitative research (COREQ) guidelines [36]. The four case studies on TB followed STROBE guidelines. Adherence to these quantitative and qualitative guidelines ensures that the research is conducted and reported to international standards and adds further credibility to the research study findings.

3.4. Comparison Groups

An important methodological consideration for real-time operational research is whether or not to have a comparison group. In the first case study on the misregistration of recurrent TB, the first published study had no comparison group. However, once guidelines had been developed and disseminated, the first study acted as a comparison for the second study to assess whether misregistration had decreased [8,10].

In the second case study, a package of counselling, HIV testing and adjunctive cotrimoxazole administered to a cohort of TB patients was compared with no package in a cohort of TB patients registered the previous year (defined as a historical control) [13]. The use of historical controls is acceptable, although it is important that the investigators clearly outline any differences in the cohort composition and/or standards of care of patients before and during the intervention that might affect the primary outcome.

Another way of using a control group is to select a concurrent comparison cohort against which to judge the intervention results. For example, a study was done in Malawi to assess TB treatment outcomes in a cohort of patients offered the package of HIV testing and adjunctive cotrimoxazole in Thyolo district in 2001 and results compared with the neighbouring Mulanje district during the same time where no such interventions were offered to registered TB patients [37]. There was a significant increase in treatment success and a significant decrease in mortality and other adverse outcomes in Thyolo than in Mulanje district, with findings comparable to those of the original study conducted in Thyolo district [13]. The use of concurrent controls is also acceptable, although care must be taken to match the situation of the intervention and comparison groups as close as possible.

Not all operational research studies need comparison groups. The third case study on screening TB patients for DM had no such group [21]. However, if the stakeholder committee had decided on two different screening methods, then a comparison study would have been needed.

3.5. Timely Collection and Sharing of Data

Consideration must be given to the timely collection, sharing and validation of data. The first two case studies from Malawi [8,10,13] and the third from India [21] used paper-based questionnaires and data collection forms for the primary data. All the investigators were in the country, and there was no problem with the sharing of data. The fourth case study, however, had investigators from several countries, and there was a need to regularly check and validate the data between the overall monitoring and evaluation coordinator based in India and the country coordinators based in Africa. Doing this with paper-based records was going to be difficult, if not impossible. In the Kenya, Malawi and Zimbabwe studies [24–26], an EpiCollect5 application (https://five.epicollect.net, accessed on 7 June 2021) was therefore used to collect the aggregate data and this was used in real-time to cross-check and validate data for the different variables and ensure that numbers added up. EpiCollect5 is a free application that can be downloaded to smartphones, and it was relatively easy to train all the data collectors in the country about how to use it.

3.6. Dissemination and Getting Research into Policy and Practice

In the four case studies, key implementers carried out the research, but the decision-makers in the Ministry of Health were involved right from the start in terms of conceptualization, methodology, analysis and interpretation of the data and the writing and editing of the final manuscript. Taking a research project from protocol to publication acts as a form of quality control, demonstrating to investigators and key decision and policymakers that the science is of a good standard and the findings reliable for making decisions [38]. The publication is important and, particularly if Open Access journals are used, allows for the widespread dissemination to national and international audiences.

Dissemination, for example, at a stakeholders' meeting where decision and policymakers are present, is another essential part of sharing the findings and persuading people to adopt the recommended changes to policy and practice. In the first three case studies, interim stakeholder meetings with programme directors were held as the studies progressed, and importantly they were also held within a few weeks or months of the studies being completed leading to important national decisions being made long before the papers were published [10,15,23]. In the fourth case study, the data were put together each month as figures, tables and a narrative and sent as monthly reports to programme directors [24–26]. The monthly deadlines for submission were never missed, which allowed confidence to be built into the system, especially for trying out and monitoring new strategies.

3.7. Research Capacity Building

Skill and experience are needed to plan and conduct real-time operational research. Over the last 12 years, we have used the SORT IT (Structured Operational Research and Training Initiative) model to build capacity in programmatic or public health officers in low- and middle-income countries to undertake and publish operational research using routinely collected data [39]. This has been remarkably successful, resulting in many high-quality observational studies being undertaken and published in open access journals and adhering to STROBE guidelines [40].

SORT IT courses are structured with three one-week modules over a fixed relatively short period of 9–12 months, and as a result, most studies use routinely collected secondary data. More thought will be needed to adapt the SORT IT model to real-time operational research. This will require longer time periods between modules to ensure that (i) patient-centred ethics approvals are obtained in time, (ii) investigators are properly trained in the collection and validation of data and (iii) sample sizes are adequate to judge whether interventions are effective.

The fourth case example [24–26] also shows how capacity can be built on the ground in existing staff working on the front-line in health facilities. The Union central monitoring and evaluation coordinator trained all existing staff in Nairobi, Lilongwe and Harare about how to use EpiCollect5, useful knowledge not only for the study but also for future public health work.

3.8. Funding

Funding is a key consideration. Operational research studies that use routinely collected secondary data are simple and relatively inexpensive to do. Operational research papers published through SORT IT courses, which included the capacity building and the publication charges, cost under 7000 euro per paper when conducted and led by the institutions without additional expertise costs [41].

Real-time operational research is likely to be more expensive. However, there are opportunities for funding. The Global Fund to fight AIDS, TB and Malaria in recent years has promoted the integration of operational research into country programmes during the funding process [42], and encourages real-time operational research for more effective uptake and use of proven interventions as well as research on the introduction and deployment of new products in the field when they become available. More efficient mechanisms, however, for accessing and deploying these funds are urgently needed.

3.9. Operational Research across the Spectrum of Disease

We have focused this perspective article on real-time operational research around TB. However, this type of research can be utilized for many other different diseases. A review of published papers through the SORT IT model between 2009 and 2018 showed that while 45% of operational research projects were on TB, the remainder were on other communicable diseases, non-communicable diseases, maternal and child health, trauma and health care emergencies and access to care [40]. The UNICEF/UNDP/World Bank/WHO Special Programme for Research and Training in Tropical Diseases (TDR) currently has a large grant from the UK National Institute for Health Research (NIHR) to undertake and build capacity in operational research around the growing threat of antimicrobial resistance (AMR). Two SORT IT courses on AMR from Africa and Asia have recently been completed with excellent publication outputs to date [43].

4. Conclusions

This perspective article defined the concept of real-time operational research. We selected four examples from the field of TB to show how this type of research can be implemented, with the findings in all four cases leading to important policy and practice changes. Important considerations about how to undertake and publish real-time operational research, build capacity and find the necessary funding are discussed. Disease control programmes, health services and health systems should include operational research as one of their core activities both to improve the delivery of established health interventions and to introduce and deploy new products and interventions as they become available. This is particularly important when health services are threatened by pandemics and epidemics.

Author Contributions: Conceptualization, A.D.H., P.T., A.M.V.K., S.S., S.D.B., I.D.R., M.K., R.Z.; methodology, A.D.H., P.T., R.Z.; resources, I.D.R.; writing—original draft preparation, A.D.H., P.T., R.Z.; writing—review and editing, A.D.H., P.T., I.M., J.M.C., H.T., K.C.T., A.M.V.K., S.S., S.D.B., I.D.R., M.K., R.Z.; funding acquisition, S.D.B., A.D.H.; All authors have read and agreed to the published version of the manuscript.

Funding: The writing and publication of this perspective article was funded by Bloomberg Philanthropies through a grant (Grant Number 78941) from Vital Strategies and the Resolve to Save Lives Initiative, New York, NY, USA.

Institutional Review Board Statement: This was a perspective paper, and as such, no ethics review was required.

Informed Consent Statement: Not applicable.

Data Availability Statement: Not applicable.

Acknowledgments: Not applicable.

Conflicts of Interest: The authors declare no conflict of interest. The funders had no role in the writing of this paper.

Disclaimer: The views expressed in this paper are those of the authors and may not necessarily reflect the views of their affiliated institutions.

References

1. Zachariah, R.; Harries, A.D.; Ishikawa, N.; Rieder, H.L.; Bissell, K.; Laserson, K.; Massaquoi, M.; Van Herp, M.; Reid, T. Operational research in low-income countries: What, why, and how? *Lancet Infect. Dis.* **2009**, *9*, 711–717. [CrossRef]
2. Harries, A.D.; Khogali, M.; Kumar, A.M.V.; Satyanarayana, S.; Takarinda, K.C.; Karpati, A.; Olliaro, P.; Zachariah, R. Building the capacity of public health programmes to become data rich, information rich and action rich. *Public Health Action* **2018**, *8*, 34–36. [CrossRef] [PubMed]
3. Remme, J.H.F.; Adam, T.; Becerra-Posada, F.; D'Arcangues, C.; Devlin, M.; Gardner, C.; Ghaffar, A.; Hombach, J.; Kengeya, J.F.K.; Mbewu, A.; et al. Defining research to improve health systems. *PLoS Med.* **2010**, *7*, e1001000. [CrossRef] [PubMed]
4. Perriens, J.H.; Colebunders, R.L.; Karahunga, C.; Willame, J.C.; Jeugmans, J.; Kaboto, M.; Mukadi, Y.; Pauwels, P.; Ryder, R.W.; Prignot, J.; et al. Increased mortality and tuberculosis treatment failure rate among human immunodeficiency virus (HIV)

seropositive compared with HIV seronegative patients with pulmonary tuberculosis treated with "standard" chemotherapy in Kinshasa, Zaire. *Am. Rev. Respir. Dis.* **1991**, *144*, 750–755. [CrossRef] [PubMed]
5. Hawken, M.; Nunn, P.; Godfrey-Faussett, P.; McAdam, K.P.W.J.; Morris, J.; Odhiambo, J.; Githui, W.; Gilks, C.; Hawken, M.; Gathua, S.; et al. Increased recurrence of tuberculosis in HIV-1-infected patients in Kenya. *Lancet* **1993**, *342*, 332–337. [CrossRef]
6. Elliott, A.M.; Halwiindi, B.; Hayes, R.J.; Luo, N.; Mwinga, A.G.; Tembo, G.; Machiels, L.; Steenbergen, G.; Pobee, J.O.M.; Nunn, P.; et al. The impact of human immunodeficiency virus on mortality of patients treated for tuberculosis in a cohort study in Zambia. *Trans. R. Soc. Trop. Med. Hyg.* **1995**, *89*, 78–82. [CrossRef]
7. Kelly, P.M.; Cumming, R.G.; Kaldor, J.M. HIV and tuberculosis in rural sub-Saharan Africa: A cohort study with two year follow-up. *Trans. R. Soc. Trop. Med. Hyg.* **1999**, *93*, 287–293. [CrossRef]
8. Harries, A.D.; Hargreaves, N.J.; Kwanjana, J.H.; Salaniponi, F.M.L. Relapse and recurrent tuberculosis in the context of a National Tuberculosis Control Programme. *Trans. R. Soc. Trop. Med. Hyg.* **2000**, *94*, 247–249. [CrossRef]
9. Harries, A.D.; Chimzizi, R.B.; Nyirenda, T.E.; van Gorkom, J.; Salaniponi, F.M. Preventing recurrent tuberculosis in high HIV-prevalent areas in sub-Saharan Africa: What are the options for tuberculosis control programmes? [Unresolved Issues]. *Int. J. Tuberc. Lung Dis.* **2003**, *7*, 616–622.
10. Harries, A.D.; Salaniponi, F.M.L. Recurrent tuberculosis in Malawi: Improved diagnosis and management following operational research. *Trans. R. Soc. Trop. Med. Hyg.* **2001**, *95*, 503–504. [CrossRef]
11. Harries, A.D.; Nyangulu, D.S.; Kang'ombe, C.; Ndalama, D.; Glynn, J.R.; Banda, H.; Wirima, J.J.; Salaniponi, F.M.; Liomba, G.; Maher, D.; et al. Treatment outcome of an unselected cohort of tuberculosis patients in relation to human immunodeficiency virus serostatus in Zomba hospital, Malawi. *Trans. R. Soc. Trop. Med. Hyg.* **1998**, *92*, 343–347. [CrossRef]
12. Wiktor, S.Z.; Sassan-Morokro, M.; Grant, A.D.; Abouya, L.; Karon, J.M.; Maurice, C.; Djomand, G.; Ackah, A.; Domoua, K.; Kadio, A.; et al. Efficacy of trimethoprim-sulphamethoxazole prophylaxis to decrease morbidity and mortality in HIV-1-infected patients with tuberculosis in Abidjan, Cote d'Ivoire: A randomised controlled trial. *Lancet* **1999**, *353*, 1469–1475. [CrossRef]
13. Zachariah, R.; Spielmann, M.P.L.; Chinji, C.; Gomani, P.; Arendt, V.; Hargreaves, N.J.; Salaniponi, F.M.; Harries, A.D. Voluntary counselling, HIV testing and adjunctive cotrimoxazole reduces mortality in tuberculosis patients in Thyolo, Malawi. *AIDS* **2003**, *17*, 1053–1061. [CrossRef] [PubMed]
14. Mwaungulu, F.B.D.; Floyd, S.; Crampin, A.C.; Kasimba, S.; Malema, S.; Kanyongoloka, H.; Harries, A.D.; Glynn, J.R.; Fine, P.E.M. Cotrimoxazole prophylaxis reduces mortality in human immunodeficiency virus-positive tuberculosis patients in Karonga District, Malawi. *Bull. World Health Organ.* **2004**, *82*, 354–363. [PubMed]
15. Harries, A.D.; Zachariah, R.; Chimzizi, R.; Salaniponi, F.; Gausi, F.; Kanyerere, H.; Schouten, E.J.; Jahn, A.; Makombe, S.D.; Chimbwandira, F.M.; et al. Operational research in Malawi: Making a difference with cotrimoxazole preventive therapy in patients with tuberculosis and HIV. *BMC Public Health* **2011**, *11*, 1–9. [CrossRef] [PubMed]
16. Stevenson, C.R.; Critchley, J.A.; Forouhi, N.G.; Roglic, G.; Williams, B.G.; Dye, C.; Unwin, N.C. Diabetes and the risk of tuberculosis: A neglected threat to public health? *Chronic Illn.* **2007**, *3*, 228–245. [CrossRef] [PubMed]
17. Jeon, C.Y.; Murray, M.B. Diabetes mellitus increases the risk of active tuberculosis: A systematic review of 13 observational studies. *PLoS Med.* **2008**, *5*, 1091–1101.
18. World Health Organization and International Union against Tuberculosis and Lung Disease. *Collaborative Framework for the Care and Control of Tuberculosis and Diabetes*; WHO: Geneva, Switzerland, 2011.
19. Li, L.; Lin, Y.; Mi, F.; Tan, S.; Liang, B.; Guo, C.; Shi, L.; Liu, L.; Gong, F.; Li, Y.; et al. Screening of patients with tuberculosis for diabetes mellitus in China. *Trop. Med. Int. Health* **2012**, *17*, 1294–1301. [CrossRef]
20. Lin, Y.; Li, L.; Mi, F.; Du, J.; Dong, Y.; Li, Z.; Qi, W.; Zhao, X.; Cui, Y.; Hou, F.; et al. Screening patients with Diabetes Mellitus for Tuberculosis in China. *Trop. Med. Int. Health* **2012**, *17*, 1302–1308. [CrossRef]
21. India Tuberculosis-Diabetes Study Group. Screening of patients with tuberculosis for diabetes mellitus in India. *Trop. Med. Int. Health* **2013**, *18*, 636–645. [CrossRef] [PubMed]
22. India Tuberculosis-Diabetes Study Group. Screening of patients with diabetes mellitus for tuberculosis in India. *Trop. Med. Int. Health* **2013**, *18*, 646–654. [CrossRef] [PubMed]
23. Kumar, A.M.V.; Satyanarayana, S.; Wilson, N.C.; Chadha, S.S.; Gupta, D.; Nair, S.; Zachariah, R.; Kapur, A.; Harries, A.D. Operational research leading to rapid national policy change: Tuberculosis-diabetes collaboration in India. *Public Health Action* **2014**, *4*, 85–88. [CrossRef]
24. Mbithi, I.; Thekkur, P.; Chakaya, J.M.; Onyango, E.; Owiti, P.; Njeri, N.C.; Kumar, A.M.V.; Satyanarayana, S.; Shewade, H.D.; Khogali, M.; et al. Assessing the Real-Time Impact of COVID-19 on TB and HIV Services: The Experience and Response from Selected Health Facilities in Nairobi, Kenya. *Trop. Med. Infect. Dis.* **2021**, *6*, 74. [CrossRef] [PubMed]
25. Thekkur, P.; Tweya, H.; Phiri, S.; Mpunga, J.; Kalua, T.; Kumar, A.M.V.; Satyanarayana, S.; Shewade, H.D.; Khogali, M.; Zachariah, R.; et al. Assessing the Impact of COVID-19 on TB and HIV Programme Services in Selected Health Facilities in Lilongwe, Malawi: Operational Research in Real Time. *Trop. Med. Infect. Dis.* **2021**, *6*, 81. [CrossRef] [PubMed]
26. Thekkur, P.; Takarinda, K.C.; Timire, C.; Sandy, C.; Apollo, T.; Kumar, A.M.; Satyanarayana, S.; Shewade, H.D.; Khogali, M.; Zachariah, R.; et al. Operational research to assess the real-time impact of COVID-19 on TB and HIV services: The experience and response from health facilities in Harare, Zimbabwe. *Trop. Med. Infect. Dis.* **2021**, *6*, 94. [CrossRef]
27. Echeverría, G.; Espinoza, W.; de Waard, J.H. How TB and COVID-19 compare: An opportunity to integrate both control programmes. *Int. J. Tuberc. Lung Dis.* **2020**, *24*, 1–4. [CrossRef] [PubMed]

28. Chiang, C.Y.; Islam, T.; Xu, C.; Chinnayah, T.; Garfin, A.M.C.; Rahevar, K.; Raviglione, M. The impact of COVID-19 and the restoration of tuberculosis services in the Western Pacific Region. *Eur. Respir. J.* **2020**, *56*, 2003054. [CrossRef] [PubMed]
29. Edginton, M.E.; Ornstein, T.; Denholm, J.; El Sony, A.; Kim, S.J.; Narain, A.; O'Brien, R. Research ethics in The Union: An 8-year review of the Ethics Advisory Group. *Public Health Action* **2013**, *3*, 346–350. [CrossRef]
30. Bah, O.M.; Kamara, H.B.; Bhat, P.; Harries, A.D.; Owiti, P.; Katta, J.; Foray, L.; Kamara, M.I.; Kamara, B.O. The influence of the Ebola outbreak on presumptive and active tuberculosis in Bombali District, Sierra Leone. *Public Health Action* **2017**, *7*, S3–S9. [CrossRef]
31. Konwloh, P.K.; Cambell, C.L.; Ade, S.; Bhat, P.; Harries, A.D.; Wilkinson, E.; Cooper, C.T. Influence of Ebola on tuberculosis case finding and treatment outcomes in Liberia. *Public Health Action* **2017**, *7*, S62–S69. [CrossRef] [PubMed]
32. Ortuno-Gutierrez, N.; Zachariah, R.; Woldeyohannes, D.; Bangoura, A.; Chérif, G.-F.; Loua, F.; Hermans, V.; Tayler-Smith, K.; Sikhondze, W.; Camara, L.-M. Upholding Tuberculosis Services during the 2014 Ebola Storm: An Encouraging Experience from Conakry, Guinea. *PLoS ONE* **2016**, *11*, e0157296. [CrossRef] [PubMed]
33. Hales, S.; Lesher-Trevino, A.; Ford, N.; Maher, D.; Ramsay, A.; Tran, N. Reporting guidelines for implementation and operational research. *Bull. World Health Organ.* **2016**, *94*, 58–64. [CrossRef]
34. Von Elm, E.; Altman, D.G.; Egger, M.; Pocock, S.J.; Gøtzsche, P.C.; Vandenbroucke, J.P. The Strengthening the Reporting of Observational Studies in Epidemiology (STROBE) statement: Guidelines for reporting observational studies. *Lancet* **2007**, *370*, 1453–1457. [CrossRef]
35. O'Brien, B.C.; Harris, I.B.; Beckman, T.J.; Reed, D.A.; Cook, D.A. Standards for reporting qualitative research: A synthesis of recommendations. *Acad. Med.* **2014**, *89*, 1245–1251. [CrossRef]
36. Tong, A.; Sainsbury, P.; Craig, J. Consolidated criteria for reporting qualitative research (COREQ): A 32-item checklist for interviews and focus groups. *Int. J. Qual. Health Care* **2007**, *19*, 349–357. [CrossRef]
37. Chimzizi, R.; Gausi, F.; Bwanali, A.; Mbalume, D.; Teck, R.; Gomani, P.; Zachariah, R.; Zuza, W.; Malombe, R.; Salaniponi, F.M.; et al. Voluntary counselling, HIV testing and adjunctive cotrimoxazole are associated with improved TB treatment outcomes under routine conditions in Thyolo District, Malawi. *Int. J. Tuberc. Lung Dis.* **2004**, *8*, 579–585. [PubMed]
38. Zachariah, R.; Tayler-Smith, K.; Ngamvithayapong-Yanai, J.; Ota, M.; Murakami, K.; Ohkado, A.; Yamada, N.; Van Den Boogaard, W.; Draguez, B.; Ishikawa, N.; et al. The published research paper: Is it an important indicator of successful operational research at programme level? *Trop. Med. Int. Health* **2010**, *15*, 1274–1277. [CrossRef]
39. Ramsay, A.; Harries, A.D.; Zachariah, R.; Bissell, K.; Hinderaker, S.G.; Edginton, M.; Enarson, D.A.; Satyanarayana, S.; Kumar, A.M.V.; Hoa, N.B.; et al. The Structured Operational Research and Training Initiative for public health programmes. *Public Health Action* **2014**, *4*, 79–84. [CrossRef]
40. Zachariah, R.; Rust, S.; Thekkur, P.; Khogali, M.; Kumar, A.M.; Davtyan, K.; Diro, E.; Satyanarayana, S.; Denisiuk, O.; van Griensven, J.; et al. Quality, Equity and Utility of Observational Studies during 10 Years of Implementing the Structured Operational Research and Training Initiative in 72 Countries. *Trop. Med. Infect. Dis.* **2020**, *5*, 167. [CrossRef]
41. Quaglio, G.L.; Ramsay, A.; Harries, A.D.; Karapiperis, T.; Putoto, G.; Dye, C.; Olesen, O.F.; Tomson, G.; Zachariah, R. Calling on Europe to support operational research in low-income and middle-income countries. *Lancet Glob. Health* **2014**, *2*, e308–e310. [CrossRef]
42. Camacho, S.; Maher, D.; Kamau, E.M.; Saric, J.; Segura, L.; Zachariah, R.; Wyss, K. Incorporating operational research in programmes funded by the Global Fund to Fight AIDS, Tuberculosis and Malaria in four sub-Saharan African countries. *Global Health* **2020**, *16*, 1–8. [CrossRef] [PubMed]
43. Tropical Medicine and Infectious Disease. Special Issue "AMR in Low and Middle Income Countries". Available online: https://www.mdpi.com/journal/tropicalmed/special_issues/AMR (accessed on 7 June 2021).

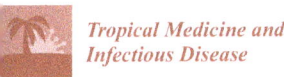

Article

Operational Research to Assess the Real-Time Impact of COVID-19 on TB and HIV Services: The Experience and Response from Health Facilities in Harare, Zimbabwe

Pruthu Thekkur [1,2,†], Kudakwashe C. Takarinda [1,3,†], Collins Timire [1,3], Charles Sandy [3], Tsitsi Apollo [3], Ajay M. V. Kumar [1,2,4], Srinath Satyanarayana [1,2], Hemant D. Shewade [1,2], Mohammed Khogali [5], Rony Zachariah [5], I. D. Rusen [6], Selma Dar Berger [1] and Anthony D. Harries [1,7,*]

1. International Union Against Tuberculosis and Lung Disease (The Union), 75006 Paris, France; Pruthu.TK@theunion.org (P.T.); kctakarinda@gmail.com (K.C.T.); collins.timire@theunion.org (C.T.); akumar@theunion.org (A.M.V.K.); SSrinath@theunion.org (S.S.); HShewade@theunion.org (H.D.S.); sberger@theunion.org (S.D.B.)
2. The Union South-East Asia Office, New Delhi 110016, India
3. AIDS and TB Department, Ministry of Health and Child Care, Causeway, Harare P.O. Box CY 1122, Zimbabwe; dr.c.sandy@gmail.com (C.S.); tsitsiapollo2@gmail.com (T.A.)
4. Yenepoya Medical College, Yenepoya, Mangalore 575018, India
5. Special Programme for Research and Training in Tropical Disease (TDR), World Health Organization, 1211 Geneva, Switzerland; khogalim@who.int (M.K.); zachariahr@who.int (R.Z.)
6. Vital Strategies, New York, NY 10005, USA; irusen@vitalstrategies.org
7. Department of Clinical Research, Faculty of Infectious and Tropical Diseases, London School of Hygiene and Tropical Medicine, London WC1E 7HT, UK
* Correspondence: adharries@theunion.org; Tel.: +44-(0)-1962-714-297
† These authors contributed equally to the work.

Abstract: When COVID-19 was declared a pandemic, there was concern that TB and HIV services in Zimbabwe would be severely affected. We set up real-time monthly surveillance of TB and HIV activities in 10 health facilities in Harare to capture trends in TB case detection, TB treatment outcomes and HIV testing and use these data to facilitate corrective action. Aggregate data were collected monthly during the COVID-19 period (March 2020–February 2021) using EpiCollect5 and compared with monthly data extracted for the pre-COVID-19 period (March 2019–February 2020). Monthly reports were sent to program directors. During the COVID-19 period, there was a decrease in persons with presumptive pulmonary TB (40.6%), in patients registered for TB treatment (33.7%) and in individuals tested for HIV (62.8%). The HIV testing decline improved in the second 6 months of the COVID-19 period. However, TB case finding deteriorated further, associated with expiry of diagnostic reagents. During the COVID-19 period, TB treatment success decreased from 80.9 to 69.3%, and referral of HIV-positive persons to antiretroviral therapy decreased from 95.7 to 91.7%. Declining trends in TB and HIV case detection and TB treatment outcomes were not fully redressed despite real-time monthly surveillance. More support is needed to transform this useful information into action.

Keywords: COVID-19; Zimbabwe; Harare; presumptive tuberculosis; tuberculosis; TB treatment outcomes; HIV; antiretroviral therapy; EpiCollect5; operational research

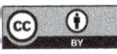

1. Introduction

In early January 2020, a new coronavirus, named severe acute respiratory syndrome coronavirus 2 (SARS-CoV-2), was linked to a series of atypical pneumonia cases reported the previous month in Wuhan city, Hubei province, China. The virus spread rapidly within China, and then onto Europe, the United States of America (USA) and the rest of the world, causing the disease known as COVID-19. On 11 March 2020, the World Health Organization (WHO) declared COVID-19 to be a global pandemic. By the end of

2020, 80 million confirmed cases and 1.8 million deaths had been reported globally to the WHO, making COVID-19 the leading cause of death among infectious diseases [1]. In April 2020, one month after the pandemic had been declared, the epicenters were China, Europe and the USA, and with large volumes of air traffic between these regions and Africa, sub-Saharan Africa was predicted to be the next region to be hard hit by COVID-19 [2,3].

At the start of the COVID-19 crisis, political attention, resources and finances were redirected within the health sector to help it grapple with the escalating numbers of COVID-19 cases. National and local lockdowns restricted movement and forced people to spend more time indoors, limiting access to health facilities. All of this raised concern that countries with high burdens of tuberculosis (TB) and human immunodeficiency virus/acquired immune deficiency syndrome (HIV/AIDS) might see interruption of health services and poor quality of care for their patients [4]. Modeling studies suggested that deaths due to HIV/AIDS and TB could increase by up to 10 and 20%, respectively, with the greatest impact on HIV resulting from interruption to antiretroviral therapy (ART) and the greatest impact on TB resulting from delayed diagnosis and treatment of new cases [5].

Similarities were drawn with the Ebola virus disease outbreak in Sierra Leone and Liberia in 2014. Through restrictions in travel, zonal quarantines and understandable community fear of health facilities, the ability of the national TB programs to diagnose TB and continue with HIV testing of their TB patients was adversely affected, and, in the case of Liberia, there was a decline in the rates of TB treatment success [6,7]. HIV testing in the general population and in health facilities decreased in both countries, although access to ART remained unaffected [8,9]. Early on in the COVID-19 pandemic, the Stop TB Partnership and WHO issued guidance about how people with TB could protect themselves and how national TB programs might adjust to COVID-19 outbreaks and national/local lockdowns [10,11]. The United Nations Joint Programme on HIV/AIDS (UNAIDS) provided similar advice and guidance to people living with HIV [12]. This global advice was augmented by urgent calls for practical planning to tackle the growing threat of COVID-19 in sub-Saharan Africa [13].

The first COVID-19 case reported to WHO by Zimbabwe was on 21 March 2020. By 15 April, Zimbabwe had reported 18 COVID-19 cases (with three deaths) [14], and the country had gone into national lockdown. The impact that this would have on public health services for the management of TB and HIV/AIDS was unknown. The Zimbabwe National TB Programme (NTP) and National HIV/AIDS Programme (NAP) began preparations for the continued delivery of TB-HIV services in this new environment of restricted movement [15]. The country also drew on the example of Guinea in West Africa, which garnered resources to weather the Ebola virus disease storm and managed to maintain TB services despite numerous obstacles [16].

The Zimbabwe NTP and NAP, working in close collaboration with the International Union Against Tuberculosis and Lung Disease (The Union), the Special Programme for Research and Training in Tropical Disease at WHO (TDR) and Vital Strategies, decided to strengthen the routine and real-time monitoring and evaluation system for TB and HIV case detection. The quarterly (3-monthly) recording and reporting system was supported in selected health facilities in the capital city of Harare by recording and reporting every month. It was hypothesized that if there were declines seen in persons presenting with presumptive TB or in numbers registered and treated for TB, or decreases in persons presenting for HIV testing or in numbers of HIV-positive persons being referred for ART, then programs could act more quickly on monthly information rather than quarterly information to reverse these trends.

The overall aim of the study was to determine the impact of the COVID-19 pandemic on TB case detection, diagnosis and treatment outcomes and on HIV testing and referral to ART through strengthened real-time surveillance. In selected health facilities in Harare, Zimbabwe, specific objectives were on a monthly basis to: (i) document the cumulative monthly increase nationally in COVID-19 cases and deaths and the effects on general health services; (ii) collect, collate and report on specific TB and HIV-related data during the

COVID-19 period (March 2020 to February 2021), (iii) document any specific programmatic responses at the national and local level to TB and HIV diagnosis and treatment during the COVID-19 period and (iv) compare the findings during the COVID-19 period with data collected and collated retrospectively during the pre-COVID-19 period (March 2019 to February 2020).

2. Materials and Methods

2.1. Study Design

This was a cohort study using programmatically collected aggregate data.

2.2. Setting

2.2.1. General Setting: Zimbabwe and Harare

Zimbabwe is a low-income country in southern Africa with an estimated population of 14.6 million in 2019 and a gross national income per capita of USD 1390 [17,18]. About 70% of the population live below the poverty line. Zimbabwe is among the top 14 countries globally with a triple burden of TB, HIV and multidrug-resistant TB [19].

Harare is the capital city with an estimated population of 1.5 million [20]. The current study took place in Harare for two main reasons. The majority of cases of COVID-19 came from this area at the onset of the pandemic, and travel around the country was extremely difficult due to quarantine and prohibited travel outside of the city during the initial lockdown. Harare city consists of 8 districts, that include 46 public health facilities, of which 44 are under the Harare City Health Department. These provide general health services integrated with TB and HIV services whilst the other two are government central hospitals which provide specialized health services. Of the 44 public health facilities under the Harare City Health Department, 13 are polyclinics which additionally provide maternity services, 29 are satellite clinics and 2 are infectious disease hospitals (of which one became reserved as the city's COVID-19 isolation center). Through stratified non-proportional sampling from each district, ten health facilities (nine polyclinics and one satellite clinic) were selected from a list of high-volume health facilities based on more than 1000 patients receiving life-long ART as a proxy for the volume of presumptive TB patients seen per year. The established staff who were already working in these sites delivering general health services and TB and HIV services assisted with the monthly collection of data.

2.2.2. TB and HIV Services

The diagnosis and treatment of TB and HIV/AIDS in Zimbabwe are the responsibility of the NTP and the NAP, respectively, under the Ministry of Health and Child Care (MO-HCC). People with symptoms suggestive of TB (typically, cough, fever, weight loss and night sweats) are classified as having presumptive TB when they attend a health facility. They are recorded as such in the presumptive TB register along with their demographic details. In the Harare city clinics, sputum samples are collected and sent to an onsite laboratory at each polyclinic, except satellite clinics that submit specimens to a laboratory at the nearest polyclinic. In the laboratories, patient details and sputum results are entered in the laboratory register. Investigations are carried out according to national and international guidelines [21,22], using the Xpert MTB/RIF assay (Cepheid, Sunnyvale, CA, USA) and/or sputum smear microscopy to establish a bacteriologically confirmed diagnosis of pulmonary TB (PTB), and results are sent back for patient tracking.

Those patients with a negative sputum result but who still have TB-related symptoms are referred to see a doctor at either of the two nearest infectious disease hospitals where clinical assessments, radiography and other circumstantial evidence are used to establish a diagnosis of clinically diagnosed PTB or extrapulmonary TB (EPTB). These patients are started on TB treatment before referral back to their initial health facility for registration and continuation of TB treatment. Patients with diagnosed TB are registered in the health facility Directly Observed Treatment (DOT) register and started on anti-TB treatment in accordance with national and international guidelines [21,22]. In the selected health facilities in Harare, patients with drug-susceptible TB (DS-TB) are treated and monitored with the standard 6-month regimens, while those with the drug-resistant disease are treated and monitored with MDR-TB regimens. Patients with drug-resistant TB were not included in this study. Treatment outcomes are monitored, recorded and reported according to international guidelines [23].

HIV testing takes place in public health facilities and is routinely offered to anyone attending for care, including TB patients, according to national and international guidelines [24–26]. HIV testing is carried out using rapid testing algorithms in line with WHO guidance, and test results are entered in the HIV Testing Services (HTS) register that is placed at all health service delivery points. Once patients are diagnosed positive for HIV, they are retested for verification of HIV diagnosis and, if confirmed HIV-positive, they are then prepared and counseled for ART and referred for immediate start of ART regardless of WHO clinical stage or CD4 cell count. Administration of an HIV screening tool for HIV risk assessment before providing a rapid HIV test and use of HIV self-testing are measures that have been scaled up recently to improve the HIV positivity yield.

There is generally good quality data capture and reporting for TB and HIV/AIDS at all levels due to regular supervision by national program supervisors.

2.2.3. Data Monitoring, Recording and Reporting for the Study in Health Facilities in Harare

Data were routinely collected daily by front-line health workers. They provided services in each of the ten health facilities in Harare using the standard MOHCC monitoring tools (presumptive TB register, sputum laboratory register, TB patient register and HTS register), most of which were paper-based. One to two weeks after the end of each month, the project country coordinator (KCT—who was appointed specifically for the study) visited each site along with his team of trained data collectors. They collated the individual data on TB and HIV variables for the previous month into monthly aggregate data, which they then entered into a proforma developed using an EpiCollect5 application (https://five.epicollect.net, accessed on 29 May 2021).

For TB treatment outcomes, the monthly cohorts of patients enrolled onto treatment eight months previously were used—this allowed for six months of treatment to be completed and a further two months for outcomes to be validated and recorded in the registers. For example, the October 2020 TB treatment outcome data were obtained for TB patients enrolled and started on treatment in February 2020. This allowed for clear separation of treatment cohorts in the pre-COVID-19 and COVID-19 periods.

National data on COVID-19 cases and deaths reported to WHO on the last day of the month were obtained from WHO situation and epidemiological reports [1].

When the prospective monthly data were collected, a schedule and the same procedures were used to collect retrospective data. For each month of the COVID-19 period (March 2020 to February 2021), data were collected on TB and HIV parameters for a matching period one year before the COVID-19 period (March 2019 to February 2020).

Once all prospective and retrospective data for the month had been entered into EpiCollect5, they were checked and validated by both the project country coordinator and the overall project monitoring and evaluation officer (PT) based at The Union. Data were then presented in a monthly report as a series of figures and tables and narrative to the directors of the NTP and NAP and to all other relevant stakeholders involved in the project. Key policy or practice changes made at the local health facility or at the national level during that month to explain and/or counteract the effects of COVID-19 on TB and HIV parameters were recorded in a narrative table within the report. These monthly reports were always sent and received by the national program staff within four weeks of closure of that month to enable timely surveillance and possible action.

2.3. Study Population

The study population included all patients presenting to TB services with presumptive TB, all TB patients registered for DS-TB treatment and all persons tested for HIV between March 2019 and February 2021; March 2020 to February 2021 was the COVID-19 period, and March 2019 to February 2020 was the pre-COVID-19 period. We also included TB patients registered for treatment eight months prior to the study period to assess treatment outcomes.

2.4. Data Variables, Sources of Data and Timing of Data Collection

Data variables for TB included aggregate numbers of patients: with presumptive PTB, stratified by male and female, adults ($\geq$15 years) and children (<15 years); who were diagnosed with bacteriologically positive PTB by either smear microscopy and/or Xpert MTB/RIF; with registered TB, stratified by bacteriologically confirmed PTB, clinically diagnosed PTB and EPTB; and with registered TB, who were newly tested for HIV in that month after being diagnosed with TB—this excluded patients who already knew they were HIV-positive or had recently been diagnosed HIV-negative. Standardized TB treatment outcomes of those patients enrolled for treatment eight months previously were collected and included—treatment success (a combination of those cured and those who completed treatment with no sputum smear examination), lost to follow-up (LTFU), died, failed treatment or not evaluated [23]. LTFU refers to a TB patient who did not start treatment or whose treatment was interrupted for two consecutive months or more. Not evaluated is an outcome given to those who transfer from one facility to another and for whom the final treatment outcome is not recorded and also to those whose outcome is not recorded and unknown to the reporting unit.

Data variables for HIV included: persons who were HIV tested at the health facilities, stratified by male and female, adults ($\geq$15 years) and children (<15 years); persons diagnosed HIV-positive; and HIV-positive persons referred to ART services.

Sources of data were the presumptive TB register, the sputum laboratory register, the TB patient register, and the HTS register. Prospective and retrospective data for the study were collected between June 2020 and March 2021.

2.5. Analysis and Statistics

Aggregate data were entered in EpiCollect5, where they were checked and validated in-country by the country coordinator and by The Union's monitoring and evaluation officer. Data were presented as frequencies and proportions, and comparisons were made between the COVID-19 period and the pre-COVID-19 period. The percentage decline in numbers during each month of the COVID-19 period was calculated relative to the numbers during the same month of the pre-COVID-19 period. The relative percentage differences observed between the first 6 months of COVID-19 (March to August 2020) and the second 6 months of COVID-19 (September 2020 to February 2021) were also calculated.

3. Results

3.1. COVID-19 Cases and Deaths and General Effects on Health Services

COVID-19 cases and deaths as reported to WHO cumulatively increased to 35,994 and 1458, respectively, during the 12 months (see Figure 1).

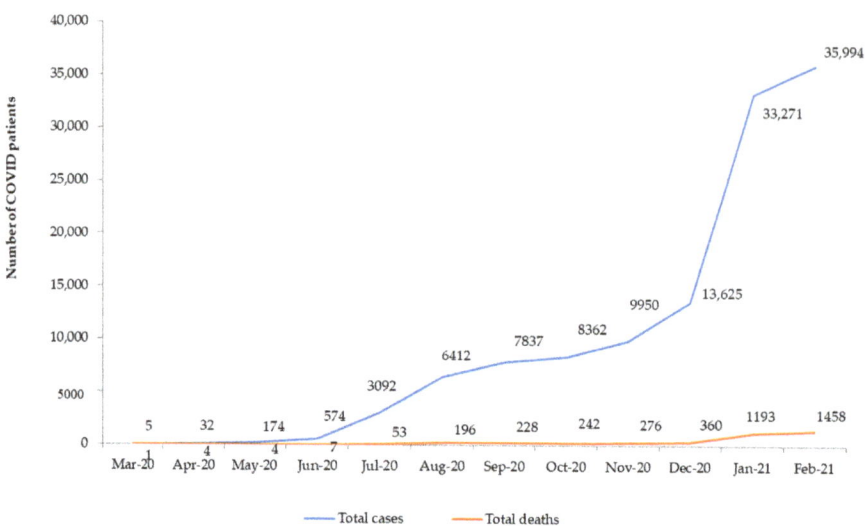

Figure 1. Cumulative number of COVID-19 cases and deaths in Zimbabwe between March 2020 and February 2021 as reported to the World Health Organization.

From a general services perspective, there had been heightened economic decline in Zimbabwe in the pre-COVID-19 period, especially towards the end of 2019 and start of 2020. This resulted in a series of health care worker strikes which affected service provision. The introduction of flexible working hours in 2020 helped to restore health service delivery. In March 2020, COVID-19 struck. There was a national lockdown between March and the end of June 2020 and again from 6 January to 28 February 2021. During lockdowns, people were not allowed to leave their places of residence, public transport ceased, there were night curfews, health facilities shortened their working hours, and some health facilities had to close due to either shortage of health care workers or if there was an outbreak of COVID-19 within the facility. Only a few patients were allowed into health facilities at a time, resulting in long waiting queues outside, which may have deterred patients from coming to the health facilities. Between July and September 2020, there was industrial strike action again in the health sector over the lack of personal protective equipment and remuneration. Locum staff brought in to fill the gaps were not familiar with programmatic activities, including recording and reporting. There was widespread community fear about contracting COVID-19 or being diagnosed with COVID-19 at health facilities during the whole period.

From a TB perspective, environmental health technicians, responsible for community follow-up of TB patients while on treatment, were repurposed to COVID-19 activities. Between 12 December 2020 and 11 January 2021, GeneXpert cartridges expired in some facilities, and during this time clinic staff did not collect sputum specimens for TB investigation.

From an HIV perspective, voluntary male medical circumcision services (VMMC), which provided HIV testing for a large number of male adolescents and men, stopped in March 2020 and remained closed for the next 12 months. There were stock-outs of HIV test kits in July 2020, which remained a challenge intermittently for the next few months.

3.2. TB Case Finding, Diagnosis and Registration

There was an overall decrease in the numbers of persons presenting with presumptive PTB (40.6%), people diagnosed with bacteriologically confirmed PTB (30.1%) and people being registered for TB treatment (33.7%) in the COVID-19 period compared to the pre-COVID-19 period (Table 1).

Table 1. Characteristics of persons with presumptive pulmonary TB and registered TB in 10 health facilities in Harare, Zimbabwe, during pre-COVID-19 and COVID-19 periods.

Numbers of Patients	Pre-COVID-19 Mar 2019–Feb 2020 N	COVID-19 Mar 2020–Feb 2021 N	Difference between Pre-COVID-19 and COVID-19 %
Presumptive pulmonary TB:	3270	1941	↓40.6
Adults (≥15 years)	3013	1849	↓38.6
Children (<15 years)	181	52	↓71.3
Male	1866	1150	↓38.4
Female	1221	782	↓36.0
Bacteriologically positive	442	309	↓30.1
Positivity rate (%)	(13.5%)	(15.9%)	↑2.4% *
Registered TB:	1078	715	↓33.7
Bacteriologically confirmed PTB	528	346	↓34.5
Clinically diagnosed PTB	465	251	↓46.0
Extrapulmonary TB	136	97	↓28.7
Eligible for being newly HIV tested	586	423	↓27.8
Newly tested for HIV (%)	(95.1%)	(90.3%)	↓4.8% *

* absolute change (increase or decrease); TB = tuberculosis; PTB = pulmonary tuberculosis; ↑ = increase; ↓ = decrease.

For presumptive PTB, the overall decrease was greater in children (71.3%) compared with adults (38.6%), but almost similar between males (38.4%) and females (36.0%). The yield of bacteriologically positive PTB in those investigated for presumptive TB increased from 13.5 to 15.9%. The decline in those diagnosed and registered with TB was worse for patients with PTB, and amongst those with pulmonary disease, it was worse for those with clinically diagnosed PTB (46.0%). The proportion of TB patients tested for HIV remained above 90%, although it declined from 95.1 to 90.3%.

The monthly numbers of persons presenting with presumptive PTB and registered TB in the pre-COVID-19 and COVID-19 periods are shown in Figure 2A,B. The footnotes for the Figures indicate the interventions that were put in place to counteract the downward trends.

Compared with the pre-COVID-19 period, the decline in presumptive TB in the first 6 months of COVID-19 (March to August 2020) was 35.8%, and this became greater in the second 6 months (September 2020 to February 2021) when the decline was 45.5%. The decline in registered TB in the first 6 months of COVID-19 was 29.9%, which also became greater in the second 6 months when the decline was 37.5%.

3.3. TB Treatment Outcomes

The overall aggregate treatment outcomes between the pre-COVID-19 and COVID-19 periods are shown in Table 2. There was a decrease in treatment success from 80.9 to 69.3%, mainly due to an increase in patients "not evaluated" (12.1%). Other program outcomes were similar between the two periods.

The monthly treatment success rates in the pre-COVID-19 and COVID-19 periods are shown in Figure 3. Interventions to reverse downward trends are indicated in the footnotes. Compared with the pre-COVID-19 period, the decline in treatment success was 14% in the first 6 months of COVID-19. This improved in the second 6 months when the decline was 7.8%. Treatment success particularly improved in January and February 2021 to 80 and 78%, respectively.

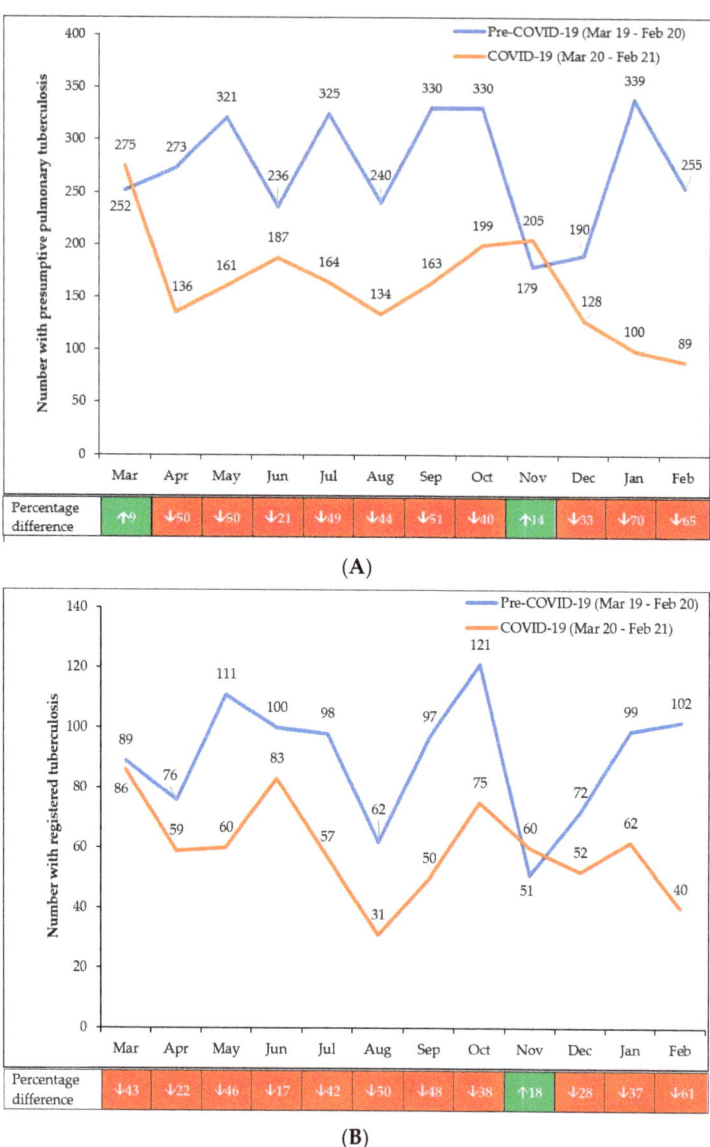

Figure 2. (**A**): Monthly numbers of persons presenting with presumptive PTB in 10 health facilities in Harare, Zimbabwe, during pre-COVID-19 and COVID-19 periods. (**B**): Monthly numbers of persons presenting with registered TB in 10 health facilities in Harare, Zimbabwe, during pre-COVID-19 and COVID-19 periods. ↑ = increase; ↓ = decrease. Interventions applied from July 2020 onwards to counteract the decline in numbers included: integrated screening of patients with respiratory symptoms for TB and COVID-19; improved contact tracing of index patients with TB and COVID-19; and strict infection control practices at health facilities which were promoted to try and encourage symptomatic patients to attend.

Table 2. Treatment outcomes of patients enrolled in TB treatment in 10 health facilities in Harare, Zimbabwe, during pre-COVID-19 and COVID-19 periods.

Treatment Outcomes in Patients Enrolled for TB Treatment	Pre-COVID-19 Mar 2019–Feb 2020 n	COVID-19 Mar 2020–Feb 2021 n	Difference between Pre-COVID-19 and COVID-19 %
Enrolled for treatment:	1210	979	
Treatment success (%)	(80.9)	(69.3)	↓11.6 *
Lost to follow-up (%)	(2.0)	(2.3)	↑0.3 *
Died (%)	(4.3)	(3.7)	↓0.6 *
Failed (%)	(0.6)	(0.4)	↓0.2 *
Not evaluated (%)	(12.2)	(24.3)	↑12.1 *

* absolute change (increase or decrease); TB = tuberculosis; ↑ = increase; ↓ = decrease; treatment outcome was considered "treatment success" when the TB patient was either cured or had "treatment completed". The success rate was calculated for the month-wise cohort of TB patients commenced on treatment eight months prior to the reporting month (this takes account of six months of treatment to be completed and another two months to finalize the recording of the final treatment outcome).

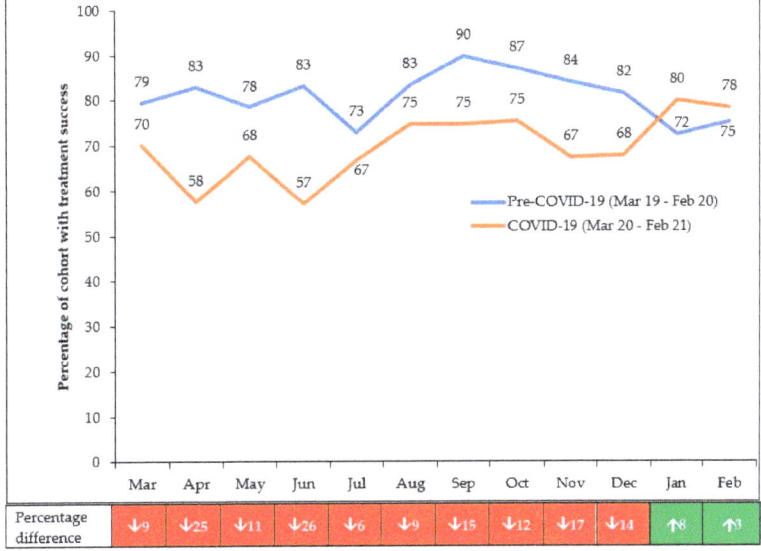

Figure 3. Treatment success amongst patients enrolled each month in 10 health facilities in Harare, Zimbabwe, during pre-COVID-19 and COVID-19 periods. Enrollment occurred eight months prior to the month of reporting (to allow for 6 months treatment and 2 months of follow-up and record the final outcome); ↑ = increase; ↓ = decrease. The interventions applied from July onwards included: medication refills given for longer periods and synchronized for TB and ART medications; attempts to reduce the outcome "not evaluated".

3.4. HIV Testing and Referral to ART

There was a large overall decrease in numbers tested for HIV between pre-COVID-19 and COVID-19 periods (Table 3). The overall decrease was greater for children (70.2%) compared with adults (62.4%) and greater for males (79.1%) compared with females (53.6%). There was a small relative increase in the HIV positivity rate from 6.0 to 8.1% and a small decrease in the referral of HIV-positive persons to ART from 95.7 to 91.7% during the COVID-19 period.

Table 3. Characteristics of persons tested for HIV and referred to antiretroviral therapy in 10 health facilities in Harare, Zimbabwe, during pre-COVID-19 and COVID-19 periods.

Characteristics	Pre-COVID-19 Mar 2019–Feb 2020 n	COVID-19 Mar 2020–Feb 2021 N	Difference between Pre-COVID-19 and COVID-19 %
Underwent HIV testing at a health facility:	51,078	18,987	↓62.8
Adults (≥15 years)	48,661	18,289	↓62.4
Children (<15 years)	2316	691	↓70.2
Male	18,278	3816	↓79.1
Female	32,706	15,171	↓53.6
Positive for HIV	3045	1547	↓36.7
HIV positivity rate (%)	(6.0%)	(8.1%)	↑2.1 *
Referred to ART (%)	(95.7%)	(91.7%)	↓4.0 *

* absolute change (increase or decrease); ↑ = increase; ↓ = decrease; ART = antiretroviral therapy.

The monthly numbers tested for HIV in the pre-COVID-19 and COVID-19 periods are shown in Figure 4.

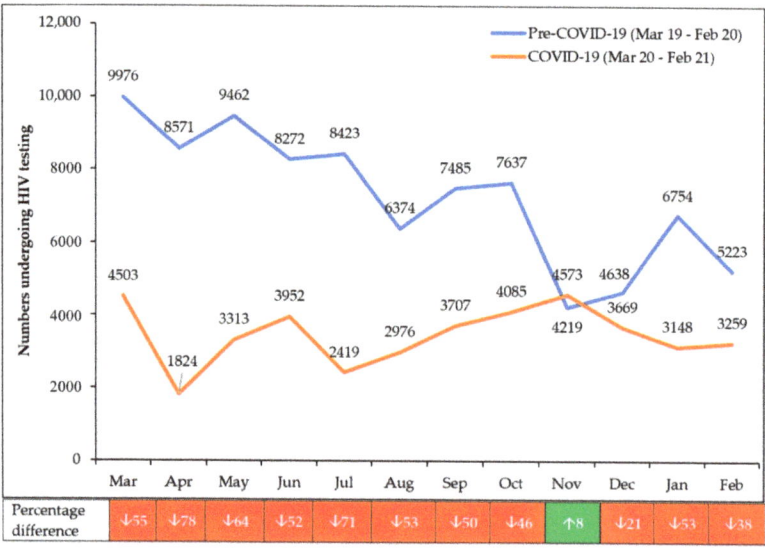

Figure 4. Monthly numbers presenting each month for HIV testing in 10 health facilities in Harare, Zimbabwe, during pre-COVID-19 and COVID-19 periods; ↑ = increase; ↓ = decrease. From August 2020 onwards, human resources support was given to the Ministry of Health by PEPFAR partners (President's Emergency Fund for AIDS Relief in Africa) by seconding direct service delivery nurses to affected sites.

The number of people being HIV tested in health facilities was already declining in the pre-COVID-19 period due to a number of factors that included: a shift from general HIV testing to more targeted HIV testing using a screening tool to identify high-risk groups, to identify those with a high lifestyle risk score assessment and to identify those who had not been tested in the previous year; promotion of HIV self-testing, with the referral of only those HIV-positive to the health facilities for confirmation of the result; and a greater focus on index partner testing. As explained in the footnotes of Figure 4, human resources support was provided to clinics from August 2020 onwards to sustain HIV testing services and ART delivery. Compared with the pre-COVID-19 period, the decline in HIV testing in the first 6 months of COVID-19 was 62.8%, which was greater than the 37.6% decline observed in the second 6 months.

4. Discussion

This is the first study in Zimbabwe to assess the impact of COVID-19 on TB and HIV services in selected health facilities in Harare, the capital city. In summary, despite attempts by the NTP, the NAP and other parts of the health sector to prepare for COVID-19 [15,27], there was a large negative impact on almost all aspects of TB case detection, diagnosis and treatment, as well as HIV testing. The referral of HIV-positive persons to ART was also affected but only to a small degree. A health service already under strain was hit hard and brought almost to its knees in the first 12 months of the COVID-19 pandemic [27].

With respect to TB program activities, the numbers of people presenting to health facilities with presumptive PTB declined considerably over the 12-month COVID-19 period. These findings were similar to those described in the early months of COVID-19 in clinics in Tehran, Iran [28] and Nigeria [29], where lockdown restrictions, transportation difficulties and community fear of health facilities were thought to hinder health facility access. There was a corresponding decline in numbers diagnosed and registered with TB, in line with reports from other countries where the decreases in TB case notifications in the early months of COVID-19 compared with previous years were 48% in clinics in China [30], 48% in clinics in Brazil [31] and 56% in India [32].

A modeling analysis at the start of the pandemic suggested that a 3-month suspension of TB services due to COVID-19 lockdown followed by ten months restoration back to normal would cause over five years an additional 1.2 million TB cases in India, 25,000 additional TB cases in Kenya and 4000 additional cases in Ukraine, mainly as a result of the accumulation of undetected TB during lockdown [33]. Unfortunately, in Zimbabwe, there was no restoration of services back to normal. On the contrary, from October 2020 to February 2021, there was a steady decline in numbers of persons with presumptive PTB and registered TB, coinciding with the expiry of cartridges for Xpert MTB/RIF assays. Sputum specimens were not collected for investigation, and patients with TB-related respiratory symptoms stayed away. The one encouraging finding was an overall increase in bacteriological positivity in the COVID-19 period compared with the previous year. There are several possible explanations that include: (i) when laboratories were functioning and reagents were available, standard laboratory operating procedures remained intact; (ii) there was selective self-referral of only those who were really sick with TB; and (iii) patients may not have had access to community TB testing services as a result of COVID-19, and therefore those with TB came to Harare city health facilities for investigation.

TB treatment success rates declined during the COVID-19 pandemic. However, there was some improvement in the second half of the year, and particularly in January and February 2021, when outcomes were better than at the corresponding times before COVID-19. The probable reason for better outcomes at this time was, as discussed earlier, a series of health care worker strikes towards the end of the pre-COVID-19 period as a result of heightened economic decline. This disrupted routine follow-up of TB patients on treatment, resulting in a high number of patients not being evaluated.

With the onset of the COVID-19 pandemic, we were concerned that COVID-19 restrictions would hinder patients collecting anti-TB medications and compromise drug adherence. However, the longer periods given between anti-TB drug refills and their synchronization with ART medication refills made things easier for patients and partly mitigated this challenge. The large proportion of patients "not evaluated" was a huge challenge, compromising the program's ability to record successful treatment outcomes. This was partly due to the environmental health technicians responsible for following up patients in the community being repurposed to COVID-19 activities. Concerted efforts, however, were made to tackle this issue, and through human resources support from PEPFAR (the President's Emergency Plan for AIDS Relief), treatment success rates considerably improved in the last two months.

With respect to HIV services, there was a significant decrease in numbers of people presenting for HIV testing, although this did improve during the latter half of the COVID-19 period. There were two main reasons for the large decline. First, the cessation of VMMC services would have resulted in a large decline in males being HIV tested during this time. Second, in April 2020, during the national lockdown, the MOHCC issued a directive for all community-based HIV testing to be temporarily halted to minimize the risk of community health workers and community members from contracting COVID-19. The improvement in the latter half of the COVID-19 period may have been due to the strong support from PEPFAR partners.

The overall reductions in HIV testing were similar to what has been observed in Europe [34], the USA [35] and Africa [36]. It is likely, though, that we have overestimated the COVID-19 impact on HIV testing because of Zimbabwe adopting a more targeted approach, promoting HIV self-testing and focusing on index HIV testing before the onslaught of COVID-19. The increase in HIV positivity observed in the COVID-19 period in our study is probably a result of this more targeted approach to identifying clients more at risk of HIV. While referrals to ART decreased in the COVID-19 period, it was encouraging to see that they were still maintained at over 90%.

There are several strengths to this study. First, the real-time monthly surveillance was embedded within the routine services of the health facilities, and there was cross-checking and validation of the data each month between the country coordinator and the overall study monitoring and evaluation officer. We believe, therefore, that the data were accurate and reflected programmatic practice in the field in Harare. Second, we used two 12-month periods to compare data, thus accounting for seasonal changes that might have affected TB case detection and HIV testing. Third, the conduct and reporting of the study were in line with the Strengthening the Reporting of Observational Studies in Epidemiology (STROBE) guidelines [37].

However, there were some limitations. Our study was limited to health facilities in Harare, and therefore may not be representative of Zimbabwe as a whole. The use of aggregate quantitative data made it impossible to understand the cascade of care for TB case detection and HIV testing during COVID-19. Further mixed-methods research with both quantitative and qualitative analysis amongst TB patients themselves, as has been conducted in Zambia [38], are needed to obtain a better idea of why patient access to health services and health service delivery was so badly affected. We only assessed referrals of HIV-positive persons to ART and did not document the initiation or retention on ART. Previous studies have suggested that ART interruption has been a problem during the COVID-19 pandemic [39]. It would have been interesting to assess this in Zimbabwe, especially as interruption to ART is thought to be one of the most important determinants of HIV-related mortality during the COVID-19 pandemic [40]. Finally, the official monthly reports to WHO of COVID-19 cases and deaths may have underestimated the true burden of COVID-19 in the country. A study on deceased people at the University Teaching Hospital morgue in Lusaka, Zambia, found that just 9% of 70 people, who were confirmed as having SARS-CoV-2 from postmortem nasopharyngeal swabs within 48 h of death, had ever been tested before death [41]. This finding is unlikely to be confined to Zambia, and large numbers of unreported cases and deaths due to COVID-19 are probably occurring in other countries in Africa.

Despite these limitations, there are some important programmatic implications from this study. First, the strengthened monthly surveillance system worked well with both NTP and HIV program directors looking each month at the monthly reports and using the data for decision making and suggesting interventions. The monthly data were also shared with the ten health facilities through the country coordinator, and this enabled the health facilities to implement interventions simultaneously. However, the monthly surveillance and the interventions applied were insufficient to reverse the direct negative effects of COVID-19 on services or the indirect effects such as industrial action and stock-outs of diagnostic tests. Given the challenges both programs faced, it is remarkable that services were able to function at all, so without monthly surveillance, it might have been much worse. The monthly surveillance as conducted in Harare required effort and external support. If this became routine as desired, the NTP would require considerable investment, probably involving electronic case-based reporting systems. Technical support by partners, who have additional human resources to help, would be vital to get activities and services back to normal.

Second, with COVID-19 likely to become endemic, there is an urgent need to bring TB case detection and treatment outcomes back to pre-COVID-19 levels. This study suggested that better contact tracing of TB patients and heightened attention to reducing the "not evaluated" category were important interventions for TB case detection and TB treatment outcomes. Support from PEPFAR partners also helped to support staff in ascertaining TB treatment outcomes. There are several other suggestions about how TB services could be sustained or improved in the face of the pandemic. These include: better integration and screening of TB and COVID-19 at the health facility and community level; sharing testing algorithms and multiplexing equipment such as GeneXpert platforms within the laboratories; having robust procurement and delivery systems to avoid reagent stock-outs; ensuring effective infection, prevention and control activities within health facilities; having longer 3-month follow-up appointments for patient check-ups and drug collection; providing health information education in health facilities and the community; and mobilizing support networks of TB survivors and TB communities [42–44]. More use of digital platforms for case finding, drug adherence, management of adverse drug reactions and training have also been recommended as a way of rapidly restoring TB diagnosis, care and prevention services [45]. The Zimbabwe NTP and MOHCC could consider which, if any, of these innovative approaches might help, and might be feasible and cost-effective to implement.

Third, HIV self-testing, index partner notification and home-based HIV testing services have allowed HIV testing numbers in the COVID-19 era to rebound in some African countries [46–48]. Zimbabwe is already moving in this direction. It is also vital to capture all HIV testing and HIV test results outside of as well as within the health sector in order to keep informed about what is happening and ensure that all HIV-infected persons are able to initiate ART. Zimbabwe again is already implementing such an approach and is tracking on a monthly basis facility and community distribution of HIV test kits, as well as numbers tested for HIV along with their results. Further deployment of electronic data capture systems will be important in this context.

Finally, the resources and funding that have been raised to fight the COVID-19 pandemic have been staggering. The proposed global financing systems that have been proposed as a way of promoting and enabling science and product development in the health sector [49] must be used and leveraged to help fight other diseases, TB and HIV/AIDS included, so that we can stay on track to deliver on the Sustainable Development Goals in 2030.

5. Conclusions

Using strengthened monthly real-time surveillance in 10 health facilities in Harare, Zimbabwe, we documented that numbers of persons with presumptive PTB and registered TB, treatment outcomes of patients enrolled on treatment and numbers being HIV tested all declined during 12 months of the COVID-19 outbreak compared with 12 months pre-COVID-19. The referral of HIV-positive persons to ART also declined, although they were maintained at high levels throughout. Despite using the monthly data, the declining trends in TB and HIV services could not be reversed because of on-going restrictions resulting from the COVID-19 pandemic combined with industrial action in the health sector and the expiry of certain diagnostic reagents. Suggestions have been made as to how to restore TB case detection and HIV testing so that TB- and HIV-related morbidity and mortality can be kept as low as possible during this difficult period.

Author Contributions: Conceptualization, P.T., K.C.T., C.T., C.S., T.A., A.M.V.K., S.S., H.D.S., M.K., R.Z., I.D.R., S.D.B. and A.D.H.; methodology, P.T., K.C.T., C.T., C.S., T.A., A.M.V.K., S.S., H.D.S., M.K., R.Z., I.D.R., S.D.B. and A.D.H.; software, P.T.; validation, P.T. and K.C.T.; formal analysis, P.T., K.C.T., C.T., C.S., T.A., A.M.V.K., S.S., H.D.S., M.K., R.Z., I.D.R., S.D.B. and A.D.H.; investigation, P.T., K.C.T. and C.T.; resources, I.D.R.; data curation, P.T., K.C.T. and A.D.H.; writing—original draft preparation, P.T., K.C.T., C.T., S.D.B. and A.D.H.; writing—review and editing, P.T., K.C.T., C.T., C.S., T.A., A.M.V.K., S.S., H.D.S., M.K., R.Z., I.D.R., S.D.B. and A.D.H.; visualization, P.T., K.C.T., C.T., S.D.B. and A.D.H.; supervision, P.T., K.C.T., C.T. and A.D.H.; project administration, S.D.B.; funding acquisition, S.D.B. and A.D.H. All authors have read and agreed to the published version of the manuscript.

Funding: This research was funded by Bloomberg Philanthropies through a grant with Vital Strategies and the Resolve to Save Lives Initiative, New York, NY, USA.

Institutional Review Board Statement: The project received ethics approval from the Medical Research Council of Zimbabwe (MRCZ/E/273) and the Ethics Advisory Group of the International Union Against Tuberculosis and Lung Disease (EAG 33/2020). As no names or other means of identifying patients during data collection were recorded and as only aggregated data were used for the study, the need for informed patient consent was waived.

Informed Consent Statement: No names or other means of identifying patients during data collection were recorded and only aggregated data were used for the study. Thus, the need for informed patient consent was waived by both of the ethics committees.

Data Availability Statement: The data that support the findings of the study are available from one of the first authors (P.T.) upon reasonable request.

Acknowledgments: The authors thank established staff working in TB and HIV control in the ten health facilities for their help in collecting the data.

Conflicts of Interest: The authors declare no conflict of interest. The funders had no role in the design of the study; in the collection, analyses, or interpretation of data; in the writing of the manuscript, or in the decision to publish the results.

References

1. World Health Organization. Coronavirus Disease (COVID-19) Weekly Epidemiological Update and Weekly Operational Update 29 December 2020. Available online: https://www.who.int/emergencies/diseases/novel-coronavirus-2019/situation-reports (accessed on 30 March 2021).
2. Gilbert, M.; Pullano, G.; Pinotti, F.; Valdano, E.; Poletto, C.; Boëlle, P.Y.; D'Ortenzio, E.; Yazdanpanah, Y.; Eholie, S.P.; Altmann, M.; et al. Preparedness and vulnerability of African countries against importations of COVID-19: A modelling study. *Lancet* **2020**, *395*, 871–877. [CrossRef]
3. Nkengasong, J.N.; Mankoula, W. Looming threat of COVID-19 infection in Africa: Act collectively, and fast. *Lancet* **2020**, *395*, 841–842. [CrossRef]
4. Pang, Y.; Liu, Y.; Du, J.; Gao, J.; Li, L. Impact of COVID-19 on tuberculosis control in China. *Int. J. Tuberc. Lung Dis.* **2020**, *24*, 545–547. [CrossRef]
5. Hogan, A.B.; Jewell, B.L.; Sherrard-Smith, E.; Vesga, J.F.; Watson, O.J.; Whittaker, C.; Hamlet, A.; Smith, J.A.; Winskill, P.; Verity, R.; et al. Potential impact of the COVID-19 pandemic on HIV, tuberculosis, and malaria in low-income and middle-income countries: A modelling study. *Lancet Glob. Health* **2020**, *8*, 1132–1141. [CrossRef]
6. Bah, O.M.; Kamara, H.B.; Bhat, P.; Harries, A.D.; Owiti, P.; Katta, J.; Foray, L.; Kamara, M.I.; Kamara, B.O. The influence of the Ebola outbreak on presumptive and active tuberculosis in Bombali District, Sierra Leone. *Public Health Action* **2017**, *7*, 3–9. [CrossRef] [PubMed]
7. Konwloh, P.K.; Cambell, C.L.; Ade, S.; Bhat, P.; Harries, A.D.; Wilkinson, E.; Cooper, C.T. Influence of Ebola on tuberculosis case finding and treatment outcomes in Liberia. *Public Health Action* **2017**, *7*, 62–69. [CrossRef]
8. Gamanga, A.H.; Owiti, P.; Bhat, P.; Harries, A.D.; Kargbo-Labour, I.; Koroma, M. The Ebola outbreak: Effects on HIV reporting, testing and care in Bonthe district, rural Sierra Leone. *Public Health Action* **2017**, *7*, 10–15. [CrossRef] [PubMed]
9. Jacobs, G.P.; Bhat, P.; Owiti, P.; Edwards, J.K.; Tweya, H.; Najjemba, R. Did the 2014 Ebola outbreak in Liberia affect HIV testing, linkage to care and ART initiation? *Public Health Action* **2017**, *7*, 70–75. [CrossRef]
10. Stop TB Partnership. TB and COVID-19. Available online: http://www.stoptb.org/covid19.asp?utm_source=The+Stop+TB+Pa (accessed on 30 March 2021).
11. World Health Organization. *World Health Organization (WHO) Information Note Tuberculosis and COVID-19*; World Health Organization: Geneva, Switzerland, 2020.
12. UNAIDS. Covid-19 and HIV. Available online: https://www.unaids.org/en/covid19 (accessed on 30 March 2021).

13. Chiang, C.Y.; Sony, A.E. Tackling the threat of COVID-19 in Africa: An urgent need for practical planning. *Int. J. Tuberc. Lung Dis.* **2020**, *24*, 541–542. [CrossRef] [PubMed]
14. World Health Organization. *Coronavirus Disease 2019 (COVID-19) Situation Report—86*; World Health Organization: Geneva, Switzerland, 2020.
15. Sandy, C.; Takarinda, K.C.; Timire, C.; Mutunzi, H.; Dube, M.; Dlodlo, R.A.; Harries, A.D. Preparing national tuberculosis control programmes for COVID-19. *Int. J. Tuberc. Lung Dis.* **2020**, *24*, 634–636. [CrossRef] [PubMed]
16. Ortuno-Gutierrez, N.; Zachariah, R.; Woldeyohannes, D.; Bangoura, A.; Chérif, G.-F.; Loua, F.; Hermans, V.; Tayler-Smith, K.; Sikhondze, W.; Camara, L.-M. Upholding Tuberculosis services during the 2014 Ebola storm: An encouraging experience from Conakry, Guinea. *PLoS ONE* **2016**, *11*, e0157296. [CrossRef]
17. Zimbabwe National Statistics Agency. *Zimbabwe Population Census, 2012*; Zimbabwe National Statistics Agency: Harare, Zimbabwe, 2013.
18. The World Bank. Zimbabwe. Available online: https://data.worldbank.org/country/ZW (accessed on 19 April 2021).
19. World Health Organization. *Global Tuberculosis Report 2020*; World Health Organization: Geneva, Switzerland, 2020.
20. Worldometer. Zimbabwe Population (2021). Available online: https://www.worldometers.info/world-population/zimbabwe-population/ (accessed on 19 April 2021).
21. Ministry of Health and Child Care (MOHCC). *Zimbabwe TB Guidelines*; MOHCC: Harare, Zimbabwe, 2010.
22. World Health Organization. *Guidelines for Treatment of Drug-Susceptible Tuberculosis and Patient Care (2017 Update)*; World Health Organization: Geneva, Switzerland, 2017.
23. World Health Organization. Definitions and Reporting Framework for Tuberculosis; 2013 Revision, Updated December 2014 and January 2020. This document Revises Previous WHO, Standard Reporting Framework for TB. Available online: https://www.who.int/tb/publications/definitions/en/#:~{}:text=2013 (accessed on 30 March 2021).
24. Ministry of Health and Child Care (MOHCC). *Operational and Service Delivery Manual for the Prevention, Care and Treatment of HIV in Zimbabwe*; MOHCC: Harare, Zimbabwe, 2017.
25. World Health Organization. Consolidated Guidelines on HIV Testing Services. Available online: https://www.who.int/publications/i/item/978-92-4-155058-1 (accessed on 30 March 2021).
26. World Health Organization. *Consolidated Guidelines on the Use of Antiretroviral Drugs for Treating and Preventing HIV Infection: Recommendations for a Public Health Approach*, 2nd ed.; World Health Organization: Geneva, Switzerland, 2016.
27. Makoni, M. COVID-19 worsens Zimbabwe's health crisis. *Lancet* **2020**, *396*, 457. [CrossRef]
28. Kargarpour Kamakoli, M.; Hadifar, S.; Khanipour, S.; Farmanfarmaei, G.; Fateh, A.; Mostafaei, S.; Siadat, S.D.; Vaziri, F. Tuberculosis under the Influence of COVID-19 Lockdowns: Lessons from Tehran, Iran. *mSphere* **2021**, *6*, e00076-21. [CrossRef] [PubMed]
29. Adewole, O.O. Impact of COVID-19 on TB care: Experiences of a treatment centre in Nigeria. *Int. J. Tuberc. Lung Dis.* **2020**, *24*, 981–982. [CrossRef]
30. Wu, Z.; Chen, J.; Xia, Z.; Pan, Q.; Yuan, Z.; Zhang, W.; Shen, X. Impact of the COVID-19 pandemic on the detection of TB in Shanghai, China. *Int. J. Tuberc. Lung Dis.* **2020**, *24*, 1122–1124. [CrossRef]
31. De Souza, C.D.F.; Coutinho, H.S.; Costa, M.M.; Magalhães, M.A.F.M.; Carmo, R.F. Impact of COVID-19 on TB diagnosis in Northeastern Brazil. *Int. J. Tuberc. Lung Dis.* **2020**, *24*, 1220–1222. [CrossRef] [PubMed]
32. Golandaj, J.A. Insight into the COVID-19 led slow-down in TB notifications in India. *Indian J. Tuberc.* **2021**, *68*, 142–145. [CrossRef]
33. Cilloni, L.; Fu, H.; Vesga, J.F.; Dowdy, D.; Pretorius, C.; Ahmedov, S.; Nair, S.A.; Mosneaga, A.; Masini, E.; Sahu, S.; et al. The potential impact of the COVID-19 pandemic on the tuberculosis epidemic a modelling analysis. *EClinicalMedicine* **2020**, *28*, 100603. [CrossRef] [PubMed]
34. Simões, D.; Stengaard, A.R.; Combs, L.; Raben, D. Impact of the COVID-19 pandemic on testing services for HIV, viral hepatitis and sexually transmitted infections in the WHO european region, March to August 2020. *Eurosurveillance* **2020**, *25*, 2001943. [CrossRef]
35. Hill, B.J.; Anderson, B.; Lock, L. COVID-19 pandemic, Pre-Exposure Prophylaxis (PrEP) Care, and HIV/STI testing among patients receiving care in three HIV epidemic priority states. *AIDS Behav.* **2021**, *1*, 1–5.
36. Ponticiello, M.; Mwanga-Amumpaire, J.; Tushemereirwe, P.; Nuwagaba, G.; King, R.; Sundararajan, R. "Everything is a Mess": How COVID-19 is impacting engagement with HIV testing services in rural southwestern uganda. *AIDS Behav.* **2020**, *24*, 3006–3009. [CrossRef] [PubMed]
37. von Elm, E.; Altman, D.G.; Egger, M.; Pocock, S.J.; Gøtzsche, P.C.; Vandenbroucke, J.P. The strengthening the reporting of observational studies in epidemiology (STROBE) statement: Guidelines for reporting observational studies. *Lancet* **2007**, *370*, 1453–1457. [CrossRef]
38. Mwamba, C.; Kerkhoff, A.D.; Kagujje, M.; Lungu, P.; Muyoyeta, M.; Sharma, A. Diagnosed with TB in the era of COVID-19: Patient perspectives in Zambia. *Public Health Action* **2021**, *10*, 141–146. [CrossRef] [PubMed]
39. Sun, Y.; Li, H.; Luo, G.; Meng, X.; Guo, W.; Fitzpatrick, T.; Ao, Y.; Feng, A.; Liang, B.; Zhan, Y.; et al. Antiretroviral treatment interruption among people living with HIV during COVID-19 outbreak in China: A nationwide cross-sectional study. *J. Int. AIDS Soc.* **2020**, *23*, e25637. [CrossRef] [PubMed]
40. Jewell, B.L.; Smith, J.A.; Hallett, T.B. Understanding the impact of interruptions to HIV services during the COVID-19 pandemic: A modelling study. *EClinicalMedicine* **2020**, *26*, 100483. [CrossRef]

41. Mwananyanda, L.; Gill, C.J.; MacLeod, W.; Kwenda, G.; Pieciak, R.; Mupila, Z.; Lapidot, R.; Mupeta, F.; Forman, L.; Ziko, L.; et al. Covid-19 deaths in Africa: Prospective systematic postmortem surveillance study. *BMJ* **2021**, *372*, n334. [CrossRef]
42. Echeverría, G.; Espinoza, W.; de Waard, J.H. How TB and COVID-19 compare: An opportunity to integrate both control programmes. *Int. J. Tuberc. Lung Dis.* **2020**, *24*, 1–4. [CrossRef] [PubMed]
43. Meneguim, A.C.; Rebello, L.; Das, M.; Ravi, S.; Mathur, T.; Mankar, S.; Kharate, S.; Tipre, P.; Oswal, V.; Iyer, A.; et al. Adapting TB services during the COVID-19 pandemic in Mumbai, India. *Int. J. Tuberc. Lung Dis.* **2020**, *24*, 1119–1121. [CrossRef] [PubMed]
44. Stop TB Partnership. One Year On, New Data Show Global Impact of COVID-19 on TB Epidemic is Worse than Expected. Available online: http://www.stoptb.org/covid19.asp (accessed on 30 March 2021).
45. Chiang, C.Y.; Islam, T.; Xu, C.; Chinnayah, T.; Garfin, A.M.C.; Rahevar, K.; Raviglione, M. The impact of COVID-19 and the restoration of tuberculosis services in the Western Pacific Region. *Eur. Respir. J.* **2020**, *56*, 2003054. [CrossRef]
46. Mhango, M.; Chitungo, I.; Dzinamarira, T. COVID-19 lockdowns: Impact on facility-based HIV testing and the case for the scaling up of home-based testing services in sub-saharan africa. *AIDS Behav.* **2020**, *24*, 3014–3016. [CrossRef]
47. Odinga, M.M.; Kuria, S.; Muindi, O.; Mwakazi, P.; Njraini, M.; Melon, M.; Kombo, B.; Kaosa, S.; Kioko, J.; Musimbi, J.; et al. HIV testing amid COVID-19: Community efforts to reach men who have sex with men in three Kenyan counties. *Gates Open Res.* **2020**, *4*, 117. [CrossRef] [PubMed]
48. Lagat, H.; Sharma, M.; Kariithi, E.; Otieno, G.; Katz, D.; Masyuko, S.; Mugambi, M.; Wamuti, B.; Weiner, B.; Farquhar, C. Impact of the COVID-19 pandemic on HIV testing and assisted partner notification services, western kenya. *AIDS Behav.* **2020**, *24*, 3010–3013. [CrossRef] [PubMed]
49. Lurie, N.; Keusch, G.T.; Dzau, V.J. Urgent lessons from COVID 19: Why the world needs a standing, coordinated system and sustainable financing for global research and development. *Lancet* **2021**, *397*, 1229–1236. [CrossRef]

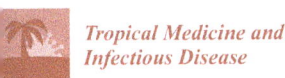
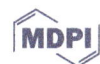

Article

Assessing the Impact of COVID-19 on TB and HIV Programme Services in Selected Health Facilities in Lilongwe, Malawi: Operational Research in Real Time

Pruthu Thekkur [1,2,†], Hannock Tweya [3,†], Sam Phiri [3], James Mpunga [4], Thokozani Kalua [5], Ajay M. V. Kumar [1,2,6], Srinath Satyanarayana [1,2], Hemant D. Shewade [1,2], Mohammed Khogali [7], Rony Zachariah [7], I. D. Rusen [8], Selma Dar Berger [1] and Anthony D. Harries [1,9,*]

1. International Union Against Tuberculosis and Lung Disease (The Union), 75006 Paris, France; Pruthu.TK@theunion.org (P.T.); akumar@theunion.org (A.M.V.K.); SSrinath@theunion.org (S.S.); HShewade@theunion.org (H.D.S.); sberger@theunion.org (S.D.B.)
2. The Union South-East Asia Office, New Delhi 110016, India
3. The Lighthouse, Kamuzu Central Hospital, Lilongwe P.O. Box 106, Malawi; htweya@lighthouse.org.mw (H.T.); samphiri@pihmalawi.com (S.P.)
4. National Tuberculosis Programme, Ministry of Health and Population, Lilongwe P.O. Box 30377, Malawi; mpungajay1@gmail.com
5. HIV/AIDS Department, Ministry of Health and Population, Lilongwe P.O. Box 30377, Malawi; thokokalua@gmail.com
6. Yenepoya Medical College, Yenepoya (Deemed to be University), University Road, Deralakatte, Mangalore 575018, India
7. Special Programme for Research and Training in Tropical Disease (TDR), World Health Organization, 1211 Geneva, Switzerland; khogalim@who.int (M.K.); zachariahr@who.int (R.Z.)
8. Vital Strategies, New York, NY 10005, USA; irusen@vitalstrategies.org
9. Department of Clinical Research, Faculty of Infectious and Tropical Diseases, London School of Hygiene and Tropical Medicine, London WC1E 7HT, UK
* Correspondence: adharries@theunion.org; Tel.: +44-(0)-1962-714-297
† Joint First Author.

Abstract: When the COVID-19 pandemic was announced in March 2020, there was concern that TB and HIV programme services in Malawi would be severely affected. We set up real-time monthly surveillance of TB and HIV activities in eight health facilities in Lilongwe to see if it was possible to counteract the anticipated negative impact on TB case detection and treatment and HIV testing. Aggregate data were collected monthly during the COVID-19 period (March 2020–February 2021) using an EpiCollect5 application and compared with monthly data collected during the pre-COVID-19 period (March 2019–February 2020); these reports were sent monthly to programme directors. During COVID-19, there was an overall decrease in persons presenting with presumptive pulmonary TB (45.6%), in patients registered for TB treatment (19.1%), and in individuals tested for HIV (39.0%). For presumptive TB, children and females were more affected, but for HIV testing, adults and males were more affected. During COVID-19, the TB treatment success rate (96.1% in pre-COVID-19 and 96.0% during COVID-19 period) and referral of HIV-positive persons to antiretroviral therapy (100% in pre-COVID-19 and 98.6% during COVID-19 period) remained high and largely unchanged. Declining trends in TB and HIV case detection were not redressed despite real-time monthly surveillance.

Keywords: COVID-19; Malawi; Lilongwe; presumptive tuberculosis; tuberculosis; TB treatment outcomes; HIV; antiretroviral therapy; EpiCollect5; operational research

1. Introduction

In early January 2020, a new coronavirus named "severe acute respiratory syndrome coronavirus 2" (SARS-CoV-2) was identified in China as the cause of a cluster of atypical pneumonia cases in Wuhan city, Hubei Province. The disease that it causes, coronavirus disease 2019 (COVID-19), then spread with frightening rapidity across the world. On 11 March 2020, the World Health Organization (WHO) declared COVID-19 to be a global pandemic. One year later, over 113 million confirmed cases of COVID-19 and 2.5 million deaths had been reported globally to WHO [1]. At the start of the pandemic, the epicentres were in China, certain European countries, and the United States. The large volumes of air traffic between these countries and Africa led to concerns that sub-Saharan Africa might be hard hit by COVID-19 [2,3].

With enormous resources and finances being redirected to enable countries to cope with the COVID-19 crisis and population lockdowns being imposed to prevent transmission of infection, there was anxiety at the beginning of the epidemic that countries with high burdens of tuberculosis (TB) and human immunodeficiency virus/acquired immune deficiency syndrome (HIV/AIDS) might not be able to provide uninterrupted and quality health care services and people-centred care to their patients [4]. It was thought that fear of COVID-19 and the inability of affected patients to move around would adversely affect health-seeking behaviour and reduce access to the diagnosis and care of TB and HIV/AIDS [5]. Modelling studies suggested that the burden of undetected TB would increase dramatically [6]. These studies further suggested that deaths due to HIV/AIDS and TB could increase by up to 10% and 20%, respectively, with the greatest impact on HIV resulting from interruption to antiretroviral therapy (ART) and the greatest impact on TB resulting from delayed diagnosis and delayed treatment of new cases [7].

Similarities were made with the Ebola virus disease outbreak in the West African countries of Sierra Leone and Liberia in 2014. The widespread travel restrictions and community fear of health facilities led to large decreases in the diagnosis of TB and, in the case of Liberia, TB treatment success rates also declined [8,9]. In both countries, HIV testing capabilities for the general population and for those in health facilities decreased, although access to ART was maintained [10,11]. Early on in the COVID-19 pandemic, The Stop TB Partnership and WHO issued guidelines about how people with TB could protect themselves and how national TB programmes might maintain services when faced with the COVID-19 crisis and population lockdowns [12,13]. The Joint United Nations Programme on HIV/AIDS (UNAIDS) provided similar guidance to people living with HIV [14]. This global advice was supported by urgent calls for practical planning to tackle the growing threat of COVID-19 in sub-Saharan Africa [5,15].

We, therefore, set up a project to measure the impact of COVID-19 on TB and HIV services in three sub-Saharan African countries, Kenya, Malawi, and Zimbabwe. This is the report from Malawi.

The first three COVID-19 cases reported to WHO by Malawi were on 2 April 2020, although the cases had been identified in-country during March. By 15 April, Malawi had reported 16 COVID-19 cases with two deaths [16]. At that time, the severity of the COVID-19 pandemic, its duration and the impact that it might have on public health services for the control of TB and HIV/AIDS was unknown.

The National TB Programme and the National HIV/AIDS Programme in Malawi, working in close collaboration with the International Union Against Tuberculosis and Lung Disease (The Union), the Special Programme for Research and Training in Tropical Disease at WHO (TDR) and Vital Strategies, therefore aimed at the early stage of the COVID-19 outbreak to strengthen routine and real-time monitoring and evaluation systems for TB and HIV case detection and disease control. In selected health facilities in Lilongwe, the capital city, the quarterly (3 monthly) recording and reporting system was augmented by monthly recording and reporting. The hypothesis was that if there were decreases in numbers of persons presenting with presumptive TB or being diagnosed, registered and treated with TB or if there were decreases in numbers presenting for HIV testing or numbers of HIV-positive persons being referred for ART, then programmes might be able to act more quickly on monthly information to reverse these trends.

The overall aim of the study was to determine the impact of the COVID-19 pandemic on TB and HIV programme services in eight selected health facilities in Lilongwe, Malawi, through strengthened real-time surveillance. Specific objectives were on a monthly basis to: (i) document the monthly increase nationally in COVID-19 cases and deaths and the effects on general health services; (ii) collect, collate, and report on specific TB- and HIV-related data during the COVID-19 period (March 2020 to February 2021); (iii) document any specific responses at the national and local level to TB and HIV diagnosis and treatment during the COVID-19 period; and (iv) compare the findings during the COVID-19 period with data collected and collated retrospectively during the pre-COVID-19 period (March 2019 to February 2020).

2. Materials and Methods

2.1. Study Design

This was a cohort study using aggregate data collected as part of programme activity.

2.2. Setting

2.2.1. General Setting: Malawi and Lilongwe

Malawi is a land-locked, low-income country in southern Africa with an estimated population of 18 million and with 84% of people living in rural areas [17]. In 2019, the gross national income per capita was USD 380 [18]. Malawi is among the top countries globally with a high burden of TB and HIV/AIDS: in 2019, there were an estimated 27,000 people with TB, of whom 13,000 were HIV positive [19], and there were 1 million people living with HIV (PLHIV) of all ages [20].

Lilongwe is the capital city with a population of about 1 million, according to the 2018 national census [17]. The current study took place in Lilongwe because, at the onset of the epidemic, the majority of cases of COVID-19 came from this city and because partial national lockdown meant it was difficult to travel outside of the city to other regions in the country. Eight health facilities were selected for the study. The selection was made based on high numbers of patients with TB and persons attending for HIV testing and because they were considered by the Lighthouse clinic, the national TB Programme and the national HIV/AIDS Programme to be representative of health facilities within Lilongwe city. The facilities included the central tertiary referral hospital, a secondary referral hospital-specific for HIV/AIDS and including TB patients, one community hospital and five health centres. All these health facilities were in the public sector domain and provided general health services integrated with TB and HIV services. The established staff providing general health and TB and HIV services were used to help with the monthly data collection.

2.2.2. TB and HIV Services

The diagnosis and treatment of TB and HIV/AIDS in Malawi are the responsibility of the National TB Programme and the Department of HIV/AIDS under the Ministry of Health. People with symptoms suggestive of TB (typically these include cough, fever, weight loss, and night sweats) are classified as having presumptive TB when they attend a health facility. Their names are recorded in the presumptive TB register, along with their demographic details. Investigations are carried out according to national and international guidelines [21,22], using sputum smear microscopy and/or the Xpert MTB/RIF (Cepheid, Sunnyvale, CA, USA) assay to establish a bacteriologically confirmed diagnosis of pulmonary TB (PTB). In patients not diagnosed by these methods, clinical assessment, radiography, and other circumstantial evidence are used to establish a diagnosis of clinically diagnosed PTB or extrapulmonary TB (EPTB). Diagnosed TB patients are registered in the TB patient register with demographic and clinical details, given a unique TB registration number and started on anti-TB treatment in accordance with national and international guidelines [21,22]. In brief, patients take their treatment under direct observation by family members or health clinic staff and come to the health facilities once a month to collect drug supplies. The same process is used at all the health facilities. In the selected health facilities in Lilongwe, patients with confirmed or presumed drug-susceptible TB are treated and monitored with the standard 6-month regimen (2 months of rifampicin/isoniazid/pyrazinamide and ethambutol followed by 4 months of rifampicin and isoniazid), and they were included in this study. Those with drug-resistant disease were not included. Treatment outcomes are monitored, recorded, and reported according to international guidelines [23].

HIV testing is institutionalized in the public health facilities, and provider-initiated counselling and testing are routinely offered to anyone attending for care according to national and international guidelines [24–26]. HIV testing is carried out using rapid testing algorithms. All people diagnosed HIV-positive are referred to ART services for immediate start of ART regardless of their WHO clinical stage or CD4-T lymphocyte cell count.

There is generally good-quality data capture and reporting for TB and HIV/AIDS at all levels due to regular supervision and checking by national programme supervisors. Some selected health facilities also benefit from additional supervision by staff of the Lighthouse clinic.

2.2.3. Data Recording and Reporting for the Study in Health Facilities in Lilongwe

Data were routinely collected on a daily basis by programme staff in each of the eight health facilities in Lilongwe using the standard existing monitoring tools (the presumptive TB register, the sputum laboratory register, and the TB patient register—in which TB treatment outcomes are recorded—and the HIV testing register), most of which were paper based. Moreover, 1–2 weeks after the end of each month, health facility staff collated individual data on TB and HIV variables for the previous month into monthly aggregate data. These were then reviewed and validated by trained data collectors, and the aggregate data were then entered into a data form developed using the EpiCollect5 application (https://five.epicollect.net, accessed on 4 May 2021). The process each month was supervised by the project country coordinator (HT—appointed for the study).

For TB treatment outcomes, the monthly cohorts of patients enrolled on anti-TB treatment 8 months previously were used—this allowed for 6 months of treatment to be completed and a further 2 months for treatment outcomes to be validated and recorded in the registers. For example, the November 2020 TB treatment outcome data were obtained for the TB patients enrolled and started on treatment in March 2020. National data on COVID-19 cases and deaths reported to WHO on the last day of each month were obtained from WHO situation and epidemiological reports [16]. At the same time as the prospective monthly data were being collected, a schedule and the same procedures were used to collect retrospective data for the previous year. Data were collected on TB and HIV parameters for each month of the COVID-19 period (March 2020 to February 2021) and were also collected for the same parameters for the pre-COVID-19 period (March 2019 to February 2020).

Once all prospective and retrospective data for the reporting month were entered into EpiCollect5, they were checked and validated by the project country coordinator and the overall project monitoring and evaluation officer (PT) based at The Union. Data were then presented in a monthly report as a series of figures and tables to the directors of the national TB programme and national HIV/AIDS programme and to all other relevant stakeholders involved in the project. Any changes made to policy and/or practice at the local health facility or at the national level during that month to counteract the negative effects of COVID-19 were recorded in a narrative table within the report. These monthly reports were always sent and received by the national programme staff within 4 weeks of closure of that month to enable timely surveillance and possible action.

2.3. Study Population

The study population included all patients presenting to the eight health facilities in Lilongwe with presumptive pulmonary TB (PTB), patients diagnosed and registered for anti-TB treatment, and all persons tested for HIV between March 2019 and February 2021: March 2020 to February 2021 was the COVID-19 period and March 2019 to February 2020 was the pre-COVID-19 period. For assessment of treatment outcomes, all TB patients enrolled on TB treatment 8 months previously were considered.

2.4. Data Variables, Sources of Data, and Timing of Data Collection

Data variables that were collected for TB included aggregate numbers of patients: with presumptive PTB, stratified by male and female, adults ($\geq$15 years) and children (<15 years); diagnosed with bacteriologically confirmed PTB by either smear microscopy and/or Xpert MTB/RIF; registered for anti-TB treatment, stratified by bacteriologically confirmed PTB, clinically diagnosed PTB, and EPTB. Standardized TB treatment outcomes of those patients enrolled for treatment 8 months previously were collected and these included treatment success (a combination of those cured with negative sputum smears and those who completed treatment with no sputum smear examination), lost to follow-up, died, failed treatment, or not evaluated [23]. Lost to follow-up is defined as a TB patient who did not start treatment or whose treatment was interrupted for 2 or more consecutive months. Not evaluated is an outcome given to TB patients where no outcome is declared. This includes those who transfer from one facility to another and for whom the final treatment outcome is not recorded. Data variables for HIV included persons who were HIV tested at the health facilities, stratified by male and female, adults ($\geq$15 years) and children (<15 years); persons diagnosed HIV-positive; and HIV-positive persons referred to ART. COVID-19 cases and deaths were those reported at the end of each month to WHO and obtained from the WHO epidemiological and situational reports.

Sources of data were the Presumptive TB Register, the Sputum Laboratory Register, the TB Patient Register, and the HIV Testing Register. Prospective and retrospective data for the study were collected between June 2020 and March 2021.

2.5. Analysis and Statistics

Data were collected in aggregate form, presented as frequencies and proportions, and comparisons were made between the COVID-19 period and the pre-COVID-19 period. The percentage decline in numbers during each month of the COVID-19 period was calculated relative to the numbers during the same month of the pre-COVID-19 period. Comparisons of percentages of persons by age, gender, and test positivity for those presenting with presumptive PTB and being HIV tested as well as the TB registration categories between the two periods were made using the chi-square test and the *p*-values presented. Furthermore, 95% confidence intervals were also presented where appropriate. The relative percentage differences observed between the first 6 months of COVID-19 (March to August 2020) and the second 6 months of COVID-19 (September 2020 to February 2021) were also calculated and presented in the narrative text.

3. Results

3.1. COVID-19 Cases and Deaths and General Effects on Health Services

COVID-19 cases and deaths as reported to WHO gradually increased to 31,798 and 1037, respectively, during the 12-month period (see Figure 1).

In terms of the general effects of COVID-19 on health services, the government of Malawi declared a national disaster in March 2020 and ordered a national lockdown. This was challenged in the High Court by the civil society, who were anxious about their livelihoods, and a partial lockdown was then put in place from 23 March to 9 October 2020. This included travel restrictions, a suspension of public meetings, health facilities being asked to restrict numbers of patients accessing the premises, and closure of some HIV testing service delivery points. In response to a dramatic increase in notified COVID-19 cases, on 17 January 2021, the government again ordered a full national lockdown (which was not challenged by civil society), and this included a night-time curfew. During these times, there was widespread community fear about contracting COVID-19 and being diagnosed with the disease, and there was a large decline in general out-patient attendances between January and February 2021.

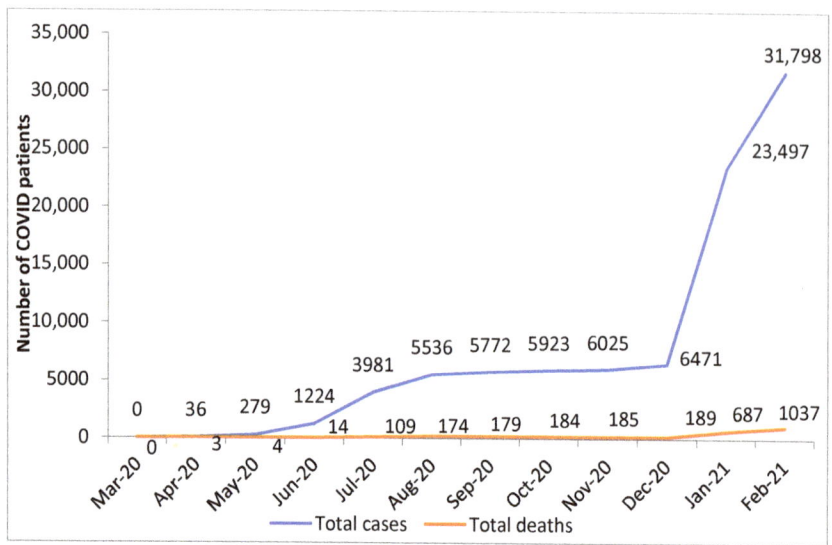

Figure 1. Cumulative number of COVID-19 cases and deaths in Malawi between March 2020 and February 2021 as reported to the World Health Organization.

3.2. TB Case Finding, Diagnosis, and Registration

There was an overall decrease in persons presenting with presumptive PTB (45.6%), being diagnosed bacteriologically positive (2.6%) and registered for TB treatment (19.1%) in the COVID-19 period compared with the pre-COVID-19 period (Table 1).

Table 1. Characteristics of persons with presumptive pulmonary TB and registered TB in eight selected health facilities in Lilongwe, Malawi, during pre-COVID-19 and COVID-19 periods.

Characteristics	Pre-COVID-19 Mar 2019 to Feb 2020 N	COVID-19 Mar 2020 to Feb 2021 N	Difference between Pre-COVID-19 and COVID-19 % (p-Value or 95%CI)
Presumptive pulmonary TB:	11,271	6137	↓ * 45.6
Adults (≥15 years)	10,657	5958	↓44.1 * (<0.001)
Children (<15 years)	484	156	↓67.8 * (<0.001)
Male	5787	3508	↓39.4 * (<0.001)
Female	5479	2628	↓52.0 * (<0.001)
Bacteriologically positive	652	635	↓2.6 * (<0.001)
Positivity rate (%)	(5.8%)	(10.3%)	↑4.5% * (3.6–5.4%)
Registered TB	1822	1474	↓19.1 *
Bacteriologically confirmed PTB	821	625	↓23.9 * (0.13)
Clinically diagnosed PTB	475	394	↓17.1 * (0.67)
Extrapulmonary TB	611	454	↓25.7 * (0.10)

* Absolute change (increase or decrease); TB = tuberculosis; PTB = pulmonary tuberculosis; CI = confidence interval.

For those with presumptive PTB, the overall decrease was greater in children (67.8%) compared with adults (44.1%) and greater in females (52.0%) compared with males (39.4%). While the absolute numbers diagnosed bacteriologically positive were almost similar in the two periods, the bacteriological positivity rate nearly doubled (from 5.8% to 10.3%). For those with registered TB, the overall decrease was almost similar between bacteriologically positive PTB (23.9%) and EPTB (25.7%) and less pronounced for clinically diagnosed PTB (17.1%).

The monthly numbers presenting with presumptive PTB and registered TB in the pre-COVID-19 and COVID-19 periods are shown in Figures 2 and 3. The TB programme attempted to keep TB services running, and from November 2020 onwards, it asked health care workers to pro-actively screen those attending outpatients for TB symptoms. Compared with the pre-COVID-19 period, the decline in presumptive PTB in the first 6 months of COVID-19 was 49.7% which was greater than the 40.0% decline in the second 6 months. The decline in registered TB in the first 6 months of COVID-19 (March 2020 to August 2020) was 22.6%, which was greater than the 15.2% decline in the second 6 months (September 2020 to February 2021).

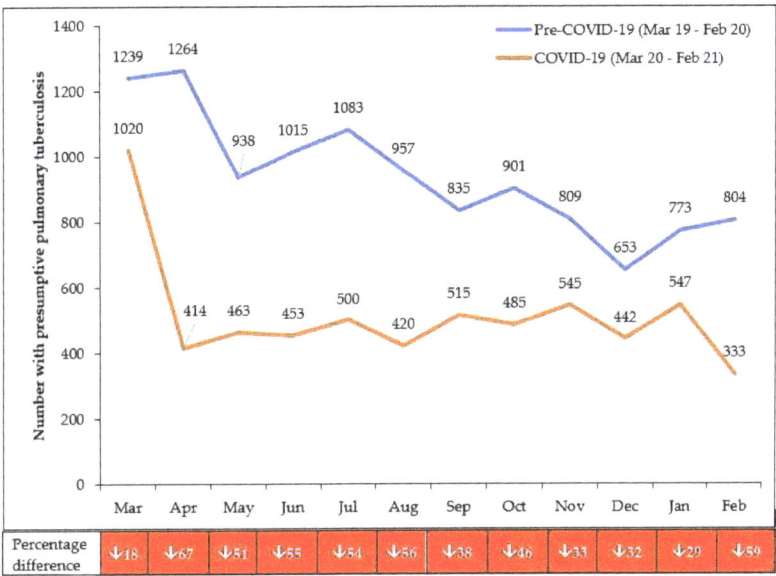

Figure 2. Numbers presenting each month with presumptive PTB in eight health facilities in Lilongwe, Malawi, during the pre-COVID-19 and COVID-19 periods. From October 2020 onwards, health workers were asked to pro-actively ask about symptoms of TB in those attending outpatient departments; there was an active tracing of patients needing to be registered.

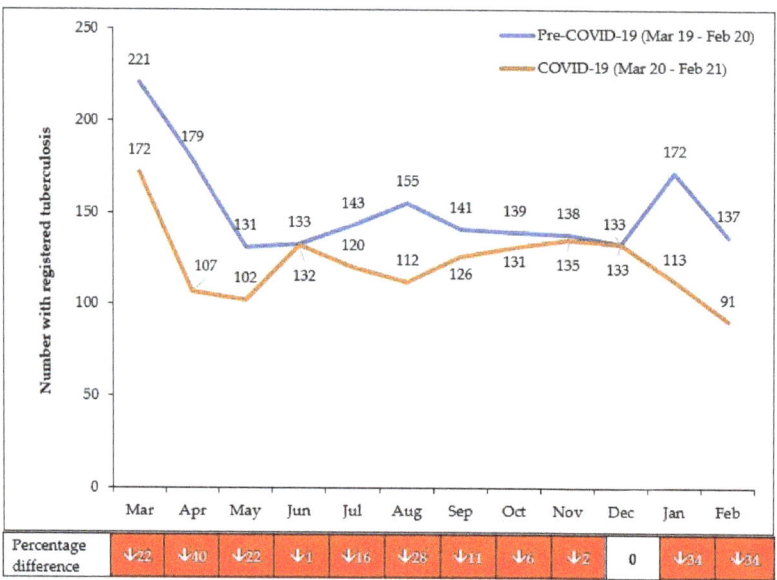

Figure 3. Numbers presenting each month with registered TB in eight health facilities in Lilongwe, Malawi, during the pre-COVID-19 and COVID-19 periods. From October 2020 onwards, health workers were asked to pro-actively ask about symptoms of TB in those attending outpatient departments; there was an active tracing of patients needing to be registered.

3.3. TB Treatment Outcomes

The overall aggregate treatment outcomes between the Pre-COVID-19 and COVID-19 periods are shown in Table 2. Treatment success was almost similar between the two periods, with small but insignificant differences in the other four adverse treatment outcomes (lost to follow-up, death, failed treatment, and not evaluated).

Table 2. Treatment outcomes of patients enrolled in TB treatment in eight selected health facilities in Malawi, during pre-COVID-19 and COVID-19 periods.

Treatment Outcomes	Pre-COVID-19 Mar 2019–Feb 2020	COVID-19 Mar 2020–Feb 2021	Difference between Pre-COVID-19 and COVID-19 % (95% CI)
Enrolled for treatment:	1915	1615	
Treatment success (%)	(96.1)	(96.0)	↓0.1 * (↓1.4 to ↓1.2)
Lost to follow-up (%)	(0.8)	(0.8)	0 (↓0.6 to ↑0.6)
Died (%)	(2.1)	(1.5)	↓0.6 * (↓1.4 to ↑0.3)
Failed (%)	(0.2)	(0.4)	↑0.2 * (↑0.6 to ↓0.2)
Not evaluated (%)	(0.9)	(1.2)	↑0.3 * (↑1.0 to ↓0.3)

* Absolute change (increase or decrease); TB = tuberculosis; CI = confidence interval; p-value for treatment outcomes = 0.25. 'Treatment success' was defined if the TB patient was either cured or had 'treatment completed'. The success rate and other treatment outcomes were calculated for the month-wise cohort of TB patients who commenced on treatment 8 months prior to the reporting month (this accounts for 6 months of treatment being completed and another 2 months for finalizing the recording of outcomes).

The monthly treatment success rates in the pre-COVID-19 and COVID-19 periods are shown in Figure 4. Treatment success was 93% or higher during the two 12-month periods as a result of active follow-up of patients and ensuring complete recording of outcomes as possible. Compared with the pre-COVID-19 period, there was an increase in treatment success in the first 6 months of COVID-19 (March 2020 to August 2020) of 0.8%, which was similar to the 0.7% increase observed in the second 6 months (September 2020 to February 2021).

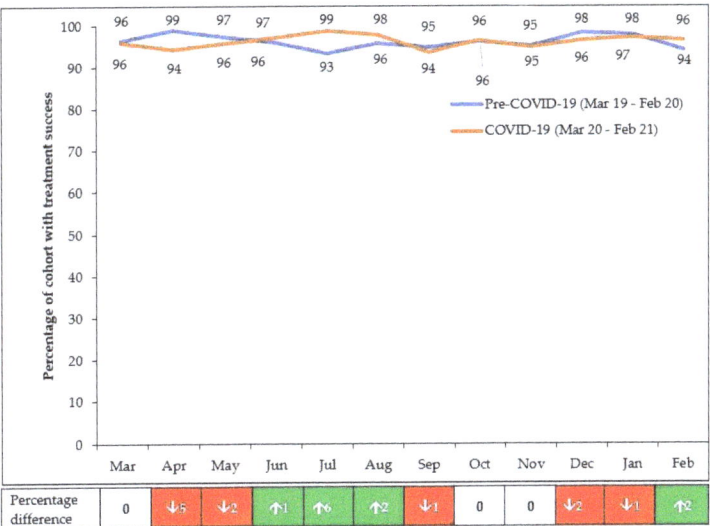

Figure 4. Treatment success amongst those enrolled each month in eight health facilities in Lilongwe, Malawi, during pre-COVID-19 and COVID-19 periods. Enrolment occurred 8 months prior to the month of reporting (to allow for 6-months treatment and 2-months to follow-up and record the final outcome).

3.4. HIV Testing at Health Facilities and Referral to ART

Results are shown in Table 3. There was an overall decrease (39.0%) in the numbers of persons tested for HIV in the COVID-19 period compared with the pre-COVID-19 period. Part of this decline was associated with increased distribution of HIV self-test kits from May 2020 onwards (where facilities then only performed confirmatory testing on those found HIV positive) and intensified use of a verbal screening tool to identify persons more likely to be HIV positive. The overall decrease in HIV testing was greater in adults (40.4%) than in children (13.5%) and greater in males (42.9%) than females (37.3%). While there was an overall decline in the number of persons diagnosed HIV positive (30.4%), the HIV positivity rate increased slightly in the COVID-19 period (0.4%), possibly as a result of the measures described above. The numbers of HIV-positive persons referred to ART was high (100%) in the pre-COVID-19 period, although this decreased slightly by 1.4% in the COVID-19 period.

Table 3. Characteristics of persons tested for HIV and referred to antiretroviral therapy in eight health facilities in Lilongwe, Malawi, during the pre-COVID-19 and COVID-19 periods.

Characteristics	Pre-COVID-19 Mar 2019 to Feb 2020 N	COVID-19 Mar 2020 to Feb 2021 N	Difference between Pre-COVID-19 and COVID-19 % (p-Value or 95%CI)
Underwent HIV testing at the facility:	210,057	128,153	↓39.0 *
Adults (≥15 years)	199,030	118,615	↓40.4 * (<0.001)
Children (<15 years)	11,027	9538	↓13.5 * (<0.001)
Male	62,896	35,944	↓42.9 * (<0.001)
Female	147,161	92,209	↓37.3 * (<0.001)
Positive for HIV	7040	4900	↓30.4 * (<0.001)
HIV-positivity rate (%)	(3.4%)	(3.8%)	↑0.4% * (0.3–0.5%)
HIV-positive persons referred to ART (%)	(100%)	(98.6%)	↓1.4% * (1.1–1.7%)

* Absolute change (increase or decrease); ART= antiretroviral therapy; CI = confidence interval.

The monthly numbers tested for HIV in the pre-COVID-19 and COVID-19 periods are shown in Figure 5. Compared with the pre-COVID-19 period, the decline in HIV testing in the first 6 months of COVID-19 (March 2020 to August 2020) was 46.4%, which was greater than the 31.1% decline observed in the second 6 months (September 2020 to February 2021).

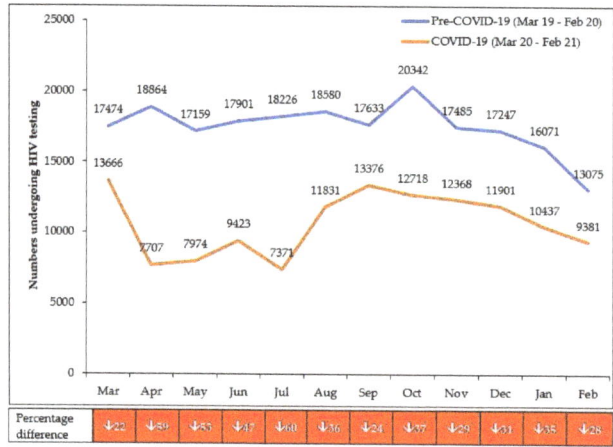

Figure 5. Numbers presenting each month for HIV testing in eight facilities in Lilongwe, Malawi, during pre-COVID-19 and COVID-19 periods. HIV services resumed after lockdown; HIV testing was also offered to contacts of HIV-positive index clients.

4. Discussion

This is the first study in Malawi to assess the impact of COVID-19 on TB and HIV services in selected health facilities in Lilongwe, the capital city. In summary, there was a large negative impact on TB case detection and HIV testing, while TB treatment outcomes for those enrolled to anti-TB treatment and the referral of HIV-positive persons to ART were essentially unaffected.

With respect to TB programme activities, the number of people presenting to health facilities with presumptive PTB declined considerably over the 12-month COVID-19 period, the negative effect being worse in the first 6 months compared with the second 6 months of the COVID-19 period. Children and women were particularly affected. There is little information in the literature to explain these findings, so the reasons have to be speculative. A qualitative study in neighbouring Zambia found that patients recently diagnosed with TB during the COVID-19 pandemic were very concerned about contracting COVID-19 during clinic visits, perceiving the disease to be highly transmissible, deadly, and without effective treatment [27]. It is possible that these concerns were felt more keenly amongst mothers and their children, thus reducing the desire of the family unit to attend health facilities. A large decline in children being admitted to and diagnosed with TB in two hospitals in Johannesburg, South Africa, during COVID-19 would support this hypothesis [28]. The decline in persons presenting with presumptive PTB was similar to what was observed in the early months of COVID-19 in clinics in Tehran, Iran [29], and Nigeria [30], where transportation difficulties, as well as community fear of health facilities, were thought to hinder health facility access.

The bacteriological positivity rate in those being investigated for presumptive PTB in our study was almost twice as high in the COVID-19 period compared with the previous year, and this may partly explain the less severe decline observed in cases diagnosed and registered with TB. This finding suggests the possibility that those with more severe symptoms and who were more likely to have TB continued trying to access health facilities and that laboratory operating procedures remained relatively intact during the COVID-19 period.

There was a decline in the number of people registered for TB treatment. These findings are also in line with reports from elsewhere where the decreases in TB case notifications in the early months of COVID-19 compared with previous years were 48% in clinics in China [31], 48% in clinics in Brazil [32], and 56% in India [33].

A recent report on 84 countries from WHO showed an overall 21% decrease in TB case notifications in 2020 compared with 2019 [34], attributed essentially to the COVID-19 pandemic. A modelling analysis at the start of the pandemic suggested that a 3-month suspension of TB services due to COVID-19 lockdown followed by 10 months restoration back to normal would cause over a 5 year period an additional 1.2 million TB cases in India, 25,000 additional TB cases in Kenya, and 4000 additional cases in Ukraine, mainly as a result of the accumulation of undetected TB during lockdown [6]. A further modelling study in high-burden, low-income, and middle-income countries predicted a 20% increase in TB mortality, with most of this occurring as a result of reductions in timely diagnosis and treatment of new cases of TB [7]. These statistics, worrying as they are, were obtained early on in the pandemic when it was hoped that service disruption would be temporary. The reality, however, is that service disruption in Malawi has continued throughout the year and is likely to continue into 2021 and beyond, with even worse impacts on the TB epidemic than originally forecasted.

On an encouraging note, however, TB treatment success rates were maintained at high levels during the COVID-19 pandemic. These high rates above 90% were surprising but were verified each month with the TB programme and the Lighthouse staff. It is possible that the smaller number of patients enrolled on treatment during the COVID-19 period made the workload of follow-up easier. At the start, we had been concerned that COVID-19 restrictions would hinder patients collecting anti-TB medications, would compromise drug adherence, and reduce the ability of TB programme staff from obtaining information about final treatment outcomes. Patients coinfected with TB and COVID-19 are at increased risk of death [35,36], and we also had concerns that there might be TB patients with undetected COVID-19, and this might increase TB treatment deaths. Fortunately, this was not the case in our study, and there was a slight decrease in the risk of death.

With respect to HIV services, there was a significant decrease in numbers presenting for HIV testing, this improving slightly during the latter half of the COVID-19 period. This is similar to the reductions in HIV testing that have been observed in Europe [37], the United States [38], and Africa [39]. The fall-off in HIV testing threatens access to diagnosis and treatment of people living with HIV that, in turn, could result in excess HIV-related deaths and ongoing transmission of HIV in the community. The increase in HIV-positivity observed in the COVID-19 period in our study is probably a result of health facility testing being more directed to targeted testing of high-risk groups and the confirmation of positive results in those identified HIV-positive through self-testing. It was encouraging to see that referrals to ART were maintained at a very high level over the whole 24 months, with only a slight decrease in the COVID-19 period. Again, this reflects the fact that any person diagnosed HIV positive is now eligible for ART.

This study had several strengths. First, the real-time monthly surveillance was embedded within the routine services of the eight health facilities. Second, there was cross-checking and validation of the data each month between the country coordinator and the overall study monitoring and evaluation officer, and we believe, therefore, that the data are accurate. Third, we used two 12-month periods to compare data, and this enabled us to account for any seasonal changes that might have affected access to health facilities, e.g., during the rainy season. Finally, the conduct and reporting of the study were in line with the Strengthening the Reporting of Observational Studies in Epidemiology (STROBE) guidelines [40].

There were, however, some limitations. Our study was limited to health facilities in Lilongwe, and therefore may not be representative of Malawi as a whole. The use of aggregate data limits our understanding of the cascade of care for TB case detection and HIV testing. We only assessed referral to ART and did not document whether ART was initiated or whether patients were retained on treatment once it had started. Previous studies have suggested that ART interruption has been a problem during the COVID-19 pandemic [41]. It would have been interesting to assess this in Malawi, especially as an interruption to ART is thought to be the most important determinant of HIV-related mortality during the COVID-19 pandemic [42]. Finally, the official monthly reports to WHO of COVID-19 cases and deaths may have underestimated the true burden of COVID-19 in the country. A study on deceased people at the University Teaching Hospital morgue in Lusaka, Zambia, found that just 9% of 70 people who were SARS-CoV-2 confirmed from postmortem nasopharyngeal swabs within 48 h of death had ever been tested before death [43]. It is likely that this type of finding is not confined to Zambia and that large numbers of unreported cases and deaths due to COVID-19 are occurring in other countries in Africa, including Malawi.

Despite these limitations, there are some important programmatic implications from this study. First, the strengthened monthly surveillance system worked well with both disease control programme directors looking each month at the monthly reports and using the data. While there were improvements in TB case detection and HIV testing in the latter half of the COVID-19 pandemic, there were still significant shortfalls in numbers, and these could not be redressed or brought back to pre-COVID-19 levels. Whether the inability to turn around this negative impact was due to ongoing anxiety and fear amongst the community about attending health facilities and/or to continued restrictions imposed by partial lockdown and then full lockdown is difficult to say and requires more in-depth mixed-methods research. Monthly surveillance required effort and external support, and while this was acknowledged to be useful during a crisis such as COVID-19, both programme directors felt it would be difficult to sustain this as a routine activity. Monthly surveillance in sentinel sites might be a less expensive way of doing this and should be considered.

Second, with COVID-19 likely to become endemic, there is an urgent need to bring TB case detection back to pre-COVID-19 levels. Several suggestions have been made about how to do this. These include: integrating TB and COVID-19 control programmes in terms of fast-tracking patients with respiratory symptoms for TB and COVID-19; screening for both diseases at community and health facility level; sharing testing algorithms and diagnostic equipment within the laboratories; ensuring effective infection, prevention, and control activities within health facilities; having longer 3-month follow-up appointments for patient check-ups and drug collection; providing health information education in health facilities and the community; and mobilizing support networks of TB survivors and TB communities [44–46]. More use of electronic platforms for case finding, drug adherence, management of adverse drug reactions, and training has also been recommended as a way of rapidly restoring TB care and prevention services [47], and Malawi could consider all of these innovative approaches.

Third, HIV self-testing and home-based HIV testing services have allowed HIV testing numbers to rebound in some other African countries [48–50]. Malawi has already moved in this direction with the scale-up of HIV self-testing and index testing, especially during the second half of the COVID-19 period. This needs to continue while at the same time ensuring that numbers and results are recorded and reported, so that HIV-infected persons in need of ART do not slip through the net.

5. Conclusions

Using strengthened monthly real-time surveillance in eight health facilities in Lilongwe, Malawi, numbers of persons with presumptive TB and registered TB, as well as numbers tested for HIV, declined during 12-months of the COVID-19 outbreak compared with 12-months pre-COVID-19. Successful TB treatment outcomes and the referral of HIV-positive persons to ART were maintained at high levels, with COVID-19 having hardly any negative impact. Unfortunately, declining trends in TB and HIV case detection were not redressed with real-time monthly surveillance. Suggestions have been made as to how to restore TB case detection and HIV testing so that TB- and HIV-related mortality can be kept as low as possible during this difficult period.

Author Contributions: Conceptualization, P.T., H.T., S.P., J.M., T.K., A.M.V.K., S.S., H.D.S., M.K., R.Z., I.D.R., S.D.B., and A.D.H.; methodology, P.T., H.T., S.P., J.M., T.K., A.M.V.K., S.S., H.D.S., M.K., R.Z., I.D.R., S.D.B., and A.D.H.; software, P.T.; validation, P.T. and H.T.; formal analysis, P.T., H.T., S.P., J.M., T.K., A.M.V.K., S.S., H.D.S., M.K., R.Z., I.D.R., S.D.B., and A.D.H.; investigation, P.T. and H.T.; resources, I.D.R.; data curation, P.T., H.T., and A.D.H.; writing—original draft preparation, P.T., H.T., S.D.B., and A.D.H.; writing—review and editing, P.T., H.T., S.P., J.M., T.K., A.M.V.K., S.S., H.D.S., M.K., R.Z., I.D.R., S.D.B., and A.D.H.; visualization, P.T., H.T., S.D.B., and A.D.H.; supervision, P.T., H.T., and A.D.H.; project administration, S.D.B.; funding acquisition, S.D.B. and A.D.H. All authors have read and agreed to the published version of the manuscript.

Funding: This research was funded by Bloomberg Philanthropies through a grant (grant number 78941) with Vital Strategies and the Resolve to Save Lives Initiative, New York, NY, USA.

Institutional Review Board Statement: The Malawi National Health Sciences Research Committee reviewed the protocol and exempted it from scientific and ethical review as they considered it to be a review of national programme data (MED/4/36c). The project received ethics approval from the Ethics Advisory Group of the International Union Against Tuberculosis and Lung Disease (EAG 33/2020). As no names or other means of identifying patients during data collection were recorded and as only aggregated data were used for the study, the need for informed patient consent was waived.

Informed Consent Statement: No names or other means of identifying patients during data collection were recorded, and only aggregated data were used for the study. Thus, the need for informed patient consent was waived by both of the ethics committees.

Data Availability Statement: The data that support the findings of the study are available from one of the first authors (P.T.) upon reasonable request.

Acknowledgments: The authors thank established staff working in TB and HIV control in the eight health facilities for their help in collecting the data.

Conflicts of Interest: The authors declare no conflict of interest. The funders had no role in the design of the study; in the collection, analyses, or interpretation of data; in the writing of the manuscript; or in the decision to publish the results.

References

1. World Health Organization. Coronavirus Disease (COVID-19) Weekly Epidemiological Update and Weekly Operational Update 29 December 2020. Available online: https://www.who.int/emergencies/diseases/novel-coronavirus-2019/situation-reports (accessed on 30 March 2021).
2. Gilbert, M.; Pullano, G.; Pinotti, F.; Valdano, E.; Poletto, C.; Boëlle, P.Y.; D'Ortenzio, E.; Yazdanpanah, Y.; Eholie, S.P.; Altmann, M.; et al. Preparedness and vulnerability of African countries against importations of COVID-19: A modelling study. *Lancet* **2020**, *395*, 871–877. [CrossRef]
3. Nkengasong, J.N.; Mankoula, W. Looming threat of COVID-19 infection in Africa: Act collectively, and fast. *Lancet* **2020**, *395*, 841–842. [CrossRef]
4. Pang, Y.; Liu, Y.; Du, J.; Gao, J.; Li, L. Impact of COVID-19 on tuberculosis control in China. *Int. J. Tuberc. Lung Dis.* **2020**, *24*, 545–547. [CrossRef]
5. Sandy, C.; Takarinda, K.C.; Timire, C.; Mutunzi, H.; Dube, M.; Dlodlo, R.A.; Harries, A.D. Preparing national tuberculosis control programmes for COVID-19. *Int. J. Tuberc. Lung Dis.* **2020**, *24*, 634–636. [CrossRef]
6. Cilloni, L.; Fu, H.; Vesga, J.F.; Dowdy, D.; Pretorius, C.; Ahmedov, S.; Nair, S.A.; Mosneaga, A.; Masini, E.; Sahu, S.; et al. The potential impact of the COVID-19 pandemic on the tuberculosis epidemic a modelling analysis. *E Clin. Med.* **2020**, *28*, 100603.
7. Hogan, A.B.; Jewell, B.L.; Sherrard-Smith, E.; Vesga, J.F.; Watson, O.J.; Whittaker, C.; Hamlet, A.; Smith, J.A.; Winskill, P.; Verity, R.; et al. Potential impact of the COVID-19 pandemic on HIV, tuberculosis, and malaria in low-income and middle-income countries: A modelling study. *Lancet Glob. Health* **2020**, *8*, e1132–e1141. [CrossRef]
8. Bah, O.M.; Kamara, H.B.; Bhat, P.; Harries, A.D.; Owiti, P.; Katta, J.; Foray, L.; Kamara, M.I.; Kamara, B.O. The influence of the Ebola outbreak on presumptive and active tuberculosis in Bombali District, Sierra Leone. *Public Health Action* **2017**, *7*, S3–S9. [CrossRef] [PubMed]
9. Konwloh, P.K.; Cambell, C.L.; Ade, S.; Bhat, P.; Harries, A.D.; Wilkinson, E.; Cooper, C.T. Influence of Ebola on tuberculosis case finding and treatment outcomes in Liberia. *Public Health Action* **2017**, *7*, S62–S69. [CrossRef] [PubMed]
10. Gamanga, A.H.; Owiti, P.; Bhat, P.; Harries, A.D.; Kargbo-Labour, I.; Koroma, M. The Ebola outbreak: Effects on HIV reporting, testing and care in Bonthe district, rural Sierra Leone. *Public Health Action* **2017**, *7*, S10–S15. [CrossRef] [PubMed]
11. Jacobs, G.P.; Bhat, P.; Owiti, P.; Edwards, J.K.; Tweya, H.; Najjemba, R. Did the 2014 Ebola outbreak in Liberia affect HIV testing, linkage to care and ART initiation? *Public Health Action* **2017**, *7*, S70–S75. [CrossRef]
12. Stop TB Partnership. TB and COVID-19. Available online: http://www.stoptb.org/covid19.asp?utm_source=The+Stop+TB+Pa (accessed on 30 March 2021).
13. World Health Organization. *World Health Organization (WHO) Information Note Tuberculosis and COVID-19*; WHO: Geneva, Switzerland, 2020.
14. UNAIDS. Covid-19 and HIV. Available online: https://www.unaids.org/en/covid19 (accessed on 30 March 2021).
15. Chiang, C.Y.; Sony, A.E. Tackling the threat of COVID-19 in Africa: An urgent need for practical planning. *Int. J. Tuberc. Lung. Dis.* **2020**, *24*, 541–542. [CrossRef] [PubMed]
16. World Health Organization. *Coronavirus Disease 2019 (COVID-19) Situation Report–86*; WHO: Geneva, Switzerland, 2020.
17. National Statistics Office. *2018 Malawi Population and Housing Census Main Report*; National Statistics Office: Lilongwe, Malawi, 2018.
18. The World Bank. Malawi. Available online: https://data.worldbank.org/country/MW (accessed on 20 April 2021).
19. World Health Organization. *Global Tuberculosis Report 2020*; World Health Organization: Geneva, Switzerland, 2020.
20. UNAIDS. UNAIDS Data 2019. Available online: https://www.unaids.org/en/resources/documents/2019/2019-UNAIDS-data (accessed on 20 April 2021).
21. Ministry of Health. *Malawi National Tuberculosis Control Programme Manual*, 7th ed.; Ministry of Health: Lilongwe, Malawi, 2012.
22. World Health Organization. *Guidelines for Treatment of Drug-Susceptible Tuberculosis and Patient Care (2017 Update)*; World Health Organization: Geneva, Switzerland, 2017.
23. World Health Organization. Definitions and Reporting Framework for Tuberculosis, 2013 Revision, Updated December 2014 and January 2020. Available online: https://www.who.int/tb/publications/definitions/en/ (accessed on 30 March 2021).
24. Ministry of Health. *Malawi Guidelines for Clinical Management of HIV in Children and Adults*, 3rd ed.; Ministry of Health: Lilongwe, Malawi, 2016.
25. World Health Organization. Consolidated Guidelines on HIV Testing Services. Available online: https://www.who.int/publications/i/item/978-92-4-155058-1 (accessed on 30 March 2021).
26. World Health Organization. *Consolidated Guidelines on the Use of Antiretroviral Drugs for Treating and Preventing HIV Infection*, 2nd ed.; Recommendations for a Public Health Approach; WHO: Geneva, Switzerland, 2016.
27. Mwamba, C.; Kerkhoff, A.D.; Kagujje, M.; Lungu, P.; Muyoyeta, M.; Sharma, A. Diagnosed with TB in the era of COVID-19: Patient perspectives in Zambia. *Public Health Action* **2021**, *10*, 141–146. [CrossRef] [PubMed]
28. Lebina, L.; Dube, M.; Hlongwane, K.; Brahmbatt, H.; Lala, S.G.; Reubenson, G.; Martinson, N. Trends in paediatric tuberculosis diagnoses in two south african hospitals early in the covid-19 pandemic. *S. Afr. Med. J.* **2020**, *110*, 1149–1150. [CrossRef]
29. Kargarpour Kamakoli, M.; Hadifar, S.; Khanipour, S.; Farmanfarmaei, G.; Fateh, A.; Mostafaei, S.; Siadat, S.D.; Vaziri, F. Tuberculosis under the Influence of COVID-19 Lockdowns: Lessons from Tehran, Iran. *mSphere* **2021**, *6*, e00076-21. [CrossRef] [PubMed]

30. Adewole, O.O. Impact of COVID-19 on TB care: Experiences of a treatment centre in Nigeria. *Int. J. Tuberc. Lung Dis.* **2020**, *24*, 981–982. [CrossRef]
31. Wu, Z.; Chen, J.; Xia, Z.; Pan, Q.; Yuan, Z.; Zhang, W.; Shen, X. Impact of the COVID-19 pandemic on the detection of TB in Shanghai, China. *Int. J. Tuberc. Lung Dis.* **2020**, *24*, 1122–1124. [CrossRef]
32. De Souza, C.D.F.; Coutinho, H.S.; Costa, M.M.; MagalhaËes, M.A.F.M.; Carmo, R.F. Impact of COVID-19 on TB diagnosis in Northeastern Brazil. *Int. J. Tuberc. Lung Dis* **2020**, *24*, 1220–1222. [CrossRef] [PubMed]
33. Golandaj, J.A. Insight into the COVID-19 led slow-down in TB notifications in India. *Indian J. Tuberc.* **2021**, *68*, 142–145. [CrossRef]
34. World Health Organization. Impact of the COVID-19 Pandemic on TB Detection and Mortality in 2020. Available online: https://cdn.who.int/media/docs/default-source/hq-tuberculosis/impact-of-the-covid-19-pandemic-on-tb-detection-and-mortality-in-2020.pdf (accessed on 30 March 2021).
35. Motta, I.; Centis, R.; D'Ambrosio, L.; García-García, J.M.; Goletti, D.; Gualano, G.; Lipani, F.; Palmieri, F.; Sánchez-Montalvá, A.; Pontali, E.; et al. Tuberculosis, COVID-19 and migrants: Preliminary analysis of deaths occurring in 69 patients from two cohorts. *Pulmonology* **2020**, *26*, 233–240. [CrossRef] [PubMed]
36. Kumar, M.S.; Surendran, D.; Manu, M.S.; Rakesh, P.S.; Balakrishnan, S. Mortality due to TB-COVID-19 coinfection in India. *Int. J. Tuberc. Lung Dis* **2021**, *25*, 250–251. [CrossRef] [PubMed]
37. Simões, D.; Stengaard, A.R.; Combs, L.; Raben, D. Impact of the COVID-19 pandemic on testing services for HIV, viral hepatitis and sexually transmitted infections in the WHO european region, March to August 2020. *Eurosurveillance* **2020**, *25*, 2001943. [CrossRef]
38. Hill, B.J.; Anderson, B.; Lock, L. COVID-19 Pandemic, Pre-exposure Prophylaxis (PrEP) Care, and HIV/STI Testing Among Patients Receiving Care in Three HIV Epidemic Priority States. *AIDS Behav* **2021**, *1*, 1–5.
39. Ponticiello, M.; Mwanga-Amumpaire, J.; Tushemereirwe, P.; Nuwagaba, G.; King, R.; Sundararajan, R. "Everything is a Mess": How COVID-19 is Impacting Engagement with HIV Testing Services in Rural Southwestern Uganda. *AIDS Behav* **2020**, *24*, 3006–3009. [CrossRef] [PubMed]
40. Von Elm, E.; Altman, D.G.; Egger, M.; Pocock, S.J.; Gøtzsche, P.C.; Vandenbroucke, J.P. The Strengthening the Reporting of Observational Studies in Epidemiology (STROBE) statement: Guidelines for reporting observational studies. *Lancet* **2007**, *370*, 1453–1457. [CrossRef]
41. Sun, Y.; Li, H.; Luo, G.; Meng, X.; Guo, W.; Fitzpatrick, T.; Ao, Y.; Feng, A.; Liang, B.; Zhan, Y.; et al. Antiretroviral treatment interruption among people living with HIV during COVID-19 outbreak in China: A nationwide cross-sectional study. *J. Int. AIDS Soc.* **2020**, *23*, e25637. [CrossRef]
42. Jewell, B.L.; Smith, J.A.; Hallett, T.B. Understanding the impact of interruptions to HIV services during the COVID-19 pandemic: A modelling study. *E Clin. Med.* **2020**, *26*, 100483. [CrossRef] [PubMed]
43. Mwananyanda, L.; Gill, C.J.; MacLeod, W.; Kwenda, G.; Pieciak, R.; Mupila, Z.; Lapidot, R.; Mupeta, F.; Forman, L.; Ziko, L.; et al. Covid-19 deaths in Africa: Prospective systematic postmortem surveillance study. *BMJ* **2021**, *372*, n334. [CrossRef]
44. Echeverría, G.; Espinoza, W.; de Waard, J.H. How TB and COVID-19 compare: An opportunity to integrate both control programmes. *Int. J. Tuberc. Lung Dis.* **2020**, *24*, 1–4. [CrossRef]
45. Meneguim, A.C.; Rebello, L.; Das, M.; Ravi, S.; Mathur, T.; Mankar, S.; Kharate, S.; Tipre, P.; Oswal, V.; Iyer, A.; et al. Adapting TB services during the COVID-19 pandemic in Mumbai, India. *Int. J. Tuberc. Lung Dis.* **2020**, *24*, 1119–1121. [CrossRef] [PubMed]
46. Stop TB Partnership. One Year on, New Data Show Global Impact of COVID-19 on TB Epidemic is Worse than Expected. Available online: http://www.stoptb.org/assets/documents/covid/TBandCOVID19_ModellingStudy_5May (accessed on 30 March 2021).
47. Chiang, C.Y.; Islam, T.; Xu, C.; Chinnayah, T.; Garfin, A.M.C.; Rahevar, K.; Raviglione, M. The impact of COVID-19 and the restoration of tuberculosis services in the Western Pacific Region. *Eur. Respir. J.* **2020**, *56*, 2003054. [CrossRef]
48. Mhango, M.; Chitungo, I.; Dzinamarira, T. COVID-19 Lockdowns: Impact on Facility-Based HIV Testing and the Case for the Scaling Up of Home-Based Testing Services in Sub-Saharan Africa. *AIDS Behav.* **2020**, *24*, 3014–3016. [CrossRef] [PubMed]
49. Odinga, M.M.; Kuria, S.; Muindi, O.; Mwakazi, P.; Njraini, M.; Melon, M.; Kombo, B.; Kaosa, S.; Kioko, J.; Musimbi, J.; et al. HIV testing amid COVID-19: Community efforts to reach men who have sex with men in three Kenyan counties. *Gates Open Res.* **2020**, *4*, 117. [CrossRef] [PubMed]
50. Lagat, H.; Sharma, M.; Kariithi, E.; Otieno, G.; Katz, D.; Masyuko, S.; Mugambi, M.; Wamuti, B.; Weiner, B.; Farquhar, C. Impact of the COVID-19 Pandemic on HIV Testing and Assisted Partner Notification Services, Western Kenya. *AIDS Behav.* **2020**, *24*, 3010–3013. [CrossRef] [PubMed]

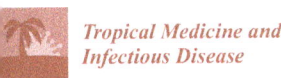
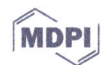

Article

Assessing the Real-Time Impact of COVID-19 on TB and HIV Services: The Experience and Response from Selected Health Facilities in Nairobi, Kenya

Irene Mbithi [1,†], Pruthu Thekkur [2,3,†], Jeremiah Muhwa Chakaya [1,4,5], Elizabeth Onyango [6], Philip Owiti [6], Ngugi Catherine Njeri [7], Ajay M.V. Kumar [2,3,8], Srinath Satyanarayana [2,3], Hemant D. Shewade [2,3], Mohammed Khogali [9], Rony Zachariah [9], I. D. Rusen [10], Selma Dar Berger [2] and Anthony D. Harries [2,11,*]

1. Respiratory Society of Kenya, Regent Court, Block A Suite A6 Hurlingham, Argwings Khodhek Road, Nairobi P.O. Box 43844-00100, Kenya; imbithi@resok.org (I.M.); chakaya.jm@gmail.com (J.M.C.)
2. International Union Against Tuberculosis and Lung Disease, 68 Boulevard Saint Michel, 75006 Paris, France; Pruthu.TK@theunion.org (P.T.); akumar@theunion.org (A.M.V.K.); SSrinath@theunion.org (S.S.); HShewade@theunion.org (H.D.S.); sberger@theunion.org (S.D.B.)
3. International Union Against Tuberculosis and Lung Disease, South-East Asia Office, C-6 Qutub Institutional Area, New Delhi 110016, India
4. Department of Medicine, Therapeutics and Dermatology, Kenyatta University, Nairobi P.O. Box 43844-00100, Kenya
5. Department of Clinical Sciences, Liverpool School of Tropical Medicine, Pembroke Place, Liverpool L3 5QA, UK
6. Division of National TB, Leprosy and Lung Disease Programme, Ministry of Health, Afya House, Cathedral Road, Nairobi P.O. Box 30016-00100, Kenya; lizonyango2004@gmail.com (E.O.); philip.owiti@gmail.com (P.O.)
7. National AIDS and STDs Control Programme, Ministry of Health, Afya House, Cathedral Road, Nairobi P.O. Box 30016-00100, Kenya; Ncatherine26@gmail.com
8. Yenepoya Medical College, Yenepoya (Deemed to be University), University Road, Deralakatte, Mangalore 575018, India
9. Special Programme for Research and Training in Tropical Disease (TDR), World Health Organization, Avenue Appia 20, 1211 Geneva, Switzerland; khogalim@who.int (M.K.); zachariahr@who.int (R.Z.)
10. Vital Strategies, 100 Broadway 4th Floor, New York, NY 10005, USA; irusen@vitalstrategies.org
11. Department of Clinical Research, Faculty of Infectious and Tropical Diseases, London School of Hygiene and Tropical Medicine, Keppel Street, London WC1E 7HT, UK
* Correspondence: adharries@theunion.org; Tel.: +44-(0)-1962-714-297
† Joint First Author.

Citation: Mbithi, I.; Thekkur, P.; Chakaya, J.M.; Onyango, E.; Owiti, P.; Njeri, N.C.; Kumar, A.M.V.; Satyanarayana, S.; Shewade, H.D.; Khogali, M.; et al. Assessing the Real-Time Impact of COVID-19 on TB and HIV Services: The Experience and Response from Selected Health Facilities in Nairobi, Kenya. *Trop. Med. Infect. Dis.* **2021**, *6*, 74. https://doi.org/10.3390/tropicalmed6020074

Academic Editors: Peter A. Leggat, John Frean and Lucille Blumberg

Received: 19 April 2021
Accepted: 6 May 2021
Published: 10 May 2021

Publisher's Note: MDPI stays neutral with regard to jurisdictional claims in published maps and institutional affiliations.

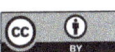

Copyright: © 2021 by the authors. Licensee MDPI, Basel, Switzerland. This article is an open access article distributed under the terms and conditions of the Creative Commons Attribution (CC BY) license (https://creativecommons.org/licenses/by/4.0/).

Abstract: There was concern that the COVID-19 pandemic would adversely affect TB and HIV programme services in Kenya. We set up real-time monthly surveillance of TB and HIV activities in 18 health facilities in Nairobi so that interventions could be implemented to counteract anticipated declining trends. Aggregate data were collected and reported monthly to programme heads during the COVID-19 period (March 2020–February 2021) using EpiCollect5 and compared with monthly data collected during the pre-COVID period (March 2019–February 2020). During the COVID-19 period, there was an overall decrease in people with presumptive pulmonary TB (31.2%), diagnosed and registered with TB (28.0%) and in those tested for HIV (50.5%). Interventions to improve TB case detection and HIV testing were implemented from August 2020 and were associated with improvements in all parameters during the second six months of the COVID-19 period. During the COVID-19 period, there were small increases in TB treatment success (65.0% to 67.0%) and referral of HIV-positive persons to antiretroviral therapy (91.2% to 92.9%): this was more apparent in the second six months after interventions were implemented. Programmatic interventions were associated with improved case detection and treatment outcomes during the COVID-19 period, suggesting that monthly real-time surveillance is useful during unprecedented events.

Keywords: COVID-19; Kenya; Nairobi; presumptive tuberculosis; tuberculosis; TB treatment outcomes; HIV; antiretroviral therapy; EpiCollect5; operational research

1. Introduction

On 11 March 2020, the World Health Organization (WHO) declared a global pandemic of coronavirus disease 2019 (COVID-19), caused by a novel coronavirus named severe acute respiratory syndrome coronavirus 2 (SARS-CoV-2). By the end of 2020, nearly 80 million cases of COVID-19 and 1.8 million deaths had been reported globally to the organization [1]. In the first few months of the global pandemic, the epicenters of the pandemic were China, Europe and the USA, and there was concern that Africa, with its large volume of air traffic connections with these countries, would be the next region hit hard by COVID-19 [2,3].

At the beginning of the COVID-19 pandemic, political attention, healthcare workers, resources and finances were directed to the health sector to enable it to cope with the looming crisis. There was also quarantine, restricted movement and increased time spent indoors by the general population. All of this led to concerns that countries with high burdens of tuberculosis (TB) and human immunodeficiency virus/acquired immune deficiency syndrome (HIV/AIDS) might be unable to provide uninterrupted and quality healthcare services to their patients [4]. It was thought that health-seeking behavior and access to care for affected patients might also be adversely affected [5].

Similarities were drawn with the Ebola virus disease outbreak in Sierra Leone and Liberia in 2014, which took the two West African countries by surprise. Through restrictions in travel, "no-touch" policies and community fear of health facilities, the ability of the national TB programmes in these countries to diagnose TB and continue with HIV testing of TB patients was adversely affected, and, in the case of Liberia, treatment success rates in TB patients declined [6,7]. HIV testing capabilities for the general population decreased in both countries, although access to antiretroviral therapy (ART) was maintained [8,9]. Early on in the COVID-19 pandemic, The Stop TB Partnership and WHO issued guidance about how people with TB could protect themselves and how national TB programmes might adapt to the COVID-19 pandemic and national lockdowns [10,11]. UNAIDS provided similar advice to people living with HIV [12]. This global advice was augmented by urgent calls for practical planning to tackle the looming threat of COVID-19 in Africa [5,13].

We, therefore, set up a pilot project to measure the burden of COVID-19 and assess its impact on TB and HIV services in three Sub-Saharan African countries, Kenya, Malawi and Zimbabwe. This is the report from Kenya.

The first COVID-19 case reported to WHO by Kenya was on the 14 March 2020. By 15 April, Kenya had reported 216 COVID-19 cases (with nine deaths) [14]. How severe the COVID-19 storm would be, how long it would last and what impact it would have on public health services for TB and HIV/AIDS, was unknown. It was felt that being prepared, however, was key to being able to cope. Guinea in West Africa, for example, weathered the Ebola virus disease storm and managed to uphold TB services during this challenging period [15].

Relevant public health authorities in Kenya (including the National Tuberculosis, Leprosy and Lung Disease Programme (NTLD-P), the National AIDS & STI Control Programme (NASCOP) and the Respiratory Society of Kenya), working in close collaboration with the International Union Against Tuberculosis and Lung Disease (The Union), the Special Programme for Research and Training in Tropical Disease at WHO (TDR) and Vital Strategies (RESOLVE) therefore aimed at the early stage of the COVID-19 pandemic to strengthen the routine and real-time monitoring and evaluation system for TB and HIV case detection. The quarterly (every three months) recording and reporting system was strengthened in selected health facilities in the capital city of Nairobi by recording and reporting on TB and HIV parameters every month. We hypothesized that if there were decreases in TB case detection, diagnosis and treatment, and reductions in persons presenting for HIV testing or those diagnosed HIV-positive being referred for ART, then programmes could act more quickly on monthly information than quarterly information to try and reverse these trends.

The overall aim of the study was to determine the impact of the COVID-19 pandemic on TB programme activities and HIV services through strengthened real-time surveillance in 18 selected health facilities in Nairobi, Kenya. The specific objectives were on a monthly basis to: (i) document the increase in nationally reported cases and deaths due to COVID-19 and its effects on general health services; (ii) collect, collate and report on specific TB and HIV-related parameters during the COVID-19 period (March 2020–February 2021), (iii) document the programmatic responses to changes in TB and HIV diagnosis and treatment during the COVID-19 period; and (iv) compare the findings with data collected and collated for the same TB and HIV parameters during the pre-COVID-19 period (March 2019–February 2020).

2. Materials and Methods

2.1. Study Design

This was a cohort study using programmatically collected aggregate data.

2.2. Setting

2.2.1. General Setting: Kenya and Nairobi

Kenya is an East African country located along the Equator. The country is bordered by Somalia, Sudan, Ethiopia, Uganda and Tanzania. In 2019, the population was estimated at almost 53 million, with 32% living in urban areas, and life expectancy at birth was estimated at 66 years [16,17]. The major drivers of the country's economy have been agriculture, fishing, forestry, education, retail trade, construction and financial services [16]. In 2019, the gross national income per capita was approximately USD 1750 [17].

Nairobi is the capital city and one of the 47 semi-autonomous counties in the country. In 2019, it had an estimated population of 4.4 million. The current study took place in the City County of Nairobi because nearly 80% of COVID-19 cases in Kenya were reported from this area at the onset of the outbreak. The County of Nairobi is divided into 10 TB control zones with just over 1000 registered health facilities [18]. To achieve good county geographical representation, two well-established facilities from each of these 10 TB control zones were purposively selected in consultation with the head of the TB Programme and the County TB and Leprosy coordinator. Selected facilities had the following on-site characteristics: TB diagnostic capability (smear microscopy and/or the Xpert MTB/RIF® assay); TB treatment and monitoring services; HIV testing and ART referral or treatment services.

The initial sites included seven hospitals, nine health centers and four dispensaries. Two of these health facilities had to be excluded before starting. One health center on the Kenyatta University Campus closed at the start of lockdown and remained closed indefinitely thereafter. One of the hospitals required its own ethics approval for the study. However, this was going to take too long and the hospital had to be excluded. This left 18 health facilities in total available for the duration of the study. The established staff who were already working in these facilities delivering TB and HIV services helped with the monthly collection of data.

2.2.2. TB and HIV Services

The diagnosis and treatment of TB and HIV/AIDS in Kenya are the responsibility of the Ministry of Health. People with symptoms suggestive of TB (cough, fever, weight loss and night sweats) are classified as having presumptive pulmonary TB (PTB). They are recorded as such when attending a health facility, along with their demographic details. Investigations are carried out according to national guidelines [19], using sputum smear microscopy and/or the Xpert MTB/RIF® assay to establish a bacteriologically confirmed diagnosis of PTB. In the other patients, clinical assessment, radiography and other circumstantial evidence are used to establish a diagnosis of clinically diagnosed PTB or extrapulmonary TB (EPTB). Patients with diagnosed TB (drug-susceptible and drug-resistant) are registered and started on anti-TB treatment in line with national and international guidelines [19,20]. Treatment outcomes are monitored, recorded and reported according to international guidelines [21].

HIV testing is institutionalized in the public health facilities and routinely offered to anyone attending for care and also to TB patients according to national and international guidelines [22,23]. HIV testing is carried out using rapid testing algorithms. Those diagnosed HIV-positive are referred to ART services for immediate start of ART regardless of WHO clinical stage or CD4 cell count.

There is generally good quality data capture and reporting for TB and HIV/AIDS at all levels due to regular supervision by county and national programme supervisors.

2.2.3. Data Monitoring, Recording and Reporting

For this study, we selected only patients with drug-susceptible TB who were treated and monitored with the standard six month regimen [19,20]. Data were routinely collected on a daily basis by healthcare workers in each study site using the standard existing monitoring tools. These included: the TB presumptive and/or the TB laboratory register for presumptive TB depending on the facility; the TB patient register for those diagnosed and registered with TB and in which TB treatment outcomes were also recorded; and the HIV Testing Services (HTS) Register in which those diagnosed HIV-positive and referred for ART were recorded. These registers were mainly paper-based. One to two weeks after the end of each month, the project country coordinator (IM—who was appointed specifically for the study) visited each site along with her team of trained data collectors. They collated the individual data on TB and HIV variables for the previous month into monthly aggregate data, which they then entered into a data form developed using an EpiCollect5 mobile application (https://five.epicollect.net, accessed on 19 April 2021).

For TB treatment outcomes, we took the monthly cohorts of patients who had been enrolled onto treatment eight months previously – this allowed for six months of treatment to be completed and a further two months for outcomes to be validated and documented in the records. Thus, for example, the August 2020 TB treatment outcome data were obtained for the TB patients enrolled and started on treatment in January 2020. National data on COVID-19 cases and deaths reported to WHO on the last day of the month were obtained from WHO situation and epidemiological reports [1]. When collecting the monthly data during the COVID-19 period, the same procedures were used to collect data for the same month one year previously (termed the pre-COVID-19 period).

Once all the data for the month had been entered into EpiCollect5, they were checked and validated by the project country coordinator and the overall project monitoring and evaluation officer (PT) based at The Union. Data were then presented in a monthly report to the heads of the NTLD-P and NASCOP and all other relevant stakeholders involved in the project. Key policy or practice changes made at the local facility, county, or national level during that month to explain and/or counteract the effects of COVID-19 on TB and HIV parameters were documented in a narrative table within the report. These monthly reports always reached the national programme staff heads within four weeks of closure of that month to enable timely surveillance and possible action.

2.3. Study Population

The study population included all patients presenting to TB services with presumptive TB, all TB patients registered for TB treatment and all persons tested for HIV in 18 health facilities in Nairobi, Kenya, between March 2019 and February 2021: the COVID-19 period was designated as March 2020 to February 2021, and the pre-COVID-19 period was designated as March 2019 to February 2020. For assessment of TB treatment outcomes, we included TB patients who started on treatment from (i) August 2018 to July 2019 (pre-COVID-19 cohort) and (ii) August 2019 to July 2020 (COVID-19 cohort).

2.4. Data Variables, Sources of Data and Timing of Data Collection

Data variables for TB included aggregate numbers of presumptive PTB patients, stratified by male and female and adults ($\geq$15 years) and children (<15 years); presumptive PTB patients who were diagnosed bacteriologically positive by either smear microscopy and/or Xpert MTB/RIF®; registered TB patients, stratified by bacteriologically confirmed PTB, clinically diagnosed PTB and EPTB; registered TB patients who were newly tested for HIV in that month after being diagnosed with TB—this excluded patients who already knew they were HIV-positive; standardized TB treatment outcomes of those patients enrolled for treatment eight months previously–these outcomes included treatment success (a combination of those cured and those who completed treatment with no sputum smear examination), lost to follow-up (LTFU), died, failed treatment or not evaluated [21]. Not evaluated is an outcome given to those who transfer from one facility to another and for whom the final treatment outcome is not recorded. Data variables for HIV included an aggregate number of persons who were HIV tested, stratified by male and female and adults ($\geq$15 years) and children (<15 years); persons diagnosed HIV-positive; HIV-positive persons referred to ART services.

Sources of primary individual data were the TB presumptive and/or TB laboratory register, the TB patient register, and the HTS register. The national COVID-19 cases and deaths reported to WHO on the last day of the month were obtained from WHO situation and epidemiological reports [1]. Aggregate data were collected from the primary data sources and uploaded to an EpiCollect5 application, where they were checked and validated, and this was carried out between June 2020 and March 2021.

2.5. Analysis and Statistics

Aggregate data were presented as frequencies and proportions, and comparisons were made between the COVID-19 period and the pre-COVID-19 period. The percentage difference (decline or increase) in numbers during each month of the COVID-19 period was calculated relative to the numbers during the same month of the pre-COVID-19 period. The relative percentage differences observed between the first six months of COVID-19 (March to August 2020) and the second six months of COVID-19 (September 2020 to February 2021) were also calculated.

3. Results

3.1. COVID-19 Cases, Deaths and General Effects on Health Services

There was a gradual increase in COVID-19 cases and deaths during the 12 months, with 105,648 cases and 1,854 deaths reported to WHO by the end of February 2021 (Figure 1).

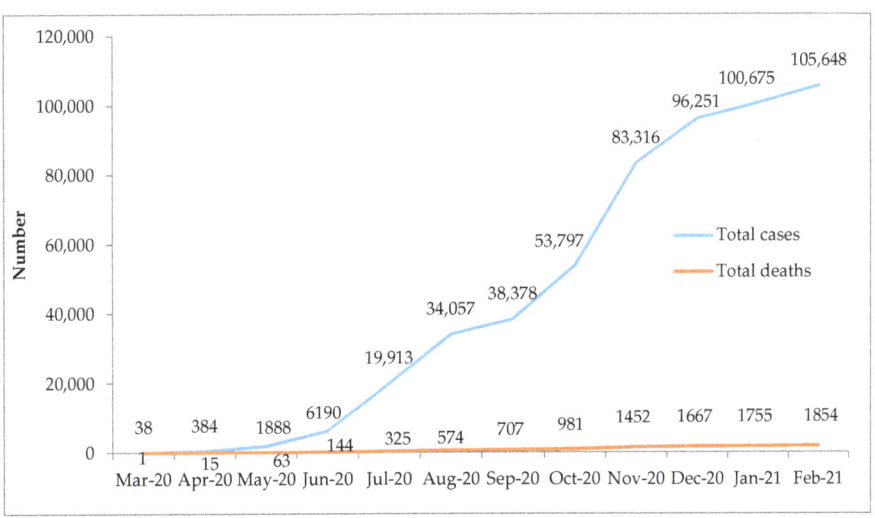

Figure 1. Cumulative number of COVID-19 cases and deaths in Kenya between March 2020 and February 2021, as reported to the World Health Organization.

In terms of general effects on services, there was a national lockdown between March 2020 and the end of June 2020. The lockdown resulted in enforced travel restrictions, shorter working hours and intermittent closures of health facilities (due to lack of personal protective equipment and sickness of healthcare workers from COVID-19). Many staff, including those working in TB and HIV, were repurposed for COVID-19 work. After the period of lockdown, there was a widespread strike by health workers, many of whom refused to come to work from November 2020 to January 2021. This resulted in some health facilities having to temporarily close down or partially close down again. There had also been previous widespread strike action in the health sector in the pre-COVID-19 period from July to October 2019. Finally, there was widespread fear and stigma about COVID-19 in the community, with people reluctant to visit health facilities due to fear of contracting COVID-19 and being diagnosed with the disease.

3.2. TB Case Finding, Diagnosis and Registration

There was an overall decrease in the aggregate numbers of persons presenting with presumptive PTB and being diagnosed and registered with TB in the COVID-19 period when compared to the pre-COVID-19 period (Table 1).

Table 1. Characteristics of persons with presumptive pulmonary TB and registered TB in 18 health facilities in Nairobi, Kenya, during pre-COVID-19 and COVID-19 periods.

Characteristics	Pre-COVID-19 Mar 2019–Feb 2020 N	COVID-19 Mar 2020–Feb 2021 n	Difference between Pre-COVID-19 and COVID-19 %
Presumptive Pulmonary TB (total)	28,038	19,295	↓31.2
Adults (≥15 years)	23,264	16,917	↓27.3
Children (<15 years)	4774	2378	↓50.2
Male	12,221	9043	↓26.0
Female	15,817	10,252	↓35.2
Bacteriologically positive	2221	1411	↓30.2
Positivity Rate (%)	(7.2%)	(7.3%)	↑0.1% *
Registered TB (Total)	3716	2676	↓28.0
Bacteriologically confirmed PTB	1985	1335	↓32.7
Clinically diagnosed PTB	1073	836	↓22.1
Extrapulmonary TB	658	505	↓23.3
Eligible for being newly HIV tested	3067	2259	↓26.3
Newly tested for HIV (%)	(94.7%)	(93.0%)	↓1.7% *

* absolute change (increase or decrease); TB = tuberculosis; PTB = pulmonary tuberculosis.

For presumptive PTB, the overall decrease was greater in children (50.2%) than in adults (27.3%) and greater in females (35.2%) than in males (26.0%). The yield of bacteriologically positive PTB in those investigated for presumptive TB increased (0.1%) marginally. For registered TB, the overall decrease was greater in bacteriologically confirmed PTB and was similar for the other two types (clinically diagnosed PTB and EPTB). The percentage of patients who were newly HIV tested out of those eligible for testing slightly decreased (1.7%).

The monthly number of people presenting with presumptive PTB and those registered for TB in the pre-COVID-19 and COVID-19 periods are shown in Figure 2A,B. The footnotes in the figures indicate the interventions put in place from August 2020 onwards to counteract the downward trends. Compared with the pre-COVID-19 period, the decline in presumptive TB in the first six months of the COVID-19 pandemic (March to August 2020) was 53.2%, which was very different to the 5.2% increase observed in the second six months (September 2020 to February 2021). The decline in registered TB in the first six months of the COVID-19 pandemic was 34.7%, which was greater than the 19.9% decrease observed in the second six months.

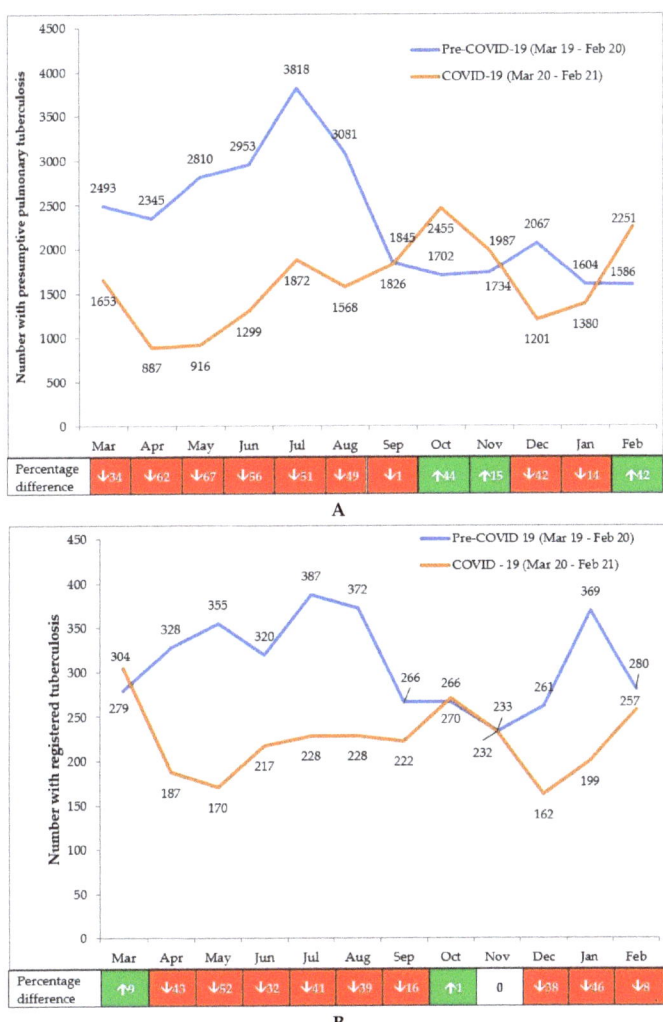

Interventions applied from August 2020 onwards to counteract the decline in numbers included: (i) integrated screening and fast-tracking of investigations for TB and COVID-19 in patients presenting with respiratory symptoms; (ii) active TB case finding in hot spots in the city; (iii) enhanced TB case finding that included screening of TB through mobile phones using a dedicated USSD dialing code, asking patients to dial into a toll-free TB screening call center staffed by healthcare workers and use of automated TB screening machines positioned at strategic spots in the community; (iv) active tracing of close contacts of index patients; and (v) improved TB screening among people living with HIV.

Figure 2. (**A**) Numbers presenting each month with presumptive PTB in 18 health facilities in Nairobi, Kenya, during pre-COVID-19 and COVID-19 periods (**B**) Numbers presenting each month with registered TB in 18 health facilities in Nairobi, Kenya, during pre-COVID-19 and COVID-19 periods.

3.3. TB Treatment Outcomes

The overall aggregate treatment outcomes between the pre-COVID-19 and COVID-19 periods are shown in Table 2. There was a slight increase in treatment success in the COVID-19 period (2.0%), mainly due to an overall decrease in patients "not evaluated" (2.2%). Other adverse programme outcomes were similar between the two periods.

Table 2. Treatment outcomes in TB patients enrolled for treatment in 18 health facilities in Nairobi, Kenya, during pre-COVID-19 and COVID-19 periods.

Treatment Outcomes in Patients Enrolled for TB Treatment	Pre-COVID-19 Mar 2019–Feb 2020 n	COVID-19 Mar 2020–Feb 2021 n	Difference between Pre-COVID-19 and COVID-19 %
Enrolled for treatment:	3640	2366	
Treatment Success (%)	(65.0)	(67.0)	↑2.0 *
Loss to Follow-up (%)	(7.3)	(7.0)	↓0.3 *
Died (%)	(4.2)	(5.0)	↑0.8 *
Failed treatment (%)	(0.8)	(0.5)	↓0.3 *
Not evaluated (%)	(22.7)	(20.5)	↓2.2 *

* absolute change (increase or decrease); TB = tuberculosis; treatment outcome was considered "treatment success" when the TB patient was either cured or had "treatment completed". The success rate was calculated for the month-wise cohort of TB patients commenced on treatment eight months before the reporting month (considering six months of treatment to be completed and another two months to finalize the recording of outcomes).

The monthly treatment success rates in the pre-COVID-19 and COVID-19 periods are shown in Figure 3. The footnotes indicate the interventions put in place from August 2020 onwards to counteract the downward trends. Compared with the pre-COVID-19 period, the decline in treatment success in the first six months of COVID-19 was 2.5%, which was very different to the 9.7% increase observed in the second six months.

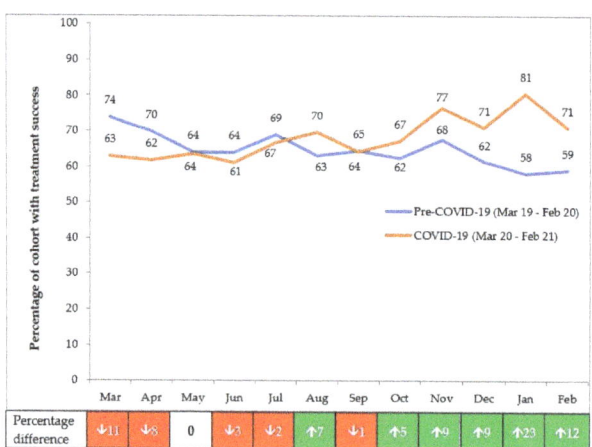

Enrollment occurred eight months before the month of reporting (to allow for six months treatment and two months to follow-up and record the final outcome); interventions applied from August 2020 onwards to counteract the decline in numbers included: (i) longer appointments for TB drug-pick-ups; (ii) phone adherence counselling; (iii) home visits for missed appointments; and (iv) attention made to reducing those "not evaluated" by proactively seeking information from the facilities to which patients were transferred.

Figure 3. Treatment success among those enrolled each month in 18 health facilities in Nairobi, Kenya, during pre-COVID-19 and COVID-19 periods.

3.4. HIV Testing Among Those Visiting the Health Facilities and Referral to ART

There was an overall aggregate decrease in numbers tested for HIV between the pre-COVID-19 and COVID-19 periods (see Table 3). The overall decrease was greater in adults (50.8%) than in children (43.0%) and almost the same between males (51.2%) and females (50.2%). There was a slight increase in the HIV-positivity rate (1.1%), and the proportion of those HIV-positive referred to ART (1.7%) in the COVID-19 period.

Table 3. Characteristics of persons tested for HIV and referred for antiretroviral therapy in 18 health facilities in Nairobi, Kenya, during pre-COVID-19 and COVID-19 periods.

Characteristics	Pre-COVID-19 Mar 2019–Feb 2020 n	COVID-19 Mar 2020–Feb 2021 N	Difference between pre-COVID-19 and COVID-19 %
People tested for HIV (Total):	150,155	74,287	↓50.5
Adults (≥15 years)	145,040	71,374	↓50.8
Children (<15 years)	5115	2913	↓43.0
Male	48,546	23,698	↓51.2
Female	101,609	50,589	↓50.2
Positive for HIV	3819	2673	↓30.0
HIV-Positivity Rate (%)	(2.5%)	(3.6%)	↑1.1 *
HIV-positive persons referred to ART (%)	(91.2%)	(92.9%)	↑1.7 *

* absolute change (increase or decrease); ART = antiretroviral therapy.

The monthly numbers tested for HIV in the pre-COVID-19 and COVID-19 periods are shown in Figure 4. Numbers were already declining in the pre-COVID period due to several factors that included: promotion of HIV self-testing, with the referral of only those HIV-positive to the health facilities for confirmation of the result; a large number of people already tested in the capital city through various testing campaigns; and more targeted testing of high-risk groups. The decline in HIV testing stabilized once COVID-19 appeared. The more targeted testing strategies and confirmation of HIV self-testing results might have explained the increase in HIV positivity from March 2020 onwards.

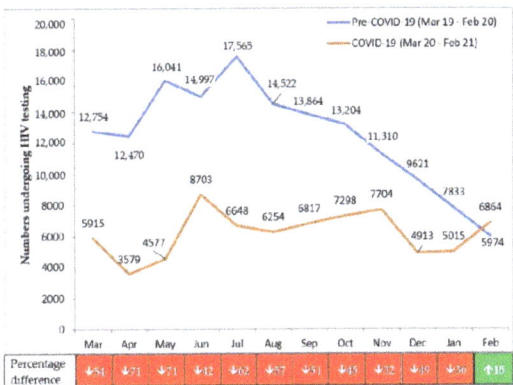

Footnotes: interventions applied from August 2020 onwards to counteract the decline in numbers included: (i) vans used to deliver HIV services to key populations in their homes; (ii) community health volunteers reaching out to people who did not know their HIV status; (iii) HIV testing of partners of infected patients was increased; (iv) longer appointments for ART drug pick-ups; (v) treatment buddies who helped with collecting medicines for children; and vi) community deliveries of ART.

Figure 4. Numbers presenting each month for HIV testing in 18 health facilities in Nairobi, Kenya, during pre-COVID-19 and COVID-19 periods.

The HIV/AIDS programme implemented several interventions from August 2020 onwards to counteract the low numbers presenting for HIV testing (see Figure 4, footnotes). Compared with the pre-COVID period, the decline in HIV-testing in the first six months of COVID-19 was 59.6%, which was greater than the 39.8% decline observed in the second six months.

4. Discussion

This is the first study in Nairobi, Kenya, to compare TB case detection, TB treatment outcomes, HIV testing and referral to ART on a month-by-month basis between the COVID-19 and pre-COVID-19 periods. There were three important findings, which require explanation and interpretation.

First, with respect to TB programme activities, there was considerable variation in TB case detection numbers during the pre-COVID-19 period. Numbers with presumptive PTB increased between April and July 2019 (the summer months), and this is in line with what usually happens each year at this particular time, both at national level and in the city county of Nairobi (source: NTLD-P). From July to October 2019, however, there was widespread strike action among the healthcare workers which severely affected health services, including TB case finding which declined dramatically. When the strike action was over, numbers with presumptive TB did not increase. There were two possible reasons for this that included (i) TB case numbers between 2018 and 2019 already being in decline, and this may have been part of the process, and (ii) community confidence in the health sector being adversely affected and taking time to pick up. In contrast, numbers with registered TB did increase, showing that the health services had returned to some degree of normality.

In spite of these pre-COVID-19 variations, there was still an overall significant decline in numbers presenting to the health facilities with presumptive PTB and in numbers being diagnosed and registered with TB in the COVID-19 period. The expected upward trend in TB case finding from April to July 2020 (the summer months) did not happen. Children and women were particularly affected, maybe because there was more difficulty for mothers and children to move around during lockdown and a heightened sense of fear for the family about accessing health facilities. The national lockdown and the ongoing challenges after lockdown, which included health facility closures and strike action in the health sector, posed ongoing problems. While numbers with presumptive TB picked up in the second six months of the COVID-19 period and particularly in the last month of the study, numbers with registered TB remained below pre-COVID-19 levels throughout this time.

These findings of declines in TB case detection are similar to reports from other health facilities and clinics in Nigeria [24], Brazil [25], China [26] and India [27]. Our study and these clinic reports align with a recent report from WHO showing an overall 21% shortfall in TB case notifications in 84 countries in 2020 compared with 2019 [28]. A modelling analysis at the start of the pandemic suggested that a three month suspension of TB services due to COVID-19 lockdown followed by ten months restoration back to normal would cause over five years an additional 25,000 TB cases and 12,500 TB deaths in Kenya, mainly as a result of the accumulation of undetected TB during lockdown [29]. A further modelling study in high-burden, low- and middle-income countries predicted a 20% increase in TB mortality, the greatest impact coming from reductions in timely diagnosis and treatment of new TB cases [30]. However, these modelling studies were done early on in the pandemic when there was hope that service disruption would be temporary. The reality is that service disruption has continued throughout the year, and has been further exacerbated by industrial action in the health sector, health facility closures and continued community fear and stigma about COVID-19.

The city of Nairobi, therefore, has done well to introduce an array of innovative measures such as integrated screening for TB and COVID-19, TB self-testing, active case finding and contact tracing to mitigate the challenges. These seem to have paid off with improvements in case detection and diagnosis in the later months of the COVID-19 period.

The measures undertaken in Nairobi are in line with those recently recommended by the Stop TB Partnership [31], which include screening patients with respiratory symptoms for both TB and COVID-19, creating, developing and supporting networks of TB survivors and TB communities and implementing real-time surveillance data.

Second, it was encouraging to see that while TB treatment success initially decreased, it then picked up to between 70% and 80% in the last four months of the study. At the start of the study, we were concerned that COVID-19 restrictions would prevent patients from collecting anti-TB medications, compromise drug adherence and reduce the ability of TB programme staff from obtaining information about final treatment outcomes. TB patients with associated COVID-19 coinfection have an increased risk of mortality [32,33]. We were worried that undetected COVID-19 in our TB patients might increase TB deaths during treatment. In the event, however, there was a minimal increase in the risk of death. The TB programme implemented patient-centered measures to help patients comply with treatment and adhere to medication, and attention was paid to reducing the "not evaluated" treatment outcome. All these measures were associated with improvements in treatment success.

Third, with respect to HIV services, there was already a marked decline in HIV testing numbers at the health facilities in the pre-COVID-19 period. While the health sector strike action between July and October 2019 played a part, there were additional explanations. HIV testing had been institutionalized in public health facilities over the years and many people visiting these facilities had already been HIV tested. NASCOP had started promoting HIV-self testing, only doing confirmatory tests in health facilities for those who had tested HIV-positive. The country was also moving towards a more targeted HIV testing approach directed at high-risk groups as recommended for Sub-Saharan Africa as a whole and for Kenya [34,35].

Despite the pre-COVID-19 decline, HIV testing numbers in health facilities remained low during the 12 months of COVID-19. The reduction in numbers is similar to the reductions in HIV testing volumes that have been documented in Europe, the USA and other countries in Africa [36–39]. The decrease in HIV testing threatens access to diagnosis and treatment, resulting in excess HIV-related deaths and ongoing transmission of HIV in the community. HIV testing started to improve in the second six months, perhaps due to implementing community outreach services for clients and the promotion of assisted partner testing as recommended nationally [40]. It was encouraging to see that referrals to ART were maintained above 90% over the 12 months, with a slight increase observed during the COVID-19 period.

There were several strengths to this study. First, we embedded monthly surveillance within the routine services of the health facilities. Second, there was cross-checking and validation of monthly data between the country coordinator and the overall study monitoring and evaluation officer. Third, we used two 12-month periods to compare data, which enabled us to account for any seasonal changes that might affect access to health facilities. Finally, the conduct and reporting of the study were in line with the Strengthening the Reporting of Observational Studies in Epidemiology (STROBE) guidelines [41].

There were, however, some limitations. Our study was limited to health facilities in Nairobi, and therefore may not be representative of Kenya as a whole. The use of aggregate data meant it was impossible to fully understand the individual cascade of care for TB case detection and HIV testing. We only assessed referral to ART and did not measure initiation and retention on ART. Previous studies have suggested that ART interruption has been a problem during the COVID-19 pandemic [42], and it would have been interesting to assess this in Kenya. We also did not assess treatment outcomes of patients with drug-resistant TB, but these patients would have been referred to other centers where the ability to track outcomes might have been difficult with COVID-19 restrictions in place. Finally, the official monthly reports to WHO of COVID-19 cases and deaths may have underestimated the actual burden, and therefore impact, of COVID-19 in the country. A seroprevalence study of anti-SARS-CoV-2 antibodies in Kenya between

April and June 2020 estimated a crude national seroprevalence of 5.6%, with levels being highest in the counties of Mombasa (8.0%) and Nairobi (7.3%) [43]. A study on deceased people at the University Teaching Hospital morgue in Lusaka, Zambia, found that only 6 (9%) of 70 people, who had SARS-CoV-2 confirmed from postmortem nasopharyngeal swabs within 48 hours of death, had ever been tested before death [44]. These data suggest that there are many unreported cases and deaths due to COVID-19, a situation likely to be present in many other African countries.

Despite these limitations, there are some important programmatic implications from this study. First, the strengthened monthly surveillance system worked well with the disease control programme heads appreciating and closely reviewing the monthly reports. Although cause and effect are difficult to infer with this type of study, the frequent access to data may have helped with the implementation of interventions on the ground to counteract declining trends in TB case detection and treatment outcomes and HIV testing. However, to continue with this system requires funding and resources, which would need to be obtained.

Second, with COVID-19 likely to become endemic, TB and COVID-19 care and treatment programmes need to think about further integration with respect to screening, laboratory infrastructure and diagnosis, contact tracing and sound infection, prevention and control measures, especially in health facility settings [45]. Resources permitting, more consideration should be given to the use of digital platforms to facilitate case finding and treatment [46]. Kenya also has a large private sector, which in the case of TB serves 20% of all patients registered and treated in the country [47], and this must not be forgotten when it comes to integration and innovation. HIV self-testing would undoubtedly fill a significant gap in clinic-based HIV testing at a time of crisis such as this [34,35], but more attention needs to be paid at the health facility level to recording and reporting on numbers self-tested along with the results.

Finally, research into improving the responses to TB and HIV/AIDS amidst the COVID-19 pandemic must continue [48]. This needs to be mainly focused on safely and effectively delivering the key programme activities and ensuring that patients can more easily access diagnostic, treatment and prevention services.

5. Conclusions

Using strengthened monthly real-time surveillance in 18 health facilities in Nairobi, Kenya, the number of people with presumptive TB and registered TB, as well as the number of people presenting for HIV testing, declined during 12 months of the COVID-19 outbreak compared with 12 months pre-COVID-19. Successful TB treatment and referral of HIV-positive persons to ART increased slightly during the COVID-19 period. Programmatic interventions on the ground were associated with an improvement in case detection and treatment outcomes in the second six months of the COVID-19 period compared to the first six months. This study strongly suggests that real-time operational research can generate useful evidence for real-time action.

Author Contributions: Conceptualization, I.M., P.T., J.M.C., E.O., P.O., N.C.N., A.M.V.K., S.S., H.D.S., M.K., R.Z., I.D.R., S.D.B., A.D.H.; methodology, I.M., P.T., J.M.C., E.O., P.O., N.C.N., A.M.V.K., S.S., H.D.S., M.K., R.Z., I.D.R., S.D.B., A.D.H.; software, P.T.; validation, I.M., P.T.; formal analysis, I.M., P.T., J.M.C., E.O., P.O., N.C.N., A.M.V.K., S.S., H.D.S., M.K., R.Z., I.D.R., S.D.B., A.D.H.; investigation, I.M., P.T.; resources, I.D.R.; data curation, I.M., P.T., A.D.H.; writing—original draft preparation, I.M., P.T., S.D.B., A.D.H.; writing—review and editing, I.M., P.T., J.M.C., E.O., P.O., N.C.N., A.M.V.K., S.S., H.D.S., M.K., R.Z., I.D.R., S.D.B., A.D.H.; visualization, I.M., P.T., S.D.B., A.D.H.; supervision, I.M., P.T., A.D.H.; project administration, S.D.B.; funding acquisition, S.D.B., A.D.H.; All authors have read and agreed to the published version of the manuscript.

Funding: This research was funded by Bloomberg Philanthropies through a grant with Vital Strategies and Resolve to Save Lives Initiative, New York, USA. The grant number is 78941.

Institutional Review Board Statement: The project received ethics approval from the Kenya Medical Research Institute (KEMRI/RES/7/3/1) and the Ethics Advisory Group of the International Union Against Tuberculosis and Lung Disease (EAG 33/2020). As no names or other means of identifying patients during data collection were recorded and only aggregated data were used for the study, the need for informed patient consent was waived.

Informed Consent Statement: No names or other means of identifying patients during data collection were recorded and only aggregated data were used for the study. Thus, the need for informed patient consent was waived by both of the ethics committees.

Data Availability Statement: The data that support the findings of the study are available from one of the first authors (P.T.) upon reasonable request.

Acknowledgments: The authors thank established staff working in TB and HIV control in the 18 health facilities with their help in collecting the data.

Conflicts of Interest: The authors declare no conflict of interests. The funders had no role in the design of the study; in the collection, analyses, or interpretation of data; in the writing of the manuscript, or in the decision to publish the results.

References

1. World Health Organization. Coronavirus Disease (COVID-19) Weekly Epidemiological Update and Weekly Operational Update 29 December 2020. Available online: https://www.who.int/emergencies/diseases/novel-coronavirus-2019/situation-reports (accessed on 30 March 2021).
2. Gilbert, M.; Pullano, G.; Pinotti, F.; Valdano, E.; Poletto, C.; Boëlle, P.Y.; D'Ortenzio, E.; Yazdanpanah, Y.; Eholie, S.P.; Altmann, M.; et al. Preparedness and vulnerability of African countries against importations of COVID-19: A modelling study. *Lancet* **2020**, *395*, 871–877. [CrossRef]
3. Nkengasong, J.N.; Mankoula, W. Looming threat of COVID-19 infection in Africa: Act collectively, and fast. *Lancet* **2020**, *395*, 841–842. [CrossRef]
4. Pang, Y.; Liu, Y.; Du, J.; Gao, J.; Li, L. Impact of COVID-19 on tuberculosis control in China. *Int. J. Tuberc. Lung Dis.* **2020**, *24*, 545–547. [CrossRef]
5. Sandy, C.; Takarainda, K.C.; Timire, C.; Mutunzi, H.; Dube, M.; Dlodlo, R.A.; Harries, A.D. Preparing national tuberculosis control programmes for COVID-19. *Int. J. Tuberc. Lung Dis.* **2020**, *24*, 634–636. [CrossRef]
6. Bah, O.M.; Kamara, H.B.; Bhat, P.; Harries, A.D.; Owiti, P.; Katta, J.; Foray, L.; Kamara, M.I.; Kamara, B.O. The influence of the Ebola outbreak on presumptive and active tuberculosis in Bombali District, Sierra Leone. *Public Health Action* **2017**, *7*, S3–S9. [CrossRef] [PubMed]
7. Konwloh, P.K.; Cambell, C.L.; Ade, S.; Bhat, P.; Harries, A.D.; Wilkinson, E.; Cooper, C.T. Influence of Ebola on tuberculosis case finding and treatment outcomes in Liberia. *Public Health Action* **2017**, *7*, S62–S69. [CrossRef]
8. Gamanga, A.H.; Owiti, P.; Bhat, P.; Harries, A.D.; Kargbo-Labour, I.; Koroma, M. The Ebola outbreak: Effects on HIV reporting, testing and care in Bonthe district, rural Sierra Leone. *Public Health Action* **2017**, *7*, S10–S15. [CrossRef]
9. Jacobs, G.P.; Bhat, P.; Owiti, P.; Edwards, J.K.; Tweya, H.; Najjemba, R. Did the 2014 Ebola outbreak in Liberia affect HIV testing, linkage to care and ART initiation? *Public Health Action* **2017**, *7*, S70–S75. [CrossRef]
10. Stop TB Partnership. TB and COVID-19. Available online: http://www.stoptb.org/covid19.asp?utm_source=The+Stop+TB+Pa (accessed on 30 March 2021).
11. World Health Organization. *World Health Organization (WHO) Information Note Tuberculosis and COVID-19*; WHO: Geneva, Switzerland, 2020.
12. UNAIDS. Covid-19 and HIV. Available online: https://www.unaids.org/en/covid19 (accessed on 30 March 2021).
13. Chiang, C.Y.; Sony, A.E. Tackling the threat of COVID-19 in Africa: An urgent need for practical planning. *Int. J. Tuberc. Lung Dis.* **2020**, *24*, 541–542. [CrossRef] [PubMed]
14. World Health Organization. *Coronavirus Disease 2019 (COVID-19) Situation Report—86*; WHO: Geneva, Switzerland, 2020.
15. Ortuno-Gutierrez, N.; Zachariah, R.; Woldeyohannes, D.; Bangoura, A.; Chérif, G.-F.; Loua, F.; Hermans, V.; Tayler-Smith, K.; Sikhondze, W.; Camara, L.-M. Upholding Tuberculosis Services during the 2014 Ebola Storm: An Encouraging Experience from Conakry, Guinea. *PLoS ONE* **2016**, *11*, e0157296. [CrossRef] [PubMed]
16. Kenya National Bureau of Statistics; Ministry of Health; National AIDS Control Council; Kenya Medical Research Institute; National Council for Population and Development; The DHF Program. *Kenya Demographic and Health Survey 2014*; Kenya National Bureau of Statistics: Nairobi, Kenya, 2015.
17. The World Bank. Kenya. Available online: https://data.worldbank.org/country/KE (accessed on 30 March 2021).
18. Global Citizen. There Are over 9000 Clinics in Kenya's Nairobi County. Only 1079 Are Legal. Available online: https://www.globalcitizen.org/en/content/kenya-illegal-health-clinics-nairobi-country/ (accessed on 30 March 2021).
19. National Tuberculosis & Lung Disease Program. *Guideline for Intergrated Tubeculosis, Leprosy & Lung Disease in Kenya*; National Tuberculosis & Lung Disease Program: Nairobi, Kenya, 2017.

20. World Health Organization. *Guidelines for Treatment of Drug-Susceptible Tuberculosis and Patient Care (2017 Update)*; World Health Organization: Geneva, Switzerland, 2017.
21. World Health Organization. Definitions and Reporting Framework for Tuberculosis; 2013 Revision, Updated December 2014 and January 2020. Available online: https://www.who.int/tb/publications/definitions/en/#:~{}:text=2013 (accessed on 30 March 2021).
22. World Health Organization. Consolidated Guidelines on HIV Testing Services. Available online: https://www.who.int/publications/i/item/978-92-4-155058-1 (accessed on 30 March 2021).
23. World Health Organization. *Consolidated Guidelines on the Use of Antiretroviral Drugs for Treating and Preventing HIV Infection. Recommendations for a Public Health Approach—Second Edition*; WHO: Geneva, Switzerland, 2016.
24. Adewole, O.O. Impact of COVID-19 on TB care: Experiences of a treatment centre in Nigeria. *Int. J. Tuberc. Lung Dis.* **2020**, *24*, 981–982. [CrossRef] [PubMed]
25. De Souza, C.D.F.; Coutinho, H.S.; Costa, M.M.; MagalhaeËes, M.A.F.M.; Carmo, R.F. Impact of COVID-19 on TB diagnosis in Northeastern Brazil. *Int. J. Tuberc. Lung Dis.* **2020**, *24*, 1220–1222. [CrossRef] [PubMed]
26. Wu, Z.; Chen, J.; Xia, Z.; Pan, Q.; Yuan, Z.; Zhang, W.; Shen, X. Impact of the COVID-19 pandemic on the detection of TB in Shanghai, China. *Int. J. Tuberc. Lung Dis.* **2020**, *24*, 1122–1124. [CrossRef] [PubMed]
27. Meneguim, A.C.; Rebello, L.; Das, M.; Ravi, S.; Mathur, T.; Mankar, S.; Kharate, S.; Tipre, P.; Oswal, V.; Iyer, A.; et al. Adapting TB services during the COVID-19 pandemic in Mumbai, India. *Int. J. Tuberc. Lung Dis.* **2020**, *24*, 1119–1121. [CrossRef]
28. World Health Organization. Impact of the COVID-19 Pandemic on TB Detection and Mortality in 2020. Available online: https://cdn.who.int/media/docs/default-source/hq-tuberculosis/impact-of-the-covid-19-pandemic-on-tb-detection-and-mortality-in-2020.pdf (accessed on 30 March 2021).
29. Cilloni, L.; Fu, H.; Vesga, J.F.; Dowdy, D.; Pretorius, C.; Ahmedov, S.; Nair, S.A.; Mosneaga, A.; Masini, E.; Sahu, S.; et al. The potential impact of the COVID-19 pandemic on the tuberculosis epidemic a modelling analysis. *EClinicalMedicine* **2020**, *28*, 100603. [CrossRef]
30. Hogan, A.B.; Jewell, B.L.; Sherrard-Smith, E.; Vesga, J.F.; Watson, O.J.; Whittaker, C.; Hamlet, A.; Smith, J.A.; Winskill, P.; Verity, R.; et al. Potential impact of the COVID-19 pandemic on HIV, tuberculosis, and malaria in low-income and middle-income countries: A modelling study. *Lancet Glob. Health* **2020**, *8*, e1132–e1141. [CrossRef]
31. Stop TB Partnership. One Year on, New Data Show Global Impact of COVID-19 on TB Epidemic is Worse than Expected. Available online: http://www.stoptb.org/assets/documents/covid/TBandCOVID19_ModellingStudy_5May (accessed on 30 March 2021).
32. Motta, I.; Centis, R.; D'Ambrosio, L.; García-García, J.M.; Goletti, D.; Gualano, G.; Lipani, F.; Palmieri, F.; Sánchez-Montalvá, A.; Pontali, E.; et al. Tuberculosis, COVID-19 and migrants: Preliminary analysis of deaths occurring in 69 patients from two cohorts. *Pulmonology* **2020**, *26*, 233–240. [CrossRef] [PubMed]
33. Kumar, M.S.; Surendran, D.; Manu, M.S.; Rakesh, P.S.; Balakrishnan, S. Mortality due to TB-COVID-19 coinfection in India. *Int. J. Tuberc. Lung Dis.* **2021**, *25*, 250–251. [CrossRef]
34. Mhango, M.; Chitungo, I.; Dzinamarira, T. COVID-19 Lockdowns: Impact on Facility-Based HIV Testing and the Case for the Scaling Up of Home-Based Testing Services in Sub-Saharan Africa. *AIDS Behav.* **2020**, *24*, 3014–3016. [CrossRef] [PubMed]
35. Odinga, M.M.; Kuria, S.; Muindi, O.; Mwakazi, P.; Njraini, M.; Melon, M.; Kombo, B.; Kaosa, S.; Kioko, J.; Musimbi, J.; et al. HIV testing amid COVID-19: Community efforts to reach men who have sex with men in three Kenyan counties. *Gates Open Res.* **2020**, *4*, 117. [CrossRef]
36. Simões, D.; Stengaard, A.R.; Combs, L.; Raben, D. Impact of the COVID-19 pandemic on testing services for HIV, viral hepatitis and sexually transmitted infections in the WHO european region, March to August 2020. *Eurosurveillance* **2020**, *25*, 2001943. [CrossRef] [PubMed]
37. Darcis, G.; Vaira, D.; Moutschen, M. Impact of coronavirus pandemic and containment measures on HIV diagnosis. *Epidemiol. Infect.* **2020**, *148*, e185. [CrossRef] [PubMed]
38. Hill, B.J.; Anderson, B.; Lock, L. COVID-19 Pandemic, Pre-exposure Prophylaxis (PrEP) Care, and HIV/STI Testing Among Patients Receiving Care in Three HIV Epidemic Priority States. *AIDS Behav.* **2021**, *25*, 1361–1365. [CrossRef] [PubMed]
39. Ponticiello, M.; Mwanga-Amumpaire, J.; Tushemereirwe, P.; Nuwagaba, G.; King, R.; Sundararajan, R. "Everything is a Mess": How COVID-19 is Impacting Engagement with HIV Testing Services in Rural Southwestern Uganda. *AIDS Behav.* **2020**, *24*, 3006–3009. [CrossRef]
40. Lagat, H.; Sharma, M.; Kariithi, E.; Otieno, G.; Katz, D.; Masyuko, S.; Mugambi, M.; Wamuti, B.; Weiner, B.; Farquhar, C. Impact of the COVID-19 Pandemic on HIV Testing and Assisted Partner Notification Services, Western Kenya. *AIDS Behav.* **2020**, *24*, 3010–3013. [CrossRef]
41. von Elm, E.; Altman, D.G.; Egger, M.; Pocock, S.J.; Gøtzsche, P.C.; Vandenbroucke, J.P. The Strengthening the Reporting of Observational Studies in Epidemiology (STROBE) statement: Guidelines for reporting observational studies. *Lancet* **2007**, *370*, 1453–1457. [CrossRef]
42. Sun, Y.; Li, H.; Luo, G.; Meng, X.; Guo, W.; Fitzpatrick, T.; Ao, Y.; Feng, A.; Liang, B.; Zhan, Y.; et al. Antiretroviral treatment interruption among people living with HIV during COVID-19 outbreak in China: A nationwide cross-sectional study. *J. Int. AIDS Soc.* **2020**, *23*, e25637. [CrossRef]
43. Uyoga, S.; Adetifa, I.M.O.; Karanja, H.K.; Nyagwange, J.; Tuju, J.; Wanjiku, P.; Aman, R.; Mwangangi, M.; Amoth, P.; Kasera, K.; et al. Seroprevalence of anti-SARS-CoV-2 IgG antibodies in Kenyan blood donors. *Science* **2021**, *371*, 79–82. [CrossRef]

44. Mwananyanda, L.; Gill, C.J.; MacLeod, W.; Kwenda, G.; Pieciak, R.; Mupila, Z.; Lapidot, R.; Mupeta, F.; Forman, L.; Ziko, L.; et al. Covid-19 deaths in Africa: Prospective systematic postmortem surveillance study. *BMJ* **2021**, *372*, n334. [CrossRef]
45. Echeverría, G.; Espinoza, W.; de Waard, J.H. How TB and COVID-19 compare: An opportunity to integrate both control programmes. *Int. J. Tuberc. Lung Dis.* **2020**, *24*, 1–4. [CrossRef]
46. Chiang, C.Y.; Islam, T.; Xu, C.; Chinnayah, T.; Garfin, A.M.C.; Rahevar, K.; Raviglione, M. The impact of COVID-19 and the restoration of tuberculosis services in the Western Pacific Region. *Eur. Respir. J.* **2020**, *56*, 2003054. [CrossRef] [PubMed]
47. Mailu, E.W.; Owiti, P.; Ade, S.; Harries, A.D.; Manzi, M.; Omesa, E.; Kiende, P.; MacHaria, S.; Mbithi, I.; Kamene, M. Tuberculosis control activities in the private and public health sectors of Kenya from 2013 to 2017: How do they compare? *Trans. R. Soc. Trop. Med. Hyg.* **2019**, *113*, 740–748. [CrossRef] [PubMed]
48. Graciaa, D.S.; Kempker, R.R.; Sanikidze, E.; Tukvadze, S.; Mikiashvili, L.; Aspindzelashvili, R.; Alkhazashvili, D.; Blumberg, H.M.; Avaliani, Z.; Tukvadze, N. TB research amidst the COVID-19 pandemic. *Int. J. Tuberc. Lung Dis.* **2021**, *25*, 167–170. [CrossRef] [PubMed]

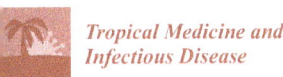 *Tropical Medicine and Infectious Disease*

Article

A Case Series Describing the Recurrence of COVID-19 in Patients Who Recovered from Initial Illness in Bangladesh

Pritimoy Das *, Syed M. Satter, Allen G. Ross, Zarin Abdullah, Arifa Nazneen, Rebeca Sultana, Nadia Ali Rimi, Kamal Chowdhury, Rashedul Alam, Shahana Parveen, Md Mahfuzur Rahman, Mohammad Enayet Hossain, Mohammed Ziaur Rahman, Razib Mazumder, Ahmed Abdullah, Mahmudur Rahman, Sayera Banu, Tahmeed Ahmed, John D. Clemens and Mustafizur Rahman

International Centre for Diarrhoeal Disease Research, Bangladesh (icddr,b), Dhaka 1212, Bangladesh; dr.satter@icddrb.org (S.M.S.); allen.ross@icddrb.org (A.G.R.); zarin.abdullah@icddrb.org (Z.A.); arifa.nazneen@icddrb.org (A.N.); rebeca@icddrb.org (R.S.); nadiarimi@icddrb.org (N.A.R.); kiachowdhury@icddrb.org (K.C.); rashedul.alam@icddrb.org (R.A.); sparveen@icddrb.org (S.P.); mf.rahman@icddrb.org (M.M.R.); enayet.hossain@icddrb.org (M.E.H.); mzrahman@icddrb.org (M.Z.R.); rmazumder@icddrb.org (R.M.); ahmed.abdullah@icddrb.org (A.A.); rahman.mahmudur@icddrb.org (M.R.); sbanu@icddrb.org (S.B.); tahmeed@icddrb.org (T.A.); jclemens@icddrb.org (J.D.C.); mustafizur@icddrb.org (M.R.)
* Correspondence: pritimoy@icddrb.org or pritimoydas@gmail.com

Abstract: To date, severe acute respiratory syndrome coronavirus-2 (SARS-CoV-2) has infected over 80 million people globally. We report a case series of five clinically and laboratory confirmed COVID-19 patients from Bangladesh who suffered a second episode of COVID-19 illness after 70 symptom-free days. The International Centre for Diarrhoeal Disease Research, Bangladesh (icddr,b), is a leading public health research institution in South Asia. icddr,b staff were actively tested, treated and followed-up for COVID-19 by an experienced team of clinicians, epidemiologists, and virologists. From 21 March to 30 September 2020, 1370 icddr,b employees working at either the Dhaka (urban) or Matlab (rural) clinical sites were tested for COVID-19. In total, 522 (38%) were positive; 38% from urban Dhaka (483/1261) and 36% from the rural clinical site Matlab (39/109). Five patients (60% male with a mean age of 41 years) had real-time reverse transcription-polymerase chain reaction (rRT-PCR) diagnosed recurrence (reinfection) of SARS-CoV-2. All had mild symptoms except for one who was hospitalized. Though all cases reported fair risk perceptions towards COVID-19, all had potential exposure sources for reinfection. After a second course of treatment and home isolation, all patients fully recovered. Our findings suggest the need for COVID-19 vaccination and continuing other preventive measures to further mitigate the pandemic. An optimal post-recovery follow-up strategy to allow the safe return of COVID-19 patients to the workforce may be considered.

Keywords: COVID-19; recurrence; reinfection; Bangladesh

1. Introduction

SARS-CoV-2, a novel enveloped RNA beta coronavirus, has manifested a variety of clinical characteristics from asymptomatic infection to severe pneumonia, vasculitis and death [1–3]. The World Health Organization (WHO) declared this disease a pandemic on 11 March 2020. As of 29 December 2020, SARS-CoV-2 infected more than 81 million people worldwide, with 1,784,533 deaths [4]. Bangladesh officially declared its first COVID-19 case on 8 March 2020 [5]. By 30 December 2020, 512,496 cases and 7531 deaths were reported in the country [6].

Direct, indirect or close contact with infected people and exposure to their saliva and respiratory droplets, which are released when an infected person coughs, sneezes, or speaks, may cause viral transmission [7]. The median incubation period of this virus is about 5 days and the infectious period duration is approximately 10 days [8,9]. A meta-analysis found that 59% of all transmission came from asymptomatic carriers [8].

WHO defines a laboratory confirmed case of COVID-19 if the patient's sample (at least a single nasopharyngeal (NP) and/or oropharyngeal swab or wash and/or lower respiratory sputum and/or endotracheal aspirate or bronchoalveolar lavage) tests positive by real-time reverse transcription-polymerase chain reaction (rRT-PCR) [10]. rRT-PCR assays only inform clinicians whether SARS-CoV-2 is present or not. However, these assays also provide quantitative data on cycle threshold (Ct) values, which are inversely related to the viral load and are not reported clinically. An advanced assay (e.g., whole genome sequencing) is required to interpret a recurrence—whether it is a relapse or a true reinfection. The effect of SARS-CoV-2 viral load on clinical outcomes and recurrence has not been extensively studied.

Generally, "relapse" may be defined as a "recurrence" with the same species and strain of a micro-organism that was present before, whereas "reinfection" is a secondary infection with a different species or strain. Reinfections with respiratory viruses may occur as a result of a weakened or waning immune response (e.g., respiratory syncytial virus), reinfection with a different genotype/species (e.g., rhinoviruses), or the viruses' high variability (e.g., influenza virus). The immunity against SARS-CoV-2 is not well established and it is uncertain how long the antibody will prevent re-infection [11]. Moreover, vaccine-induced protective immunity may differ from natural immunity due to the immune-evasion strategies of wild-type viruses [12]. However, there is some evidence of persistence of neutralizing antibodies in COVID-19 patients with natural infection for the first few months (~8 months) [13,14]. The immune response following a natural infection is thought to be incomplete, and reinfections are likely [15]. One should not confuse relapse with "long COVID" which refers to symptoms of COVID-19 that continue after the typical convalescence period. According to some reports, about 10% of people who tested positive for SARS-CoV-2 had one or more symptoms for more than 12 weeks [16].

Reinfection with SARS-CoV-2 is rare but possible, according to recent studies. Positive RT-PCR results in patients who recovered from initial illness have been reported in a number of countries [17]. In August 2020, a reinfection case was confirmed in Hong Kong in a patient with clearly different genome sequences [18]. Three confirmed reinfection cases were also reported from Nevada, USA [19], Belgium [20] and Ecuador [21].

There are some anecdotal reports of reinfection/relapse from Bangladesh. Among the positive COVID-19 staff cases from the International Centre for Diarrhoeal Disease Research, Bangladesh (icddr,b), the investigators noticed that some patients who clinically recovered from their illness (RT-PCR negative) were found to be RT-PCR positive for SARS-CoV-2 a second time. The aim of our study was to investigate suspected cases of reinfection or relapse excluding long COVID. We explored the clinico-epidemiological data of recurrent COVID-19 cases in Bangladesh and correlated these findings with their RT-PCR test results and whole genome sequencing.

2. Materials and Methods

2.1. Study Design and Setting

We conducted a case series of icddr, b staff between March and September 2020 where the community transmission of SARS-COV-2 was established.

2.2. Study Population and Procedure

The International Centre for Diarrhoeal Disease Research, Bangladesh (icddr,b) is a leading public health research institution in South Asia with approximately 4000 staff. Since 21 March 2020, all staff with clinical features (fever, cough, cold or respiratory distress) of COVID-19 were instructed to contact the icddr,b Staff Clinic. The staff clinic doctors advised any suspected staff member to undertake a nasopharyngeal swab for a COVID-19 test using RT-PCR. Some high-risk staff, such as staff nurses collecting NP swabs and laboratory personnel working with SARS-CoV-2, were also advised to undertake routine COVID-19 tests.

When a patient was RT-PCR positive, staff clinic doctors advised patients for home isolation if the condition was not severe enough for hospitalization. The staff clinic also prescribed and distributed medicines for each COVID-19 positive patient. Along with severe cases, less severe cases were also admitted to the isolation center of icddr,b if the staff member had difficulty with home isolation. All positive cases were advised to have a repeat test on day 14 and every week thereafter until tested negative.

The WHO criteria [22] for withdrawing from isolation for symptomatic patients as: 10 days after symptom onset, plus at least three additional days without symptoms (including fever and respiratory symptoms); and for asymptomatic cases: 10 days after a positive test for SARS-CoV-2. Based on the WHO case criteria and recent publications [23], we set the following criteria for selecting patients to investigate for reinfection: (1) an initial SARS-CoV-2 PCR-confirmed diagnosis; (2) followed by clinical recovery and with at least one negative SARS-CoV-2 PCR result; (3) followed by a confirmed SARS-CoV-2 PCR positive result from a single nasopharyngeal swab test with clinical symptoms at least 28 days after the previous SARS-COV-2 negative PCR result. The WHO clinical progression scale [24] specific for COVID-19 was used for clinical classification and assessing disease severity.

2.3. Laboratory Investigations

All participants submitted a single nasopharyngeal swab that was collected by trained nurses in viral transportation media. The specimens were transported to the laboratory in coolers within an hour of collection. RNA was extracted from the nasopharyngeal samples using QiaAmp Viral RNA Mini kit (Qiagen, Hilden, Germany). A final volume of 60 microliters of RNA was eluted from a 140-microliter sample. RNA was tested for SARS-CoV-2 by real-time reverse transcription polymerase chain reaction (rRT-PCR) targeting ORF1ab- and N-gene specific primers and probes following the protocol of Chinese Center for Disease Control and Prevention (briefly as China CDC). A positive case was determined if the CT values of two targets (ORF1ab and N) were <37 in the same specimen. If CT values of any sample were 37−40 or a single target was positive, it was resampled and retested. If the CT values were still 37−40 and the amplification curves had obvious peaks, the sample was considered positive. We did repeat tests for all second-time positives to confirm that they were not false-positive cases. If a single target was positive in the repeat test, it was determined to be positive. The complete sequencing of positive isolates from the first and second episodes of each case was conducted using the Illumina NextSeq 500 platform. The RNA libraries were prepared using the Illumina TruSeq Stranded Total RNA Gold Library kit (Illumina, San Diego, CA, USA) following the manufacturer's instructions. The normalized pooled library was sequenced employing the Illumina NextSeq v2.5 sequencing kit (Illumina, San Diego, CA, USA). Additionally, all samples were tested for common respiratory viruses including: influenza A and B viruses, respiratory syncytial virus (RSV), parainfluenza (1, 2, 3), human metapneumovirus (hMPV), and adenovirus using real-time PCR following standard procedure [25,26].

3. Results

From 21 March to 30 September 2020, among the 3056 icddr,b employees working at Dhaka and Matlab centers, 1370 were tested for COVID-19 and 522 (38%) tested positive. Within this period, eight patients (1.5%) had recurrent episodes of COVID-19 infection. Three were excluded due to a short gap (less than 28 days) between previous PCR negativity and subsequent PCR positivity and the absence of any clinical sign/symptoms during their first episode of COVID-19 positivity. None of them had a history of compromised immunity. Of the five remaining patients who fulfilled our criteria for selecting patients to investigate for reinfection, 60% were male. All five cases were 35 to 49 years old with a mean age of 41 years (Table 1). All five cases perceived that the second episode, which occurred after a long recovery time, was a COVID-19 reinfection.

Table 1. Clinical characteristics of the COVID-19 cases for both their first and second episodes of illness.

Patients Characteristics			First Episode			Clinically Symptom Free Days	Second Episode				
Case #	Past Medical History	Illness Onset Date (D1)	Clinical Feature	Treatment	First Clinical Recovery		Illness Onset Date	Clinical Feature	Treatment	Duration of Illness in Days	Outcome
1	HTN	D1 13 May	Fever, cough	Home isolation, A+D+I+Z+VD	D15	98	D112 2 September	Fever, cough, cold	Home isolation, D+I+Z+VD	18	Recovered
2	None	D1 19 May	Malaise	Home isolation, A+Z+HQ	D10	92	D 101 27 August	Sore throat, fever, cough, headache	Home isolation, D+Z+VD	21	Recovered
3	HTN	D1 28 May	F, H, S	Home isolation, D+I+Z+VD	D8	70	D77 12 August	F, C, Low oxygen saturation, pneumonic features in CT scan	Moxifloxacin, Amoxycillin with Clavulanic acid, P, F	12	Recovered
4	Asthma	D1 1 June	Fever	Home isolation, D+I+Z+VD	D6	85	D90 29 August	Fever, cold	Home isolation, D+I+Z	9	Recovered
5	HTN, HT	D1 7 May	Fever, cough	Home isolation, A+Z+HQ	D2	131	D135 18 September	S, H, Chest pain, Hospitalized	Home isolation, D+I+VD+R	6	Recovered

Note: for all patients, we considered the starting date of the illness (first day of symptom onset) as "Day One" (D1). Sign-symptoms: F = fever; H = headache; A = anosmia; J = joint pain; M = malaise; C = dry cough; S = sore throat; HTN = hypertension; DM = diabetes; HT = hypothyroidism; RhA = rheumatoid arthritis. Medications: A = azithromycin 500 mg tablet, once daily for 5 days; D = doxycycline 100 mg capsule, twice daily for 5 days; H = hydroxychloroquine 200 mg tablet, first day—two tab stat., from second day onwards—twice daily for 10 days; Z = zinc 20 mg tablet, twice daily for 14 days; VD = vitamin D3 2000 IU, one tablet on every alternate day for one month; M = montelukast 10 mg tablet, once daily for 10 days; R = rivaroxaban 10 mg tablet, once daily for 45 days; I = ivermectin 6 mg tablet, two tablets on day one only; amoxycillin with clavulanic acid (625 mg), eight hourly for 7 days; moxifloxacin, 400 mg tablet once daily for 7 days; P = tablet prednisolone for two weeks, starting at 16 mg daily for three days and then tapered dose; F = favipiravir 200 mg tablet, 1600 mg twice daily on day 1, 600 mg twice daily on day 2–10.

The clinical course of the patients over time (onset of symptoms, severity, duration, recovery time) and PCR results are illustrated in Figure 1. Figure 1 clearly demarcates two episodes of COVID-19 illness.

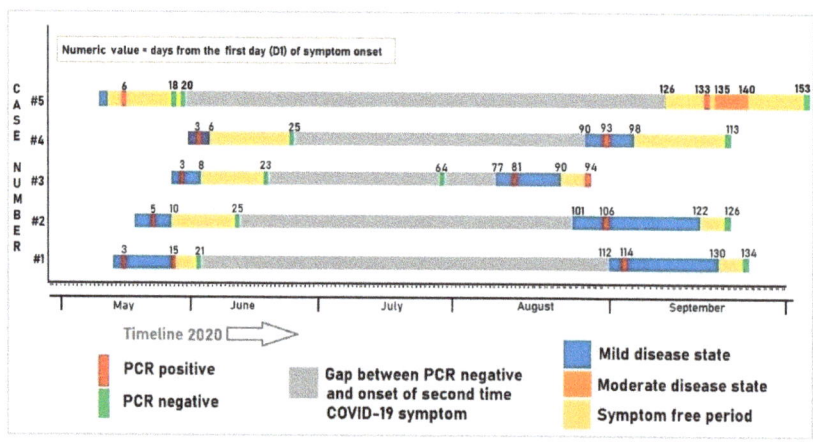

Figure 1. Clinical course and the corresponding PCR test results of the five patients with recurrent episodes of COVID-19 infection.

3.1. Case Series

3.1.1. Case 1

The first case presented with fever and a cough starting on 13 May (D1; D = day). The nasopharyngeal swab was drawn on 16 May, and the RT-PCR test was COVID-19 positive. The patient had a history of hypertension for three years. The patient reported no contact with suspected cases. He was advised to home isolate and was treated with azithromycin, ivermectin, doxycycline and zinc tablets (Table 1). He became asymptomatic on D15. On 3 June, his RT-PCR was negative. After a 98-day asymptomatic period, he developed a fever, dry cough and cold on 2 September, and tested positive a second time on 4 September. Case 1 reported attending a meeting at his office and also shopping at a nearby wet market for fish and other groceries in the 14 days before the onset of the second time illness. Although the case reported wearing a mask and using hand sanitizer during these outside visits, he states that these visits may have been the source of COVID-19 exposure. His symptoms persisted for 18 days before full clinical recovery and his RT-PCR was negative 22 days after the second onset of symptoms (24 September). He was well aware of COVID-19 as he read extensively about the infection from different online materials. In terms of vaccination, he was hopeful, assuming that it would continue to reduce the risk of COVID-19 and its severity. His test results are summarized in Table 2.

Table 2. Laboratory findings of the COVID-19 cases for both first and second episodes of illness.

Case #	First Episode			Gap between PCR Negative and PCR Positive Dates (days)	Second Episode				
	RT-PCR for SARS-CoV-2				RT-PCR for SARS-CoV-2			Other Investigations	
	Positive		Negative		Positive		Negative		
	Days from Symptom Onset	CT Value	PCR-Negative Day		Days from the first episode onset date	CT Value	PCR-Negative Day	Other Respiratory Viruses *	Other
1	D3 D15	38.3 33.7	D21	93	D114	34.8	D134	Negative	Chest X-ray-Normal D-Dimer-Normal
2	D5	21.7	D25	81	D106	34.8	D126	Influenza H3	ECG, BP normal
3	D3	34.5	D23	58	D81 D94	24.7 33.8	-	Negative	Ground glass appearance in CT scan chest, CRP level raised
4	D3	16.1	D25	68	D93	33.2	D113	Influenza H3	-
5	D6	36.8	D18, D20	115	D133	36.6	D153	Negative	ECG, Chest X-ray, D-Dimer all normal

* Influenza virus A and B, respiratory syncytial virus (RSV), parainfluenza (1, 2, 3), human metapneumovirus (hMPV), and adenovirus.

3.1.2. Case 2

The second case was a research assistant. She reported malaise on 19 May (D1). Two days later, her RT-PCR test was found to be positive. She had no other comorbidity. She went only to her workplace in the past 14 days before the onset of symptoms. The patient reported no contact with suspected cases. She was advised to home isolate. Her ECG, blood pressure and oxygen saturation were within normal limits. She became asymptomatic after D10 (27 May). She was tested again on D25 (12 June) and her RT-PCR test was negative. Case 2 reported that she went to the office regularly after being PCR negative. She used public transportation to and from work as well as on field trips. After a 92-day asymptomatic period, she developed a sore throat, fever, dry cough and a headache on 27 August. She was retested on 1 September and was found to be RT-PCR positive for the second time. No family members or any close contacts were positive for coronavirus within this time frame. She reported that she might have unknowingly been exposed to someone who is COVID-19 positive while traveling or engaging with patients and their caregivers at her workstation. For the second episode of illness, she was again treated at home with oral medication (Table 1). Her symptoms persisted for 21 days and her RT-PCR test was found to be negative on 21 September (Table 1). Influenza H3 coinfection was discovered in her second respiratory specimen. Since she received basic biosafety training from her office, she was well aware of COVID-19 transmission including person-to-person infection and through respiratory droplets in the air. She also shared an interest in the COVID-19 vaccine, which she hopes would benefit both her family and community.

3.1.3. Case 3

Case three was a hypertensive physician who reported a fever, headache and sore throat on 28 May (D1). Two days later, his PCR sample was found to be positive. He was isolated at home. Four days later, he became symptom-free. On 19 June, his follow-up sample was found negative. He was asymptomatic for the next 70 days. He reported fever, cold and low oxygen saturation (self-reported at 93%) on 12 August, and again was found to be PCR positive on 16 August. The case reported that within the past 14 days of his second episode, he had interaction with two COVID-19 relatives. During this second episode, he was tested for CBC, CRP, D-Dimer, LDH, a CT scan, and an echocardiogram. All were within normal limits except that a ground-glass appearance was evident on the chest CT and the CRP was elevated. After 12 days of illness, he became asymptomatic on 24 August (D90). On 29 August (D94) his PCR test was found to be positive. He was advised to isolate for another week without additional treatment and no further PCR testing was recommended. He reported having direct contact with COVID-19 positive patients and visiting them in the hospital is the riskiest way to acquire COVID-19 infection compared to exposure to an open environment like a wet market or workplace. He has a very positive attitude towards vaccinations.

3.1.4. Case 4

Case four was an account officer with a history of recurrent asthma. He developed a fever on 1 June (D1) and tested positive for COVID-19 on 3 June. His fever subsided after three days. His next scheduled PCR test was negative on 25 June. Due to the nature of the job, case 4 reported that he frequently went to his office in the preceding 14 days using office transportation and also visited local markets for shopping. Eighty-five days after the relief of symptoms, he reported fever and cough on 29 August and was found PCR positive on 1 September. The staff clinic prescribed ivermectin, doxycycline, zinc for the second illness. His fever subsided 3 days after onset, but a dry cough persisted for seven days. On 21 September, his scheduled PCR test was negative. During his second episode, he was co-infected with influenza H3. His detailed treatment history and laboratory findings are depicted in Tables 1 and 2. He had a basic understanding of how the virus spreads. For COVID-19 prevention, he emphasized handwashing with soap or sanitizer on a regular basis, maintaining social distance, and wearing a mask outside. He desired to get a COVID-19 vaccine as soon as possible to protect himself and safeguard his family.

3.1.5. Case 5

Case five was a young doctor working at the Matlab hospital. She reported to the staff clinic on 9 May with a sore throat and cough starting on 7 May 2020. Both her father and son were previously diagnosed as COVID-19-positive and she was a close contact. On 12 May, her PCR test result was found positive. She was isolated at home and treated with azithromycin, hydroxychloroquine and zinc tablets. Fourteen days after initial positivity, consecutive tests, 24 h apart, were found to be negative. After a prolonged asymptomatic period (113 days), she was tested again, given she was unknowingly in close contact with a COVID-19-positive nurse at work in the preceding week. On 16 September, she tested positive for a second time. Two days after the second diagnosis, she reported a very severe headache, chest pain and a sore throat. She measured her oxygen saturation and it was low (90%). She was subsequently admitted to icddr,b hospital on 20 May. Her ECG, Chest X-ray, and D-dimer levels were tested and found to be within normal limits. As her symptoms improved over the day, she was discharged in the evening on the same date for home isolation. She also self-medicated with rivaroxaban tablets for the prevention of thrombotic events. She reported relief from symptoms on 23 September. Her follow-up PCR test conducted after 21 days was negative on 6 October. She reported that overconfidence, accompanied by carelessness, was the primary reason for getting the infection from a contaminated surface, or direct or indirect interaction with a COVID-19 positive individual. She reported that taking precautions such as using masks, gloves, hand sanitization, and maintaining a safe distance can reduce some risk of this infection. She was very enthusiastic about the COVID-19 vaccination because she thought it would minimize the risk of getting this disease.

4. Discussion

We reported a case series of five clinically and laboratory confirmed COVID-19 patients suffering a second episode of COVID-19 after a gap of over 70 days free of symptoms. The recurrent cases had largely mild symptoms in both the first and second episodes of illness (only one case had moderate symptoms during their second episode). Most of the samples had high CT values (>30) indicating a low viral load. Whole genome sequencing is essential for determining true reinfections; however, our attempt failed due to low viral loads in collected NP swabs. Therefore, it is still unclear whether these were due to true reinfections or possible persistent low-level of infection sustained by viable viral particles or extra viral RNA. Nevertheless, our small case series indicates that symptomatic SARS-CoV-2 recurrence can possibly occur among individuals who recovered from their initial illness.

Our institute data showed that approximately 1% of all staff to date had the second episode of COVID-19. The proportion of recurrent RNA positivity after recovering from COVID-19 in our study was lower than that reported by Camilla et al. (2020) in a meta-analysis, where the proportion was reported between 7 and 23% [17]. Several factors might explain the low percentage. Firstly, we followed a strict case definition for a patient to be included in our investigation with a combination of clinical symptoms, PCR positivity, at least a one-month gap between a negative test report and the reappearance of COVID-19 symptoms followed by the presence of viral RNA in a second PCR test. Secondly, we could not actively monitor and follow-up all first-time positive cases in person because of resource constraints, and the follow-up system depended on the passive reporting of symptoms by the staff to the clinic. As most employees worked from home, they were probably reluctant to report symptoms to the staff clinic in order to avoid social stigma [27]. Thus, we might have missed many mild to moderate symptomatic recurrences of COVID-19 among our study population. Thirdly, there is a high probability of asymptomatic reinfection [28] which was not captured in our surveillance system. Hence, the actual number of recurrences of SARS-CoV-2 RNA positivity in our population may have been underestimated. Consensus criteria for deciding true SARS-CoV-2 reinfection should be set as new findings accumulate. Finally, our cohort did not include a collection of blood samples to describe the immunological profile that could allow us to evaluate the immune status of the cases.

The protective role and longevity of antibody responses to the virus remain unanswered. Some recent reports suggest that neutralizing antibodies against the virus remain relatively stable for several months after infection. In line with another case series [29], it is not clear whether the virus can persist in some COVID-19 patients for a longer period and transmit to close contacts and later reappear as an apparent second illness with COVID-like symptoms. Therefore, we should still advise our staff to maintain social distance, wear masks and self-isolate as much as possible to prevent reinfection. Bangladesh has received 9 million doses of the COVID-19 vaccine, Covishield (AstraZeneca) from the Serum Institute of India and vaccinated a total of 3,682,152 individuals as of 7 March 2021 (Health Bulletin of DGHS, 7 March 2021). Given the global spread of new variants, it is yet to be explored whether mass vaccination against existing strains can reduce the incidence rate to sufficient levels required to halt the pandemic.

Two of our patients showed concomitant influenza virus infection during their second COVID-19 episode. Both SARS-CoV-2 and influenza virus have common signs and symptoms, so it is likely that many patients with respiratory tract symptoms can be co-infected with influenza (H3). The influenza positive cases were clinically indistinguishable from the other three cases. The role of influenza in altering the clinical course of COVID-19 is unclear, thus further studies will be required to explore the pros/cons of co-infection.

Most of our cases reported mild symptoms. The immunological memory against SARS-CoV-2 is not well established and it is uncertain whether the first infection can prevent re-infection [11]. Limited data suggest that SARS-CoV-2-specific $CD4^+/CD8^+$ T cells can persist for up to 3–5 months and IgG to the spike protein up to eight months in COVID-19 patients [13,14]. If true, all of our initial cases may have developed immunological memory which may have partially protected them during their second illness.

Though our study was based on systematically collected data and prospectively investigated by an experienced group of clinicians, epidemiologists, and virologists, it had several limitations. Firstly, we tried to compare whole genome sequence data obtained from the first and second episodes from individual cases. However, only two complete sequences (with 99% coverage) were recovered from the 10 isolates (Supplementary Figure S1). Therefore, we could not determine whether the virus detected was identical or a different variant. Secondly, we could not conclude whether these cases were true reinfections or just relapsed cases. It is possible that the virus in the first episode diminished in the upper respiratory tract, became PCR negative, but was sustained in other parts of the body such as the pharynx, trachea, lungs, heart, kidneys, intestines, brain, genitals, or in body fluids such as the cerebrospinal fluid, semen and breast milk [30]. A systematic review showed that the virus could be sustained in other samples, such as the stool, for a longer period of time after the nasopharyngeal swab was negative [31]. Natural infection should, in theory, offer a degree of protection against future reinfection. However, in reality, this is not always achieved, given the differences in innate immunity and host genetics. Influenza vaccines that include previous variants may not protect against a new variant, so reinfection is likely. A lack of acquired immunity may partially explain the observed COVID-19 recurrence, but further immunogenetic studies examining innate, acquired and concomitant immunity are required.

Active case finding and isolation, quarantine, regular hand washing, wearing face masks, cough etiquette, avoiding public meetings, and maintaining physical distancing are the steps of choice in the absence of necessary vaccination coverage. The efficacy of such initiatives, however, is largely dependent on public willingness to cooperate and their perceptions of risk towards COVID-19 [32]. All our COVID-19 positive cases were well aware of the coronavirus disease: how it spreads and what preventive measures should ideally be maintained to minimize the risk. Our findings support a previous study conducted in ten countries, including Asia, which found that people who had personal and direct experience with COVID-19 had significantly higher risk perceptions [33]. Although our whole genome sequencing was inconclusive, all five cases believed their second episode of the illness was reinfection because their sufferings were identical to (or even worse than) the first. Epidemiologically, they had the potential exposures before the second episode, and clinically their signs and symptoms were also compatible with COVID-19 infection.

5. Conclusions

Our findings suggest the need for the COVID-19 vaccination to halt community transmission as well as to continue all preventive measures such as mask, hand wash and social distancing. Additionally, an optimal post-recovery follow-up strategy to allow the safe return of COVID-19 patients to the workforce may be considered.

Supplementary Materials: The following are available online at https://www.mdpi.com/2414-6366/6/2/41/s1, Figure S1: Phylogenetic tree based on the SARS-CoV-2 genome, demonstrated homology between the icddr,b SARS-CoV-2 genomes (case numbers 2 and 4) and other reported SARS-CoV-2 genomes from Bangladesh retrieved from the GISAID database.

Author Contributions: Study conceptualization: P.D., S.M.S., R.M., M.R. (Mustafizur Rahman), M.R. (Mahmudur Rahman); literature research: P.D., M.R. (Mustafizur Rahman), M.R. (Mahmudur Rahman), R.M.; data collection: P.D., S.M.S., Z.A., A.N., R.S., N.A.R., K.C., R.A., S.P.; data analysis: P.D., M.M.R., A.A.; results interpretation: P.D., M.R., A.G.R., M.Y.H., M.Z.R.; manuscript writing: P.D., S.M.S., M.R. (Mustafizur Rahman), M.R. (Mahmudur Rahman), A.G.R.; manuscript review: J.D.C., A.G.R., R.M., S.B., T.A., M.R. (Mustafizur Rahman); coordination: M.R. (Mustafizur Rahman). All authors have read and agreed to the published version of the manuscript.

Funding: The case report is a part of "COVID-19 testing and tracing in Bangladesh" study funded by the Bill and Melinda Gates Foundation (Investment ID INV-017556).

Institutional Review Board Statement: This study is in line with the ethical statement of institutional review board of icddr,b (PR-21010, ACT-01108).

Informed Consent Statement: Informed consent was obtained from all subjects involved in the study.

Data Availability Statement: Data cannot be shared publicly because they are confidential. Data are available from the respective department of icddr,b for researchers who meet the criteria for access to confidential data.

Acknowledgments: icddr,b acknowledges with gratitude the commitment of the Bill and Melinda Gates Foundation to its research efforts. icddr,b is grateful to the Governments of Bangladesh, Canada, Sweden and the UK for providing core support. We are grateful to our study participants for their time and cooperation.

Conflicts of Interest: The authors declare no conflict of interest.

References

1. Cheng, Z.J.; Shan, J. 2019 Novel Coronavirus: Where We Are and What We Know. *Infection* **2020**, *48*, 155–163. [CrossRef]
2. Huang, C.; Wang, Y.; Li, X.; Ren, L.; Zhao, J.; Hu, Y.; Zhang, L.; Fan, G.; Xu, J.; Gu, X.; et al. Clinical Features of Patients Infected with 2019 Novel Coronavirus in Wuhan, China. *Lancet* **2020**, *395*, 497–506. [CrossRef]
3. Leung, C. Clinical Features of Deaths in the Novel Coronavirus Epidemic in China. *Rev. Med. Virol.* **2020**, *30*, e2103. [CrossRef] [PubMed]
4. Worldometer Coronavirus Update (Live): Cases and Deaths from COVID-19 Virus Pandemic. Available online: https://www.worldometers.info/coronavirus/ (accessed on 29 December 2020).
5. Bangladesh Preparedness and Response Plan for COVID-19. 2020. Available online: http://www.mohfw.gov.bd/index.php?option=com_docman&task=doc_download&gid=23359&lang=en (accessed on 26 January 2021).
6. COVID-19. Available online: http://dashboard.dghs.gov.bd/webportal/pages/covid19.php (accessed on 29 December 2020).
7. Transmission of SARS-CoV-2: Implications for Infection Prevention Precautions. Available online: https://www.who.int/news-room/commentaries/detail/transmission-of-sars-cov-2-implications-for-infection-prevention-precautions (accessed on 6 March 2021).
8. Johansson, M.A.; Quandelacy, T.M.; Kada, S.; Prasad, P.V.; Steele, M.; Brooks, J.T.; Slayton, R.B.; Biggerstaff, M.; Butler, J.C. SARS-CoV-2 Transmission From People Without COVID-19 Symptoms. *JAMA Netw. Open* **2021**, *4*, e2035057. [CrossRef] [PubMed]
9. McAloon, C.; Collins, Á.; Hunt, K.; Barber, A.; Byrne, A.W.; Butler, F.; Casey, M.; Griffin, J.; Lane, E.; McEvoy, D.; et al. Incubation Period of COVID-19: A Rapid Systematic Review and Meta-Analysis of Observational Research. *BMJ Open* **2020**, *10*, e039652. [CrossRef]
10. World Health Organization. *Laboratory Testing for Coronavirus Disease 2019 (COVID-19) in Suspected Human Cases*; World Health Organization: Geneva, Switzerland, 2020; pp. 1–7. Available online: https://www.who.int/publications/i/item/10665-331501 (accessed on 26 January 2021).
11. Grifoni, A.; Weiskopf, D.; Ramirez, S.I.; Mateus, J.; Dan, J.M.; Moderbacher, C.R.; Rawlings, S.A.; Sutherland, A.; Premkumar, L.; Jadi, R.S.; et al. Targets of T Cell Responses to SARS-CoV-2 Coronavirus in Humans with COVID-19 Disease and Unexposed Individuals. *Cell* **2020**, *181*, 1489–1501.e15. [CrossRef] [PubMed]
12. Jeyanathan, M.; Afkhami, S.; Smaill, F.; Miller, M.S.; Lichty, B.D.; Xing, Z. Immunological Considerations for COVID-19 Vaccine Strategies. *Nat. Rev. Immunol.* **2020**, *20*, 615–632. [CrossRef]
13. Iyer, A.S.; Jones, F.K.; Nodoushani, A.; Kelly, M.; Becker, M.; Slater, D.; Mills, R.; Teng, E.; Kamruzzaman, M.; Garcia-Beltran, W.F.; et al. Persistence and Decay of Human Antibody Responses to the Receptor Binding Domain of SARS-CoV-2 Spike Protein in COVID-19 Patients. *Sci. Immunol.* **2020**, *5*, eabe0367. [CrossRef] [PubMed]
14. Wajnberg, A.; Amanat, F.; Firpo, A.; Altman, D.R.; Bailey, M.J.; Mansour, M.; McMahon, M.; Meade, P.; Mendu, D.R.; Muellers, K.; et al. Robust Neutralizing Antibodies to SARS-CoV-2 Infection Persist for Months. *Science* **2020**, *370*, 1227–1230. [CrossRef]
15. Goldman, J.D.; Wang, K.; Röltgen, K.; Nielsen, S.C.A.; Roach, J.C.; Naccache, S.N.; Yang, F.; Wirz, O.F.; Yost, K.E.; Lee, J.Y.; et al. Reinfection with SARS-CoV-2 and Failure of Humoral Immunity: A Case Report. *medRxiv* **2020**. [CrossRef]

16. The Prevalence of Long COVID Symptoms and COVID-19 Complications—Office for National Statistics. Available online: https://www.ons.gov.uk/news/statementsandletters/theprevalenceoflongcovidsymptomsandcovid19complications (accessed on 7 March 2021).
17. Mattiuzzi, C.; Henry, B.M.; Sanchis-Gomar, F.; Lippi, G. Sars-Cov-2 Recurrent Rna Positivity after Recovering from Coronavirus Disease 2019 (COVID-19): A Meta-Analysis. *Acta Biomed.* **2020**, *91*, e2020014. [CrossRef] [PubMed]
18. To, K.K.-W.; Hung, I.F.-N.; Ip, J.D.; Chu, A.W.-H.; Chan, W.-M.; Tam, A.R.; Fong, C.H.-Y.; Yuan, S.; Tsoi, H.-W.; Ng, A.C.-K.; et al. COVID-19 Re-Infection by a Phylogenetically Distinct SARS-Coronavirus-2 Strain Confirmed by Whole Genome Sequencing. *Clin. Infect. Dis.* **2020**. [CrossRef]
19. Tillett, R.L.; Sevinsky, J.R.; Hartley, P.D.; Kerwin, H.; Crawford, N.; Gorzalski, A.; Laverdure, C.; Verma, S.C.; Rossetto, C.C.; Jackson, D.; et al. Genomic Evidence for Reinfection with SARS-CoV-2: A Case Study. *Lancet Infect. Dis.* **2020**. [CrossRef]
20. Van Elslande, J.; Vermeersch, P.; Vandervoort, K.; Wawina-Bokalanga, T.; Vanmechelen, B.; Wollants, E.; Laenen, L.; André, E.; Van Ranst, M.; Lagrou, K.; et al. Symptomatic SARS-CoV-2 Reinfection by a Phylogenetically Distinct Strain. *Clin. Infect. Dis.* **2020**. [CrossRef]
21. Prado-Vivar, B.; Becerra-Wong, M.; Guadalupe, J.J.; Marquez, S.; Gutierrez, B.; Rojas-Silva, P.; Grunauer, M.; Trueba, G.; Barragan, V.; Cardenas, P. COVID-19 Re-Infection by a Phylogenetically Distinct SARS-CoV-2 Variant, First Confirmed Event in South America. *SSRN Electron. J.* **2020**. [CrossRef]
22. Criteria for Releasing COVID-19 Patients from Isolation. Available online: https://www.who.int/news-room/commentaries/detail/criteria-for-releasing-COVID-19-patients-from-isolation (accessed on 9 November 2020).
23. Tomassini, S.; Kotecha, D.; Bird, P.W.; Folwell, A.; Biju, S.; Tang, J.W. Setting the Criteria for SARS-CoV-2 Reinfection—Six Possible Cases. *J. Infect.* **2021**, *82*, 282–327. [CrossRef] [PubMed]
24. Marshall, J.C.; Murthy, S.; Diaz, J.; Adhikari, N.; Angus, D.C.; Arabi, Y.M.; Baillie, K.; Bauer, M.; Berry, S.; Blackwood, B.; et al. A Minimal Common Outcome Measure Set for COVID-19 Clinical Research. *Lancet Infect. Dis.* **2020**, *20*, e192–e197. [CrossRef]
25. Homaira, N.; Luby, S.P.; Hossain, K.; Islam, K.; Ahmed, M.; Rahman, M.; Rahman, Z.; Paul, R.C.; Bhuiyan, M.U.; Brooks, W.A.; et al. Respiratory Viruses Associated Hospitalization among Children Aged <5 Years in Bangladesh: 2010–2014. *PLoS ONE* **2016**, *11*, e0147982. [CrossRef]
26. Das, P.; Sazzad, H.M.S.; Aleem, M.A.; Rahman, M.Z.; Rahman, M.; Anthony, S.J.; Lipkin, W.I.; Gurley, E.S.; Luby, S.P.; Openshaw, J.J. Hospital-Based Zoonotic Disease Surveillance in Bangladesh: Design, Field Data and Difficulties. *Philos. Trans. R. Soc. B Biol. Sci.* **2019**. [CrossRef] [PubMed]
27. Mahmud, A.; Islam, M.R. Social Stigma as a Barrier to Covid-19 Responses to Community Well-Being in Bangladesh. *Int. J. Community Well-Being* **2020**. [CrossRef]
28. Iwasaki, A. What Reinfections Mean for COVID-19. *Lancet Infect. Dis.* **2020**, *21*, 3–5. [CrossRef]
29. Zheng, K.I.; Wang, X.B.; Jin, X.H.; Liu, W.Y.; Gao, F.; Chen, Y.P.; Zheng, M.H. A Case Series of Recurrent Viral RNA Positivity in Recovered COVID-19 Chinese Patients. *J. Gen. Intern. Med.* **2020**, *35*, 2205–2206. [CrossRef] [PubMed]
30. Trypsteen, W.; Van Cleemput, J.; van Snippenberg, W.; Gerlo, S.; Vandekerckhove, L. On the Whereabouts of SARS-CoV-2 in the Human Body: A Systematic Review. *PLoS Pathog.* **2020**, *16*, e1009037. [CrossRef] [PubMed]
31. Van Doorn, A.S.; Meijer, B.; Frampton, C.M.A.; Barclay, M.L.; de Boer, N.K.H. Systematic Review with Meta-Analysis: SARS-CoV-2 Stool Testing and the Potential for Faecal-Oral Transmission. *Aliment. Pharmacol. Ther.* **2020**, *52*, 1276–1288. [CrossRef] [PubMed]
32. Asefa, A.; Qanche, Q.; Hailemariam, S.; Dhuguma, T.; Nigussie, T. Risk Perception Towards COVID-19 and Its Associated Factors Among Waiters in Selected Towns of Southwest Ethiopia. *Risk Manag. Healthc. Policy* **2020**, *13*, 2601–2610. [CrossRef]
33. Dryhurst, S.; Schneider, C.R.; Kerr, J.; Freeman, A.L.J.; Recchia, G.; van der Bles, A.M.; Spiegelhalter, D.; van der Linden, S. Risk Perceptions of COVID-19 around the World. *J. Risk Res.* **2020**, *23*, 994–1006. [CrossRef]

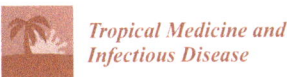

Communication

Malaria in the Time of COVID-19: Do Not Miss the Real Cause of Illness

Johannes Jochum [1,*], Benno Kreuels [1], Egbert Tannich [2], Samuel Huber [3], Julian Schulze zur Wiesch [3], Stefan Schmiedel [3], Michael Ramharter [1] and Marylyn M. Addo [3]

1. Department of Tropical Medicine, Bernhard Nocht Institute for Tropical Medicine & I. Department of Medicine, University Medical Center Hamburg-Eppendorf, 20359 Hamburg, Germany; b.kreuels@uke.de (B.K.); ramharter@bnitm.de (M.R.)
2. National Reference Centre for Tropical Pathogens, Bernhard Nocht Institute for Tropical Medicine, 20359 Hamburg, Germany; tannich@bnitm.de
3. I. Department of Medicine, University Medical Center Hamburg-Eppendorf, 20246 Hamburg, Germany; s.huber@uke.de (S.H.); j.schulze-zur-wiesch@uke.de (J.S.z.W.); s.schmiedel@uke.de (S.S.); m.addo@uke.de (M.M.A.)
* Correspondence: j.jochum@uke.de; Tel.: +49-40428180

Abstract: We report a case of *Plasmodium falciparum* malaria in a patient asymptomatically co-infected with severe acute respiratory syndrome coronavirus 2 (SARS-CoV-2). In the current ongoing coronavirus pandemic, co-infections with unrelated life-threatening febrile conditions may pose a particular challenge to clinicians. The current situation increases the risk for cognitive biases in medical management.

Keywords: severe acute respiratory syndrome coronavirus 2; plasmodium falciparum; differential diagnosis; cognitive bias; diagnostic reasoning

---

Since the end of 2019, the global outbreak of coronavirus disease 2019 (COVID-19) has spread rapidly and represents a major challenge to many healthcare systems worldwide [1]. In this situation, co-infections and comorbidities pose a particular challenge to clinicians, as the current focus on COVID-19 management may, on the one hand, lead to inappropriate diagnostics and management of other medical conditions, and on the other hand, to the risk of propagation of severe acute respiratory syndrome coronavirus 2 (SARS-CoV-2) within hospitals. Here, we describe a case of acute falciparum malaria and concurrent SARS-CoV-2 infection, illustrating the challenges in diagnostic reasoning during the current pandemic.

A 61-year-old female patient presented at the emergency department of the University Medical Center Hamburg-Eppendorf on 22 March 2020 with a fever of 40.2 °C, myalgia, and diarrhea. All symptoms had been present for four days. Nine days before presentation, she had returned from a two-week journey to Cameroon. She reported no chronic medical conditions or regular medication. Due to her recent air travel, fever and the ongoing pandemic with COVID-19, she was tested for SARS-CoV-2. Reverse transcription PCR of an oropharyngeal swab turned out positive and the patient was admitted to the COVID-19 isolation ward. Auscultation, lung ultrasound, and chest X-ray revealed no findings consistent with an atypical pneumonia (Figure 1). Laboratory results showed severe thrombocytopenia of 23,000/μL and C-reactive protein of 103 mg/L (Table 1). These results were considered atypical for a clinically mild case of COVID-19, given the available data [2]. Therefore, differential diagnoses were sought.

Prior to admission, the patient herself had already initiated presumptive treatment for malaria with atovaquone-proguanil due to her recent travel and lack of chemoprophylaxis. As history and laboratory findings were, indeed, compatible with malaria, we performed a microscopic examination of the patient's blood. A thin blood film was found to be positive for *Plasmodium falciparum* with an asexual parasitemia of 4% (Figure 2). Treatment with

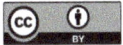

atovaquone-proguanil was continued and all clinical symptoms subsided on day three after admission. Two sets of blood cultures and PCR diagnostic for influenza remained negative. Although the detection of SARS-CoV-2 was confirmed in a subsequent sample, the patient never experienced respiratory symptoms during the follow-up of one month.

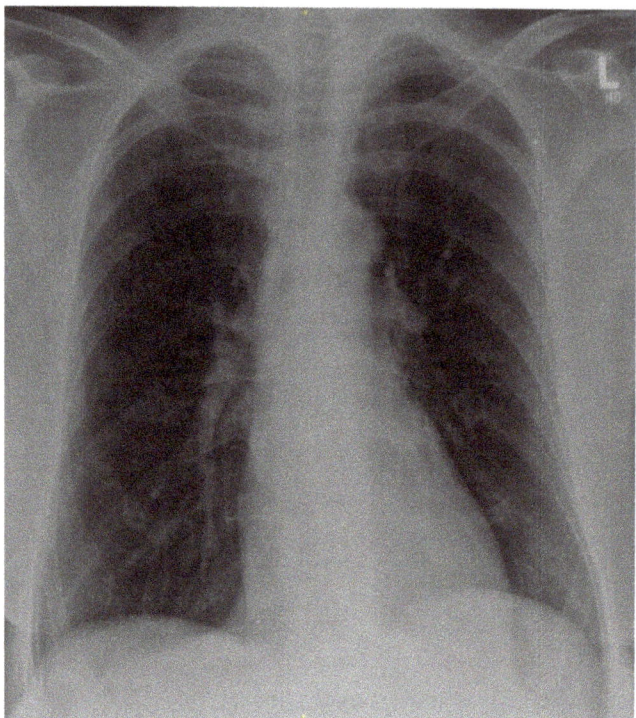

Figure 1. Supine chest X-ray at the time of admission without evidence of pneumonic consolidations or ground glass opacities. Courtesy of Prof. Gerhard Adam, Department of Diagnostic and Interventional Radiology and Nuclear Medicine, University Medical Center Hamburg-Eppendorf, Hamburg.

Table 1. Laboratory values of the patient on admission, 4 days after onset of symptoms.

Laboratory Parameter and Unit	Patient Value	Reference Range
Leucocyte count/µL	2700	3800–11,000
Hemoglobin g/dL	13.9	12.3–15.3
Platelet count/µL	23,000	150,000–400,000
Total bilirubin mg/dL	1.5	0.3–1.2
Alanine aminotransferase U/L	40	<35
Aspartate aminotransferase U/L	36	<35
Lactate dehydrogenase U/L	358	120–246
Creatinine mg/dL	0.67	0.55–1.02
C-reactive protein mg/L	103	<5

Due to its increasingly wide spread distribution in the population, COVID-19 may be encountered as a co-infection with any other classical disease. Dual infection with SARS-CoV-2 and malaria have been reported recently, with most patients being free of respiratory symptoms attributable to SARS-CoV-2 [3,4]. It is of importance not to miss such co-infections to avoid in-hospital spread of SARS-CoV-2 infection with the potential for high mortality in other hospitalized patients. At the same time, it is important not to narrow the spectrum of differential diagnoses of febrile conditions despite the ongoing COVID-19 pandemic. When patient load is high and staff are in short supply, it is tempting to be satisfied with an initial diagnosis, particularly when this diagnosis is consistent with the current outbreak. The pandemic situation contributes to the risk for cognitive biases during the medical management, in particular, availability bias and premature closure [5,6].

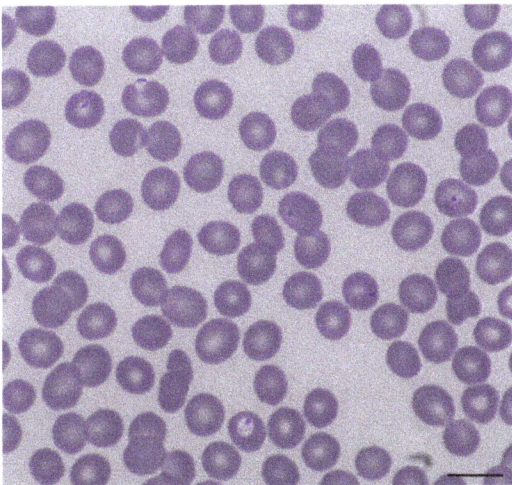

Figure 2. Thin blood film with *Plasmodium falciparum* trophozoites, *Giemsa* stain, original magnification 1000×. Scale bar: 10 μm

Importantly, only one day after admission of our patient, we received a telephone call by a desperate man who was denied a medical evaluation when he developed a high fever after travel to Ghana. His family doctor, as well as the local hospital, judged this to likely be COVID-19 and recommended home isolation—advice that has potentially fatal consequences. Subsequently, this patient was also admitted to hospital with *Plasmodium falciparum* malaria. The two patients illustrate the currently increased risk of missing life-threatening differential diagnoses with the requirement of a specific therapy beyond giving antibiotics for suspected sepsis. This becomes even more relevant when international travel is relaunched and is an important lesson for future outbreaks.

Author Contributions: Conceptualization, J.J., M.R., and M.M.A.; writing—original draft preparation, J.J. writing—review and editing, J.J., B.K., E.T., S.H., J.S.z.W., S.S., M.R. and M.M.A.; supervision, M.R. and M.M.A. All authors have read and agreed to the published version of the manuscript.

Funding: This research received no external funding.

Institutional Review Board Statement: Not applicable.

Informed Consent Statement: Obtained.

Data Availability Statement: Not applicable.

Acknowledgments: We thank Gerhard Adam, Department of Diagnostic and Interventional Radiology and Nuclear Medicine, University Medical Center Hamburg-Eppendorf, Hamburg, for providing the chest X-ray image of the patient.

Conflicts of Interest: The authors declare no potential conflict of interest.

References

1. World Health Organization. Coronavirus Disease 2019 (COVID-19) Epidemiological Update 28.09.2020. Available online: https://www.who.int/docs/default-source/coronaviruse/situation-reports/20200928-weekly-epi-update.pdf?sfvrsn=9e354665_4 (accessed on 29 September 2020).
2. Guan, W.J.; Ni, Z.Y.; Hu, Y.; Liang, W.H.; Ou, C.Q.; He, J.X.; Zhong, N.S. Clinical characteristics of Coronavirus disease 2019 in China. *N. Engl. J. Med.* **2020**, *382*, 1708–1720. [CrossRef] [PubMed]
3. Sardar, S.; Sharma, R.; Alyamani, T.Y.M.; Aboukamar, M. COVID-19 and *Plasmodium* vivax malaria co-infection. *IDCases* **2020**, *21*, e00879. [CrossRef]
4. Correia, M.J.; Frade, L.; Guerreiro, R.; Araujo, I.; Baptista, T.; Fonseca, C.; Mansinho, K. A patient with severe malaria and COVID-19: How do you tell the difference between these infections? *Eur. J. Case Rep. Intern. Med.* **2020**, *7*, 002007. [CrossRef] [PubMed]
5. Saposnik, G.; Redelmeier, D.; Ruff, C.C.; Tobler, P.N. Cognitive biases associated with medical decisions: A systematic review. *BMC Med. Inform. Decis. Mak.* **2016**, *16*, 138. [CrossRef] [PubMed]
6. Norman, G.R.; Monteiro, S.D.; Sherbino, J.; Ilgen, J.S.; Schmidt, H.G.; Mamede, S. The causes of errors in clinical reasoning: Cognitive biases, knowledge deficits, and dual process thinking. *Acad. Med.* **2017**, *92*, 23–30. [CrossRef] [PubMed]

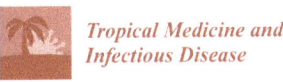

Communication

If Not COVID-19 What Is It? Analysis of COVID-19 versus Common Respiratory Viruses among Symptomatic Health Care Workers in a Tertiary Infectious Disease Referral Hospital in Manila, Philippines

Kristal An Agrupis [1,2], Annavi Marie G. Villanueva [1,2,*], Ana Ria Sayo [3], Jezreel Lazaro [3], Su Myat Han [2], Alyannah C. Celis [1], Shuichi Suzuki [1,2], Ann Celestyn Uichanco [3], Jocelyn Sagurit [3], Rontgene Solante [3], Lay-Myint Yoshida [4], Koya Ariyoshi [2,4] and Chris Smith [2,5]

1. San Lazaro Hospital, Nagasaki University Collaborative Research Office, Manila 1003, Philippines; agrupiskristalan@gmail.com (K.A.A.); anyacloud23@gmail.com (A.C.C.); suzuki_shuichi@nagasaki-u.ac.jp (S.S.)
2. School of Tropical Medicine and Global Health, Nagasaki University, Nagasaki 852-8102, Japan; pearl.june@gmail.com (S.M.H.); koya.ariyoshi@gmail.com (K.A.); christopher.smith@lshtm.ac.uk (C.S.)
3. Adult Infectious Disease and Tropical Medicine Department, San Lazaro Hospital, Manila 1003, Philippines; anariasayo@yahoo.com (A.R.S.); jez_lazaro@yahoo.com (J.L.); acpuichanco@gmail.com (A.C.U.); berewmd@yahoo.com.ph (J.S.); rontgenesolante@gmail.com (R.S.)
4. Institute of Tropical Medicine, Nagasaki University, Nagasaki 852-8523, Japan; lmyoshi@nagasaki-u.ac.jp
5. Faculty of Infectious and Tropical Diseases, London School of Hygiene and Tropical Medicine, London WC1E 7HT, UK
* Correspondence: agvillanueva@up.edu.ph

Abstract: The COVID-19 global pandemic is entering its second year. In this short report we present additional results as a supplement to our previous paper on COVID-19 and common respiratory virus screening for healthcare workers (HCWs) in a tertiary infectious disease referral hospital in Manila, Philippines. We sought to understand what etiologic agents could explain the upper/lower respiratory tract infection-like (URTI/LRTI-like) symptoms exhibited by 88% of the 324 HCWs tested. Among the patients who had URTI/LRTI-like symptoms, only seven (2%) were positive for COVID-19, while 38 (13%) of the symptomatic participants were identified positive for another viral etiologic agent. Rhinovirus was the most common infection, with 21 (9%) of the symptomatic participants positive for rhinovirus. Based on these results, testing symptomatic HCWs for common respiratory illnesses in addition to COVID-19 should be considered during this time of global pandemic.

Keywords: COVID-19; respiratory viruses; coinfections; health care workers; Philippines; rhinovirus

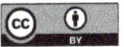

1. Introduction

The COVID-19 global pandemic is caused by the novel severe acute respiratory syndrome coronavirus 2 (SARS-CoV-2) and continues into a second year [1]. In the Philippines, around ~552,000 cases have been recorded, ~11,500 (2%) of whom have died, as of 15 February 2021 [2]. HCWs remain at high risk of acquiring the infection as they attend hospitalized COVID-19 patients. In the months that followed the first confirmed case of COVID-19 in the Philippines, recorded in San Lazaro Hospital (SLH) [3], there has been an increasing national trend of confirmed cases. The influx of patients has placed an enormous workload on hospitals, and consequently to HCWs. Mandatory quarantine/isolation of HCWs suspected of exposure has strained hospital workforces; specifically, HCWs experiencing a high-risk exposure to a confirmed case, or presenting with influenza-like-illness (ILI), are required to undergo at least two weeks of quarantine/isolation away from the hospital. The resulting reduction in the HCW workforce causes extended work hours for the remaining available staff, and inevitable "shift fatigue" [4] accompanied with increased fear and anxiety in working with COVID-19 patients.

We have reported that at SLH in Manila only 2% of HCWs were positive for SARs-CoV-2 as screened by RT-PCR (8 out of 324 HCWs screened) [5]. At that time, the criteria for screening were: (1) a history of close contact or high-risk exposure with a confirmed COVID-19 case or (2) the development of COVID-related signs and symptoms. Of the 324 HCWs, 88% had upper/lower respiratory tract infection-like (URTI/LRTI-like) illness such as fever, cough, sore throat, runny nose, shortness of breath, and loss of smell and taste. The small percentage of SARs-CoV-2 positivity suggests the possibility of underlying infections other than SARs-CoV-2.

SARS-CoV-2 is projected to circulate in the population indefinitely [6], and thus is likely to continue to cocirculate with common respiratory viruses. Although there is limited data on the prevalence of common respiratory viral infections in the Philippines, the Department of Health reports that acute respiratory infections consistently top the leading causes of morbidity in the country [7]. COVID-19 resides in the respiratory tract of the human host, and commonly exhibits URTI/LRTI-like symptoms, which overlap with those of common respiratory viral infections [8]. Because of the relatively small proportion of confirmed COVID-19 among HCWs described above [5], we sought to investigate whether HCWs who presented with these symptoms could be explained by other common respiratory viral etiologic agents.

2. Materials and Methods

HCW participants were tested for the presence of the following respiratory viruses: COVID-19, influenza A and B, human metapneumovirus (HMPV), respiratory syncytial virus (RSV), parainfluenza types 1 to 4, coronavirus 229E, coronavirus OC43, rhinovirus, adenovirus, and bocavirus.

Viral RNA from nasopharyngeal and oropharyngeal swab specimens were extracted using a QIAamp Viral RNA Mini Kit (Qiagen, Hilden, Germany), following the manufacturer's instructions [9]. Real-time PCR was performed to detect SARS-CoV-2 viral RNA using Corman et al. [10] and Nao et al. [11] protocols. Multiplex and hemi-nested multiplex PCR was done to test for the presence of the genetic materials from 13 other respiratory viruses, based on the protocol by Yoshida et al. [12]. Amplicons were visualized in 2% agarose gel.

We limited our analysis to those who exhibited URTI/LRTI-like symptoms. We categorized participants as "having URTI/LRTI-like symptoms" when they exhibited at least one of the following: fever, cough, sore throat, runny nose, shortness of breath, or loss of smell and taste. The epidemiological and clinical characteristics of these HCWs were compared between those who tested positive for the respiratory viral panels other than COVID-19 and those who tested negative for any of the panel of tests. The values were expressed as absolute numbers and percentages for categorical variables, and mean with standard deviation (SD) and median for continuous variables. Fisher's exact test and chi-square test were used to test for associations between categorical variables, and the Mann–Whitney test was used to compare discrete variables between classifications of categorical variables. A p-value of ≤ 0.05 was considered statistically significant. Stata SE ver. 16.1 (StataCorp 2019, College Station, TX, USA) was used for all analyses.

3. Results

Our previous publication detailed the epidemiological and clinical characteristics of the 324 HCW staff tested for SARS-CoV-2 at SLH in Manila [5]. Here we subjected the same group to a panel of respiratory viral tests from March 20 to 20 April 2020. Out of 324, 286 (88%) presented with URTI/LRTI-like symptoms. A summary of those who tested positive for at least one of the viral panels, including SARS-CoV-2, is shown in Table 1. Among those who exhibited URTI/LRTI-like symptoms, only 2% (7 out of 286) were confirmed to have SARS-COV-2 infection. Specifically, five tested positive for only

SARS-CoV-2 (2%) and two others had coinfections with two or more viruses: one with influenza A (0.4%), and another with influenza A and parainfluenza 1 (0.4%). Twenty-one (9%) of the participants were infected with rhinovirus—19 with rhinovirus alone (7%) and two with bocavirus coinfection (0.7%)—making it the most common infection of those who exhibited URTI/LRTI-like symptoms (55% out of those who yielded positive results). Other viruses that tested positive were influenza A (0.7%) and B (0.7%), bocavirus (0.4%), parainfluenza 1 (0.4%), adenovirus (0.7%), and coinfections of adenovirus and bocavirus (0.7%). Coinfection was observed in six HCW samples (2%). Overall, 38 (13%) of the participants who presented with URTI/LRTI-like symptoms were identified with a viral etiologic agent. HMPV, RSV, Parainfluenza 2 to 4, coronavirus 229E, and coronavirus OC43 were not detected in any of the samples.

Table 1. Summary of the positive test results of viral panels (including SARS-CoV-2) tested among HCWs suspected of having COVID-19 and presented with URTI/LRTI-like symptoms, San Lazaro Hospital, March–April 2020 (N = 286).

Viral Etiologic Agents	Infected HCWs (n, %)
SARS-CoV-2	5 (1.7)
Rhinovirus	19 (6.5)
Influenza A	2 (0.7)
Influenza B	2 (0.7)
Human bocavirus	1 (0.4)
Parainfluenza 1	1 (0.4)
Adenovirus	2 (0.7)
Coinfections *	
SARS-CoV-2 + Influenza A + Parainfluenza 1	1 (0.4)
SARS-CoV-2 + influenza A	1 (0.4)
Adenovirus + Bocavirus	2 (0.7)
Rhinovirus + Bocavirus	2 (0.7)
Total	**38 (13.3)**

* Coinfection—sample tested positive for more than one etiologic agent.

Excluding SARS-CoV-2 from the analysis (Table 3), most participants who tested positive for the respiratory viral panel (N = 36) belonged to a young age group (39% were 20–29 years old, and 33% were 30–39 years old), were female (67%), and worked as nurses (67%). Other health care workers infected were six nursing aides (17%), four radiology technicians (11%), and two medical doctors (6%). The most common respiratory symptoms exhibited by those who tested positive were sore throat (71%), cough (50%), and runny nose (43%); while nonrespiratory symptoms were predominantly headache (58%), myalgia (33%), and fatigue (19%). Only headache showed significant association with being positive for the respiratory viruses tested ($p = 0.04$).

Table 2. Comparison of characteristics and signs and symptoms of HCWs suspected to have COVID-19 who tested positive and negative for the additional respiratory viral panel *.

Characteristics	Positive (N = 36) (n, %)	Negative (N = 280) (n, %)	p-Value
Age (years)			
mean (SD)	35 (11.1)	36 (8.4)	
median (range)	30.5 (23–63)	33 (24–61)	0.14
Age group (years)			
20–29	14 (38.9)	72 (25.7)	
30–39	12 (33.3)	124 (44.3)	
40–49	4 (11.1)	62 (22.1)	
50–59	4 (11.1)	20 (7.1)	
60–69	2 (5.6)	2 (0.7)	

Table 3. Comparison of characteristics and signs and symptoms of HCWs suspected to have COVID-19 who tested positive and negative for the additional respiratory viral panel *.

Characteristics	Positive (N = 36) (n, %)	Negative (N = 280) (n, %)	p-Value
Sex			
Female	24 (66.7)	186 (66.4)	
Male	12 (33.3)	94 (33.6)	1
Occupation			
Nurse	24 (66.7)	175 (62.5)	0.03
Medical doctor	2 (5.6)	34 (12.1)	
Nursing aide	6 (16.7)	6 (16.7)	
Radiology technician	4 (11.1)	2 (0.7)	
Laboratory personnel	0	9 (3.2)	
Admission/reception staff	0	4 (1.4)	
Level of exposure			
Low risk	28 (77.8)	195 (69.6)	0.3
High risk	8 (22.2)	85 (30.4)	
URTI/LRTI-like symptoms			
Fever	1 (2.8)	2 (0.7)	0.3
Cough	18 (50)	138 (50.4)	1
Sore throat	25 (71.4)	188 (68.6)	0.7
Runny nose	15 (42.9)	108 (39.4)	0.7
Shortness of breath	2 (5.7)	26 (9.6)	0.4
Loss of smell	3 (11.5)	7 (3.2)	0.1
Loss of taste	1 (3.9)	8 (3.7)	1
Comorbidities			
Asthma	2 (5.6)	20 (7.1)	1
Cancer	0	2 (0.7)	1
Chronic liver disease	0	1	0.4
Diabetes	1 (12.5)	5 (13.9)	0.92
Heart disease	2 (5.6)	6 (2.1)	0.2
Hypertension	8 (22.2)	58 (20.7)	0.8
Obesity	6 (16.7)	50 (17.9)	1
No comorbidities	20 (55.6)	172 (61.4)	0.5
Duration between onset of symptoms and swab collection			
mean (SD)	8 (5.4)	9 (8.1)	
median	7	6	0.5

* HCWs who tested positive for covid-19 were excluded from the analysis.

4. Discussion

In the present study more health care workers exhibiting URTI/LRTI-like symptoms tested positive for common respiratory viruses, particularly rhinoviruses [13], than pandemic-related COVID-19. Our results are comparable to the outcome of an earlier study from China which tested clinically suspected COVID-19 patients for SARS-CoV-2 and other respiratory viruses. Their findings showed that 1% were positive for SARS-CoV-2, with an overall detection rate of other respiratory pathogens of 10%, and rhinovirus also being the most common underlying virus (3%). However, the coinfection rate was higher at 12% [14]. Notably, coinfections in our samples were observed more commonly with bocavirus (four samples that had coinfections with other respiratory viruses). Two (<1%) confirmed SARS-CoV-2 positive samples also had coinfections. Reported rates of coinfection of SARS-CoV-2 and other respiratory viruses range from 1% to 20% [15–17].

Among those who had coinfections, only one HCW yielded positive results for three etiologic agents (SARS-CoV-2, Influenza A and Parainfluenza (1); a 48-year-old, male who was tested on the fifth day of illness. He was categorized as low-risk exposure and presented with fever, sore throat, cough, fatigue and loss of appetite.

The signs and symptoms exhibited by those who tested positive for respiratory viruses other than COVID-19 were indistinguishable from those observed among persons who tested positive for SARS-CoV-2 [5]. Based upon symptoms alone it is a challenge to identify patients with acute respiratory illness (ARI) and COVID-19, primarily because their presenting signs and symptoms are almost similar at the outset. In the context of HCWs who are attending to COVID-19 patients in a developing country like the Philippines, where hospitals are usually understaffed, it is crucial to clarify the actual infection rate of SARS-CoV-2 and other respiratory viruses. At the moment, for HCWs presenting with mild symptoms who tested negative for SARS-CoV-2, for example, this guides decisions regarding continuing quarantine versus allowing to work. In addition to relieving the burden of "shift fatigue" among HCWs, a definitive diagnosis of "something other than COVID-19" should also help alleviate unnecessary anxiety. A limitation of this study is that we tested for an incomplete panel of viruses, and no bacterial pathogens. Subclinical viral infection is common, particularly rhinovirus, among healthy individuals [18], and it is possible that the symptoms of the HCWs in our study could be explained by other causative agents than those in the respiratory viral panel we tested. Further studies could test for an expanded range of pathogens relevant to respiratory illness.

5. Conclusions

Although COVID-19 is a serious concern, our study showed that it was not the main pathogen responsible for respiratory tract infections among HCWs. Symptoms associated with SARS-CoV-2 and other respiratory viral etiologies are frequently shared. While it is important to continue regular screening and testing for COVID-19 among this high-risk population, efforts should also focus on ensuring that HCWs have access to rapid molecular tests for other common respiratory illnesses.

Author Contributions: Conceptualization, K.A.A., C.S., A.M.G.V., and S.S.; data curation, A.M.G.V., S.M.H, and C.S.; formal analysis, K.A.A., A.M.G.V, S.M.H., and C.S.; funding acquisition, C.S. and K.A.; investigation, A.M.G.V., S.S., A.R.S., J.L., A.C.U., J.S., and A.C.C.; methodology, A.M.G.V., C.S., K.A., and L.-M.Y.; project administration, S.S., A.M.G.V., A.R.S., J.L., A.C.U., J.S., and R.S.; supervision, K.A., L.-M.Y., and C.S.; visualization, K.A.A. and C.S.; writing—original draft, K.A.A. and C.S.; writing—review and editing, K.A.A., A.M.G.V., A.R.S., J.L., S.M.H., A.C.C., S.S., A.C.U., J.S., R.S., L.-M.Y., K.A., and C.S. All authors have read and agreed to the published version of the manuscript.

Funding: This work was partly funded by Nagasaki University (salary support for K.A.A., A.M.G.V., S.M.H., S.S., A.C.C., K.A., L.-M.Y., and C.S.).

Institutional Review Board Statement: This study was conducted according to the guidelines of the Declaration of Helskinki, and approved by the San Lazaro Hospital—Research Ethics and Review Unit (Ref: SLH-RERU-2020-022-I) and the School of Tropical Medicine and Global Health, Nagasaki University Ethical Committee (NU_TMGH_2020_119_1).

Informed Consent Statement: Informed consent was obtained from all subjects involved in the study.

Conflicts of Interest: The authors declare no conflict of interest. The funder of the study did not play any role in the conceptualization and design of the study, collection, analysis and interpretation of data, writing of the manuscript or in the decision to publish the results.

References

1. World Health Organization. *Coronavirus disease 2019 (COVID-19) Situation Report—52*; WHO: Manila, Philippines, 8 September 2020.
2. Department of Health—Philippines. DOH COVID-19 Bulletin # 339 | Department of Health Website. Available online: https://doh.gov.ph/covid19casebulletin339 (accessed on 12 March 2021).
3. Edrada, E.; Lopez, E.; Villarama, J.; Salva, V.E.; Dagoc, B.; Smith, C.; Sayo, A.; Verona, J.; Trifalgar-Arches, J.; Lazaro, J.; et al. First COVID-19 Infections in the Philippines: A case report. *Trop. Med. Health* **2020**, *48*. [CrossRef] [PubMed]

4. Beresford, L. Shift Fatigue in Healthcare Workers. Available online: https://www.the-hospitalist.org/hospitalist/article/125427/shift-fatigue-healthcare-workers (accessed on 26 January 2021).
5. Villanueva, A.; Lazaro, J.; Sayo, A.; Myat Han, S.; Ukawa, T.; Suzuki, S.; Takaya, S.; Telan, E.; Solante, R.; Ariyoshi, K.; et al. COVID-19 Screening for Healthcare Workers in a Tertiary Infectious Diseases Referral Hospital in Manila, the Philippines. *Am. J. Trop. Med. Hyg.* **2020**, *103*. [CrossRef]
6. Kissler, S.; Tedijanto, C.; Goldstein, E.; Grad, Y.; Lipsitch, M. Projecting the transmission dynamics of SARS-CoV-2 through the postpandemic period. *Science* **2020**. [CrossRef]
7. Department of Health—Philippines. Morbidity | Department of Health Website. Available online: https://doh.gov.ph/morbidity (accessed on 12 March 2021).
8. Guan, W.; Ni, Z.; Hu, Y.; Liang, W.; Ou, C.; He, J.; Liu, L.; Shan, H.; Lei, C.; Hui, D.; et al. Clinical Characteristics of Coronavirus Disease 2019 in China. *N. Engl. J. Med.* **2020**, *382*. [CrossRef] [PubMed]
9. QIAGEN. QIAamp Viral RNA Mini Handbook—QIAGEN. Available online: https://www.qiagen.com/us/resources/resourcedetail?id=c80685c0-4103-49ea-aa72-8989420e3018$\langle$=en (accessed on 23 January 2021).
10. Corman, V.; Landt, O.; Kaiser, M.; Molenkamp, R.; Meijer, A.; Chu, D.; Bleicker, T.; Brünink, S.; Schneider, J.; Schmidt, M.; et al. Detection of 2019 novel coronavirus (2019-nCoV) by real-time RT-PCR. *Euro Surveill.* **2020**, *25*. [CrossRef] [PubMed]
11. Nao, N.S.K.; Katano, H. Detection of Second Case of 2019-nCoV Infection in Japan. Available online: https://www.niid.go.jp/niid/images/vir3/nCoV/method-niid-20200123-2_erratum.pdf\T1\textgreater{} (accessed on 21 January 2021).
12. Yoshida, L.; Suzuki, M.; Yamamoto, T.; Nguyen, H.; Nguyen, C.; Nguyen, A.; Oishi, K.; Vu, T.; Le, T.; Le, M.; et al. Viral pathogens associated with acute respiratory infections in central vietnamese children. *Pediatric Infect. Dis. J.* **2010**, *29*. [CrossRef] [PubMed]
13. Jacobs, S.; Lamson, D.; St George, K.; Walsh, T. Human rhinoviruses. *Clin. Microbiol. Rev.* **2013**, *26*. [CrossRef] [PubMed]
14. Si, Y.; Zhao, Z.; Chen, R.; Zhong, H.; Liu, T.; Wang, M.; Song, X.; Li, W.; Ying, B. Epidemiological surveillance of common respiratory viruses in patients with suspected COVID-19 in Southwest China. *BMC Infect. Dis.* **2020**, *20*, 1–7. [CrossRef] [PubMed]
15. Burrel, S.; Hausfater, P.; Dres, M.; Pourcher, V.; Luyt, C.; Teyssou, E.; Soulié, C.; Calvez, V.; Marcelin, A.; Boutolleau, D. Co-infection of SARS-CoV-2 with other respiratory viruses and performance of lower respiratory tract samples for the diagnosis of COVID-19. *Int. J. Infect. Dis.* **2021**, *102*. [CrossRef] [PubMed]
16. Wee, L.; Ko, K.; Ho, W.; Kwek, G.; Tan, T.; Wijaya, L. Community-acquired viral respiratory infections amongst hospitalized inpatients during a COVID-19 outbreak in Singapore: Co-infection and clinical outcomes. *J. Clin. Virol.* **2020**, *128*. [CrossRef] [PubMed]
17. Kim, D.; Quinn, J.; Pinsky, B.; Shah, N.; Brown, I. Rates of Co-infection Between SARS-CoV-2 and Other Respiratory Pathogens. *JAMA* **2020**, *323*. [CrossRef]
18. Yoshida, L.; Suzuki, M.; Nguyen, H.; Le, M.; Dinh, V.T.; Yoshino, H.; Schmidt, W.; Nguyen, T.; Le, H.; Morimoto, K.; et al. Respiratory syncytial virus: Co-infection and paediatric lower respiratory tract infections. *Eur. Respir. J.* **2013**, *42*. [CrossRef] [PubMed]

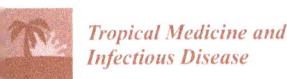

Case Report

SARS-CoV-2 Infection and CMV Dissemination in Transplant Recipients as a Treatment for Chagas Cardiomyopathy: A Case Report

Sarah Cristina Gozzi-Silva [1,2,*], Gil Benard [1], Ricardo Wesley Alberca [1], Tatiana Mina Yendo [1], Franciane Mouradian Emidio Teixeira [1,2], Luana de Mendonça Oliveira [1], Danielle Rosa Beserra [1], Anna Julia Pietrobon [1,2], Emily Araujo de Oliveira [1,2], Anna Cláudia Calvielli Castelo Branco [1,2], Milena Mary de Souza Andrade [1], Iara Grigoletto Fernandes [1], Nátalli Zanete Pereira [1], Yasmim Álefe Leuzzi Ramos [1], Julia Cataldo Lima [1], Bruna Provenci [3], Sandrigo Mangini [3], Alberto José da Silva Duarte [1] and Maria Notomi Sato [1,2]

Citation: Gozzi-Silva, S.C.; Benard, G.; Alberca, R.W.; Yendo, T.M.; Teixeira, F.M.E.; Oliveira, L.d.M.; Beserra, D.R.; Pietrobon, A.J.; Oliveira, E.A.d.; Branco, A.C.C.B.; et al. SARS-CoV-2 Infection and CMV Dissemination in Transplant Recipients as a Treatment for Chagas Cardiomyopathy: A Case Report. *Trop. Med. Infect. Dis.* 2021, 6, 22. https://doi.org/10.3390/tropicalmed6010022

Received: 16 January 2021
Accepted: 8 February 2021
Published: 10 February 2021

Publisher's Note: MDPI stays neutral with regard to jurisdictional claims in published maps and institutional affiliations.

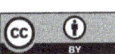

Copyright: © 2021 by the authors. Licensee MDPI, Basel, Switzerland. This article is an open access article distributed under the terms and conditions of the Creative Commons Attribution (CC BY) license (https://creativecommons.org/licenses/by/4.0/).

1. Laboratory of Dermatology and Immunodeficiencies (LIM-56), Institute of Tropical Medicine of School of Medicine of São Paulo (FMUSP), 05403-000 São Paulo, Brazil; bengil60@gmail.com (G.B.); ricardowesley@usp.br (R.W.A.); tatiana.yendo@gmail.com (T.M.Y.); franciane.mteixeira@usp.br (F.M.E.T.); luana.mendonca@usp.br (L.d.M.O.); daniellerb@usp.br (D.R.B.); pietrobonaj@usp.br (A.J.P.); emilyaraujo@hotmail.com (E.A.d.O.); annabranco@usp.br (A.C.C.C.B.); milena_mary@hotmail.com (M.M.d.S.A.); iaragf@usp.br (I.G.F.); natalli@usp.br (N.Z.P.); yasmim.leuzzi@usp.br (Y.Á.L.R.); juliacataldolima@hotmail.com (J.C.L.); adjsduar@usp.br (A.J.d.S.D.); marisato@usp.br (M.N.S.)
2. Institute of Biomedical Sciences, University of São Paulo, 05508-000 São Paulo, Brazil
3. Instituto do Coração (Incor), Hospital das Clínicas, School of Medicine of University of São Paulo (HCFMUSP), 05403-900 São Paulo, Brazil; bruna_provenci@hotmail.com (B.P.); sanmangini@ig.com.br (S.M.)
* Correspondence: sarahgozzi@usp.br

Abstract: Coronavirus disease 2019 (COVID-19) is caused by severe acute respiratory syndrome coronavirus 2 (SARS-CoV-2). COVID-19 has infected over 90 million people worldwide, therefore it is considered a pandemic. SARS-CoV-2 infection can lead to severe pneumonia, acute respiratory distress syndrome (ARDS), septic shock, and/or organ failure. Individuals receiving a heart transplantation (HT) may be at higher risk of adverse outcomes attributable to COVID-19 due to immunosuppressives, as well as concomitant infections that may also influence the prognoses. Herein, we describe the first report of two cases of HT recipients with concomitant infections by SARS-CoV-2, *Trypanosoma cruzi*, and cytomegalovirus (CMV) dissemination, from the first day of hospitalization due to COVID-19 in the intensive care unit (ICU) until the death of the patients.

Keywords: SARS-CoV-2; COVID-19; heart transplant; CMV; Chagas disease; infection; severity

1. Introduction

Coronavirus disease 2019 (COVID-19), an infectious respiratory disease caused by severe acute respiratory syndrome coronavirus 2 (SARS-CoV-2), has spread on a pandemic scale since the first case was reported in Wuhan, China, in 2019 [1]. Most patients with the disease have mild-to-moderate symptoms; however, approximately 15% develop severe pneumonia, while approximately 5% develop acute respiratory distress syndrome (ARDS), septic shock, and/or organ failure [2]. Lymphopenia is a recurrent feature in these patients, with a significant reduction in CD4+ T cells, CD8+ T cells, B cells, and natural killer (NK) cells [3], increasing the susceptibility of patients to severe illness and co-infection [4]. In fact, co-infections are associated with worsening of the clinical condition [5].

Chagas disease (CD) is a zoonosis whose etiologic agent is the protozoan *Trypanosoma cruzi*. It is estimated that 6–8 million people worldwide are infected [6]. CD has two distinct phases: an acute one, which is rare, with a strong production of type 1 cytokines, and a chronic phase, which develops in 30–40% of CD cases. The chronic phase of CD can be characterized by cardiomyopathy, arrhythmias, megaviscera, and, more rarely, polyneuropathy and stroke [7]. TCD4+ and TCD8+ lymphocytes are the main cells responsible for controlling parasitic infection. However, the immune response also contributes to tissue damage and pathology [8].

Chagasic cardiomyopathy represents the main cause of mortality from this disease, which can lead to heart failure, whose indication for treatment, especially in endemic countries, may include heart transplantation (HT) as a strategy to curb the evolution of this complication [6,9]. However, the immunosuppression and possible reactivation of the causative agent *T. cruzi* following HT require intensive clinical care and laboratory monitoring [10].

Other infections such as that caused by cytomegalovirus (CMV), a herpes virus that infects up to 60–100% of people in adulthood, are associated with transplant complications [11]. Primary CMV infection is generally asymptomatic in immunocompetent individuals, with the virus generating a latent infection. On the contrary, in immunocompromised and immunosuppressed populations, such as solid organ transplantation, hematopoietic stem cell transplantation, and HIV/AIDS patients, CMV reactivation is responsible for significant morbidity and mortality [12]. Although reactivation of infections such as CMV and CD are often described in transplant recipients, there are no reports of concomitant infection by *T. cruzi*, CMV, and SARS-CoV-2 in the context of HT in the literature to date.

Therefore, in this report, we investigated the progress of two patients who underwent HT at the Heart Institute of Hospital das Clínicas (Incor) and were subsequently transferred to the special intensive care unit (ICU) of the Hospital das Clínicas (Hospital das Clínicas, Faculty of Medicine, University of São Paulo-HCFMUSP) due to SARS-CoV-2 infection. These patients were diagnosed with COVID-19 by nasopharyngeal detection of SARS-CoV-2 RNA using reverse transcriptase polymerase chain reaction (RT-PCR). In addition, during hospitalization, CMV dissemination was evidenced by quantitative DNA detection in the blood. We describe herein the laboratory data from the first day of hospitalization due to COVID-19 until the death of the patients.

The baseline characteristics of these two patients, as well as their past clinical data, are summarized in Table 1.

Table 1. Patients' characteristics, comorbidities, treatment, and complications.

	Patient 1	Patient 2
Sex	Female	Male
Age	55	62
Positive SARS-CoV-2 RT-PCR date	1 June 2020	29 June 2020
Heart transplant date	2 May 2020	5 December 2019
Death date	30 days	207 days
Days between positive SARS-CoV-2 diagnosis and death	47 days	21 days
Complications during ICU stay	ARDS due to COVID–19; heart transplant rejection, disseminated cytomegalovirus; aggravated chronic kidney disease and pressure ulcer	ARDS due to COVID–19, disseminated cytomegalovirus and pancytopenia due to hemophagocytosis
Previous comorbidities	Dilated cardiomyopathy of Chagas etiology, hypothyroidism by thyroidectomy by nodule 10 years ago	Cardiomyopathy of Chagas etiology, disseminated cytomegalovirus, deep vein thrombosis, systemic arterial hypertension, diabetes, dyslipidemia, and chronic renal failure

Table 1. Cont.

	Patient 1	Patient 2
Previous use of medications	Carvedilol, losartan, furosemide, levothyroxine, isosorbide, and hydralazine	Unknown
Medicines used during ICU stay	Methylprednisolone, azathioprine, anti-thymocyte globulin, cyclosporine, tacrolimus, meropenem, linezolid, micafungin, vancomycin, polymyxin B, tigecycline, amikacin, fluconazole, ganciclovir, and hydrocortisone	Meropenem, colistin, linezolid fluconazole, amikacin, cyclosporine, azathioprine, and prednisone

ARD, acute respiratory distress syndrome; COVID-19, coronavirus disease 2019; ICU, intensive care unit; SARS-CoV-2, severe acute respiratory syndrome coronavirus 2.

2. Case Report

2.1. Patient 1

Female, 55 years old, presenting positive serology for CD since 2015, received HT on 2 May as a treatment for Chagas cardiomyopathy (Figure 1A) and underwent immunosuppressive therapy with methylprednisolone and azathioprine. Post-transplantation, she developed pneumonia, treated with meropenem and linezolid, and a remittent *Candida tropicalis* infection, treated with micafungin, with improvement. However, on 29 May, she developed dyspnea and desaturation, with a chest tomography suggestive of COVID-19. Her polymerase chain reaction (PCR) for SARS-CoV-2 was positive on 1 June.

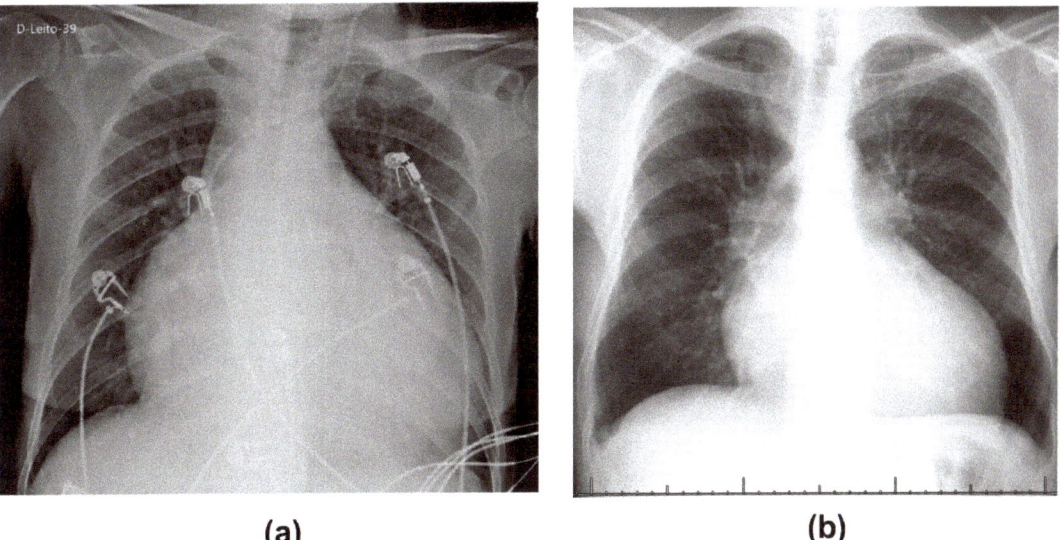

Figure 1. Chest X-ray of (**a**) patient 1 from May 2020 and (**b**) patient 2 from June 2015, taken just before heart transplantation, showing the Chagasic cardiomyopathy.

On 3 June, she was transferred to the ICU specialized for treatment of severe SARS-CoV-2 infections. Laboratory analyses then showed that the patient had a reduced number of erythrocytes and hemoglobin level, and these reductions became more accentuated by day 33 in the ICU (Figure 2A,B). On this same day, the number of neutrophils peaked (Figure 2D). From the 4th to the 16th day in ICU, important lymphopenia developed (Figure 2F), resulting in an increase in the neutrophil-to-lymphocyte ratio in the same period (Figure 2H). Additionally, from the eighth day onward, she presented severe thrombocytopenia that persisted until death (Figure 2I).

Throughout the ICU hospitalization period, there were sustained high levels of creatinine, urea, D-dimer, C-reactive protein (CRP), and lactate dehydrogenase (Figure 2J,K,N,S,W). On the 32nd day, she presented a sharp increase in prothrombin time and activated partial thromboplastin time.

The cardiac function markers of creatine kinase myocardial band (CK-MB) and troponin remained elevated from the first days of ICU admission until death (Figure 2U,X). On the day of admission to the ICU, the N-terminal pro b-type natriuretic peptide (NT pro-BNP) was 70,000 pg/mL (reference value of <125 pg/mL) (Figure 2V). On the third day of hospitalization, NT pro-BNP (155,117 pg/mL) and troponin (0.28 ng/mL, reference value of <0.014 ng/mL) peaked, being related to the period in which she presented signs of graft rejection, which was treated with pulse methylprednisolone, thymoglobulin, and plasmapheresis. In addition, disseminated CMV infection was diagnosed (RT-PCR viral loads of 122 IU/mL on day 10 and 54 IU/mL on day 19 of hospitalization), for which she received ganciclovir.

After 47 days after diagnosis of SARS-CoV-2, the patient died (18 July) due to multiple organ dysfunctions associated with COVID-19.

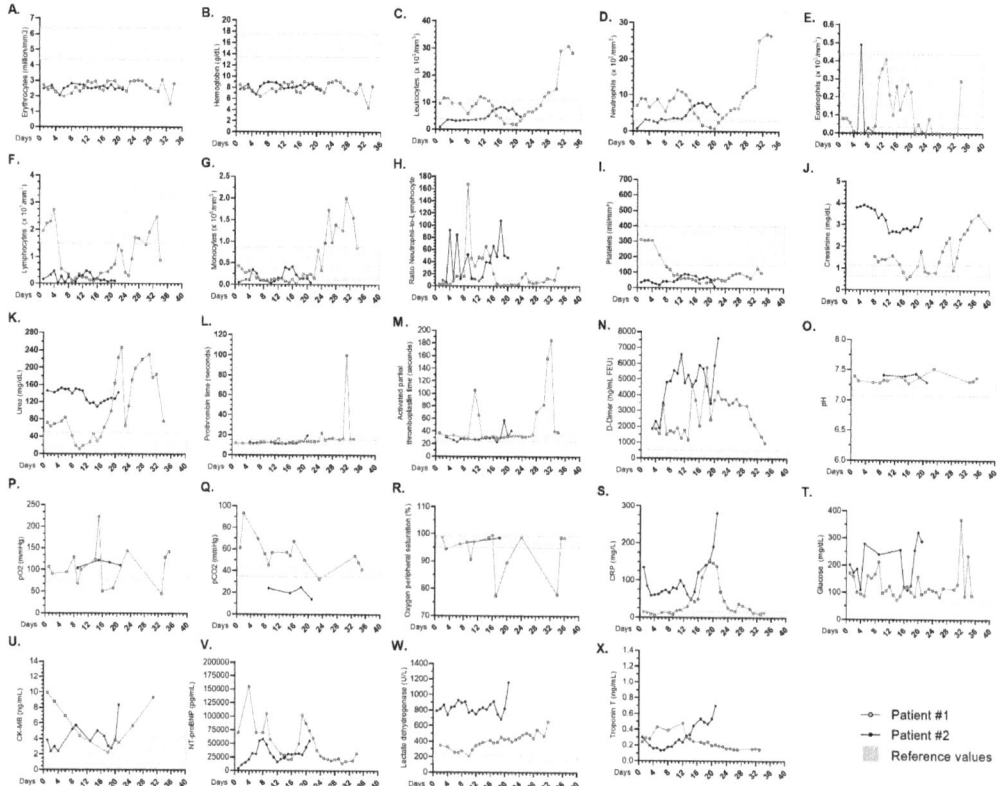

Figure 2. Daily clinical features of patients, from the first day of hospitalization in the ICU until death. Blood levels of (**A**) erythrocytes, (**B**) hemoglobin, (**C**) leukocytes, (**D**) neutrophils, (**E**) eosinophils, (**F**) lymphocytes, (**G**) monocytes, (**H**) neutrophil-to-lymphocyte ratio, (**I**) platelets, (**J**) creatinine, (**K**) urea, (**L**) prothrombin time, (**M**) activated partial thromboplastin time, (**N**) D-dimer, (**O**) pH, (**P**) pO2, (**Q**) pCO2, (**R**) oxygen peripheral, (**S**) CPR, (**T**) glucose, (**U**) CK-MB, (**V**) NT-proBNP, (**W**) lactate dehydrogenase, and (**X**) troponin T. Gray boxes represent the reference values.

2.2. Patient 2

Male, 62 years old, previously diagnosed with CD, received HT on 5 December 2019 as treatment for Chagas cardiomyopathy (Figure 1B). He underwent immunosuppressive therapy with cyclosporine, azathioprine, and prednisone. During postoperative hospitalization he presented Chagas reactivation characterized by skin biopsy and humoral graft rejection, being treated with plasmapheresis and methylprednisolone.

The patient was admitted to the ICU of the Hospital das Clínicas on 8 June, presenting cellulitis, deep vein thrombosis, and Chagas reactivation (a lower limb chagoma). The latter was treated with benznidazol. During hospitalization, he tested positive for PCR of SARS-CoV-2 on 29 June. He developed ARDS and septic and cardiogenic shock, which were the causes of his death.

Throughout the ICU hospitalization period, he maintained decreased levels of erythrocytes, hemoglobin, and lymphocytes (Figure 2A,B,F), as well as a high neutrophil/lymphocyte ratio (Figure 2H). From the 12th day, the number of platelets decreased and continued until the time of death (Figure 2I). The values of creatinine, urea, and glucose also remained high throughout the hospitalization period (Figure 2J,K,T). In addition, disseminated CMV (viral loads of 711 IU/mL detected on the 28th day and 1477 IU/mL on the 35th day of hospitalization) was diagnosed and treated with ganciclovir.

One day before death, the following laboratory parameters peaked: D-dimer (7612 ng/mL FEU, reference value of <500 ng/mL FEU), CRP (280.6 ng/mL, reference value of 0.300 ng/mL), CK-MB (8.38 ng/mL, reference value of 0.10–4.94 ng/mL), NT pro-BNP (55,393 pg/mL), lactate dehydrogenase (1161 U/L, reference value of 135–225 U/L), and troponin (0.701 ng/mL) (Figure 2N,S,U–X).

On 20 July, 36 days after admission to the ICU and 21 days after a positive COVID-19 diagnosis, the patient died.

3. Discussion

Herein, we described the first report of triple infection (SARS-CoV-2 infection, *T. cruzi* infection, and CMV dissemination) in HT recipients. Patients received HT as a form of treatment for Chagas cardiomyopathy.

We described the laboratory data from the first day of hospitalization in the ICU due to COVID-19 until the time of death. Both patients were admitted to a referral center for treatment for COVID-19 in the metropolitan region of São Paulo, a city in southeastern Brazil. We hypothesize that the triple infection by SARS-CoV-2 and CMV may have been an important cause of death and of the worsening in CD patients with HT. To date, there have been no similar reports of patients presenting these three concomitant infectious diseases and HT receptors.

COVID-19 infection among transplant recipients increases the potential for developing severe illness [13] and may vary between different organ transplants [14,15].

SARS-CoV-2 entry´s receptor angiotensin converting enzyme 2 (ACE2) and transmembrane protease serine 2 (TMPRSS2) are expressed in different tissues, such as the lungs, heart, liver, kidneys, testicles, thyroid, and adipose tissue [16]. Some patients with COVID-19 develop severe disease characterized by respiratory distress syndrome and systemic manifestations. This condition has been associated with the dysregulated release of pro-inflammatory cytokines, termed "cytokine storm," which may induce multi-organ failure [1,17].

The use of immunosuppressants and post-surgical opportunistic infections can also lead to damage of multisystem organs or even death [18]. There is a therapeutic paradox here, because while insufficient immunosuppression results in graft loss due to rejection, excessive immunosuppression can result in serious infection, including SARS-COV-2 [13], besides contributing to the reactivation of pathogens [19].

Long-term administration of immunosuppressants to solid organ transplant (SOT) receptors to reduce the risk of graft rejection may increase the risk of respiratory infections [20], although there is no clear clinical evidence of increased morbidity/mortality in SARS-CoV-2 infection [21].

Fernandez-Ruiz and collaborators [22] described a cohort of SOT receptors affected by COVID-19, 44% of whom were kidney transplant recipients, 33.3% liver transplant recipients, and 22.2% heart transplant recipients. The lethality rate was 27.8%, suggesting that SARS-CoV-2 infection had a severe course in SOT recipients.

Recently, we described the first patients with CD affected by SARS-CoV-2. The CD patients presented an increase in COVID-19 laboratory hallmarks and a rapid disease progression. Despite the efforts of the health staff, both patients died [3].

HT may be associated with the reactivation of pathogens, as reported in CD [10]. In a Brazilian cohort, the reactivation rate of Chagas disease after heart transplantation was reported to be 38.8% [23]. This fact made HT as a treatment for Chagas cardiomyopathy initially controversial. However, currently, especially in endemic countries, it is the most viable therapeutic option for patients with end-stage heart failure [24]. We hypothesize that, in the cases presented here, HT followed by reactivation of CD conferred an additional risk factor for the worsening of COVID-19.

Transplant recipients are also commonly affected by CMV reactivation, being associated with significant morbidity and mortality [12] that may worsen the infectious condition of COVID-19 [25]. In SOT, risk factors include the use of immunosuppressants for transplantation, advanced age, acute rejection, and other concomitant infections [11], with all these characteristics being present in both patients described herein. In the present report, we observed that immunosuppression may have contributed to the susceptibility to superinfections and more severe clinical manifestations in individuals undergoing HT.

Since overactivated immune responses can be one of the causes of organ damage, the anti-inflammatory effects of immunosuppression can be protective, reducing the cytokine storm related to complications in COVID-19 [26]. In this context, it has been described that immunosuppressive therapy with calcineurin inhibitors in patients with solid organ transplantation or systemic rheumatic diseases promotes a clinical course in SARS-CoV-2 infection, which is generally mild, and with an apparently low risk of superinfection [27]. In addition, immunosuppression has not been evaluated as a risk factor for SARS or MERS [28].

However, in the present case report, we observed that immunosuppression may have contributed to the susceptibility to SARS-CoV-2 infection, the reactivation of pathogens, and more serious clinical manifestations in individuals undergoing HT. Corroborating our findings, it was shown that patients with COVID-19 and cancer, due to their systemic immunosuppressive condition caused by malignancy and anticancer treatments, such as chemotherapy, had an increased risk of SARS-CoV-2 infection and a worse prognosis [29]. It has also been reported that chronic use of corticosteroids prior to SARS-CoV-2 contamination is associated with critical disease outcomes, including a high risk of death [30].

These contradictory observations show that knowledge about the relationship between COVID-19 and the patient's immune condition is limited. Further studies are needed to elucidate the immune responses and prognosis of COVID-19.

In general, HT in patient 1 proved to be successful for the treatment of Chagas cardiomyopathy, with no reactivation of the pathogen. However, after SARS-CoV-2 infection, she presented graft rejection, treated with methylprednisolone, thymoglobulin, and plasmapheresis. There is a description in eye transplantation that COVID-19 infection can compromise the balance of immunoregulatory responses that allow graft survival, contributing to rejection in individuals infected with SARS-CoV-2 [31]. Thus, this change in the balance of attenuation of the immune response, such as a reduction in the number of regulatory T cells (Tregs) [32], may favor direct cardiotoxic action and multiple organ dysfunction.

During postoperative hospitalization, patient 2 presented Chagas reactivation, evidenced by skin biopsy, indicating that the CD was not completely controlled. In addition, it is important to consider that immunosuppressive therapy can contribute to the reactivation of CD [33]. After HT, the patient presented graft rejection and was treated with plasmapheresis and methylprednisolone. With this, before the SARS-CoV-2 infection, the patient was already weakened and died 21 days after the infection, in relation to patient 1 who died after 47 days of infection.

4. Conclusions

This report highlights the first case of an association between COVID-19, CD, and CMV dissemination in HT recipients. The patients had rapid disease progression to death. We believe that HT and the usage of immunosuppressive drugs, as well as immunosuppression generated by concomitant infections, may be an important risk factor for the development of severe COVID-19, especially in endemic areas with underreported CD infection.

Author Contributions: Conceptualization, S.C.G.-S., G.B., and R.W.A.; investigation, S.C.G.-S., G.B., R.W.A., T.M.Y., F.M.E.T., L.d.M.O., D.R.B., A.J.P., E.A.d.O., A.C.C.C.B., M.M.d.S.A., I.G.F., N.Z.P., Y.Á.L.R., J.C.L., B.P., and S.M.; resources, M.N.S. and A.J.d.S.D.; writing—original draft preparation, S.C.G.-S., G.B., and R.W.A.; writing—review and editing, S.C.G.-S., G.B., and R.W.A.; visualization, S.C.G.-S., G.B., R.W.A., T.M.Y., F.M.E.T., L.d.M.O., D.R.B., A.J.P., E.A.d.O., A.C.C.C.B., M.M.d.S.A., I.G.F., N.Z.P., Y.Á.L.R., J.C.L., B.P., S.M., A.J.d.S.D., and M.N.S.; supervision, M.N.S.; funding acquisition, A.J.d.S.D. and M.N.S. All authors have read and agreed to the published version of the manuscript.

Funding: This research was funded by Fundação de Amparo à Pesquisa (FAPESP), grant numbers 2019/22448-0, 19/02679-7, 2017/18199-9, 2018/18230-6, and 2019/26928-6. Coordenação de Aperfeiçoamento de Pessoal de Nível Superior, CAPES:88887.503842/2020-00.

Institutional Review Board Statement: This study was approved by the local ethics committee (HCFMUSP n° 30800520.7.0000.0068-2020) and was carried out in accordance with the 2013 revision of the Declaration of Helsinki.

Informed Consent Statement: Informed consent was obtained from all of the subjects involved in the study.

Data Availability Statement: The laboratory data and imaging exams presented herein came from Hospital das Clinicas, Faculty of Medicine, University of São Paulo (HCFMUSP) with prior approval for their use.

Conflicts of Interest: The authors declare no conflict of interest.

References

1. Huang, C.; Wang, Y.; Li, X.; Ren, L.; Zhao, J.; Hu, Y.; Zhang, L.; Fan, G.; Xu, J.; Gu, X.; et al. Clinical Features of Patients Infected with 2019 Novel Coronavirus in Wuhan, China. *Lancet* **2020**, *395*, 497–506. [CrossRef]
2. Cao, X. COVID-19: Immunopathology and Its Implications for Therapy. *Nat. Rev. Immunol.* **2020**, *20*, 269–270. [CrossRef]
3. Yendo, T.M.; Ramos, Y.; Álefe, L.; Fernandes, I.G.; Oliveira, L.D.M.; Teixeira, F.M.E.; Beserra, D.R.; De Oliveira, E.A.; Gozzi-Silva, S.; Andrade, M.M.D.S.; et al. Case Report: COVID-19 and Chagas Disease in Two Coinfected Patients. *Am. J. Trop. Med. Hyg.* **2020**, *103*, 2353–2356. [CrossRef]
4. Netea, M.G.; Giamarellos-Bourboulis, E.J.; Domínguez-Andrés, J.; Curtis, N.; van Crevel, R.; van de Veerdonk, F.L.; Bonten, M. Trained Immunity: A Tool for Reducing Susceptibility to and the Severity of SARS-CoV-2 Infection. *Cell* **2020**, *181*, 969–977. [CrossRef]
5. Qin, C.; Zhou, L.; Hu, Z.; Zhang, S.; Yang, S.; Tao, Y.; Xie, C.; Ma, K.; Shang, K.; Wang, W.; et al. Dysregulation of Immune Response in Patients with COVID-19 in Wuhan, China. *Clin. Infect. Dis.* **2020**, *71*, 762–768. [CrossRef]
6. Álvarez-Hernández, D.-A.; Franyuti-Kelly, G.-A.; Díaz-López-Silva, R.; González-Chávez, A.-M.; González-Hermosillo-Cornejo, D.; Vázquez-López, R. Chagas Disease: Current Perspectives on a Forgotten Disease. *Rev. Médica del Hosp. Gen. México* **2018**, *81*, 154–164. [CrossRef]
7. Pérez-Molina, J.A.; Molina, I. Chagas Disease. *Lancet* **2018**, *391*, 82–94. [CrossRef]
8. Boscardin, S.B.; Torrecilhas, A.C.T.; Manarin, R.; Revelli, S.; Rey, E.G.; Tonelli, R.R.; Silber, A.M. Chagas' Disease: An Update on Immune Mechanisms and Therapeutic Strategies. *J. Cell. Mol. Med.* **2010**, *14*, 1373–1384. [CrossRef] [PubMed]
9. Fiorelli, A.I.; Santos, R.H.B.; Oliveira, J.L.; Lourenço-Filho, D.D.; Dias, R.R.; Oliveira, A.S.; Da Silva, M.F.A.; Ayoub, F.L.; Bacal, F.; Souza, G.E.C.; et al. Heart Transplantation in 107 Cases of Chagas' Disease. *Transplant. Proc.* **2011**, *43*, 220–224. [CrossRef] [PubMed]

10. Gray, E.B.; La Hoz, R.M.; Green, J.S.; Vikram, H.R.; Benedict, T.; Rivera, H.; Montgomery, S.P. Reactivation of Chagas Disease among Heart Transplant Recipients in the United States, 2012–2016. *Transpl. Infect. Dis.* **2018**, *20*, e12996. [CrossRef]
11. Azevedo, L.S.; Pierrotti, L.C.; Abdala, E.; Costa, S.F.; Strabelli, T.M.V.; Campos, S.V.; Ramos, J.F.; Latif, A.Z.A.; Litvinov, N.; Maluf, N.Z.; et al. Cytomegalovirus Infection in Transplant Recipients. *Clinics* **2015**, *70*, 515–523. [CrossRef]
12. Stern, L.; Withers, B.; Avdic, S.; Gottlieb, D.; Abendroth, A.; Blyth, E.; Slobedman, B. Human Cytomegalovirus Latency and Reactivation in Allogeneic Hematopoietic Stem Cell Transplant Recipients. *Front. Microbiol.* **2019**, *10*, 1186. [CrossRef] [PubMed]
13. Nacif, L.S.; Zanini, L.Y.; Waisberg, D.R.; Pinheiro, R.S.; Galvão, F.; Andraus, W.; D'albuquerque, L.C. COVID-19 in Solid Organ Transplantation Patients: A Systematic Review. *Clinics* **2020**, *75*, e1983. [CrossRef] [PubMed]
14. Pereira, M.R.; Mohan, S.; Cohen, D.J.; Husain, S.A.; Dube, G.K.; Ratner, L.E.; Arcasoy, S.; Aversa, M.M.; Benvenuto, L.J.; Dadhania, D.M.; et al. COVID-19 in Solid Organ Transplant Recipients: Initial Report from the US Epicenter. *Am. J. Transplant.* **2020**, *20*, 1800–1808. [CrossRef] [PubMed]
15. Heimbach, J.K.; Taner, T. SARS-CoV-2 Infection in Liver Transplant Recipients: Collaboration in the Time of COVID-19. *Lancet Gastroenterol. Hepatol.* **2020**, *5*, 958–960. [CrossRef]
16. Lin, L.; Lu, L.; Cao, W.; Li, T. Hypothesis for Potential Pathogenesis of SARS-CoV-2 Infection-a Review of Immune Changes in Patients with Viral Pneumonia. *Emerg. Microbes Infect.* **2020**, *9*, 727–732. [CrossRef]
17. Jose, R.J.; Manuel, A. COVID-19 Cytokine Storm: The Interplay between Inflammation and Coagulation. *Lancet Respir. Med.* **2020**, *8*, e46–e47. [CrossRef]
18. Schrem, H.; Barg-Hock, H.; Strassburg, C.P.; Schwarz, A.; Klempnauer, J. Aftercare for Patients with Transplanted Organs. *Dtsch. Aerzteblatt Online* **2009**, *106*, 148–156. [CrossRef] [PubMed]
19. Varani, S.; Landini, M. Cytomegalovirus-Induced Immunopathology and Its Clinical Consequences. *Herpesviridae* **2011**, *2*, 6. [CrossRef]
20. Paulsen, G.C.; Danziger-Isakov, L. Respiratory Viral Infections in Solid Organ and Hematopoietic Stem Cell Transplantation. *Clin. Chest Med.* **2017**, *38*, 707–726. [CrossRef] [PubMed]
21. Ning, L.; Liu, L.; Li, W.; Liu, H.; Wang, J.; Yao, Z.; Zhang, S.; Zhao, D.; Nashan, B.; Shen, A.; et al. Novel Coronavirus (SARS-CoV-2) Infection in a Renal Transplant Recipient: Case Report. *Am. J. Transplant.* **2020**, *20*, 1864–1868. [CrossRef] [PubMed]
22. Fernández-Ruiz, M.; Andrés, A.; Loinaz, C.; Delgado, J.F.; López-Medrano, F.; San Juan, R.; González, E.; Polanco, N.; Folgueira, M.D.; Lalueza, A.; et al. COVID-19 in Solid Organ Transplant Recipients: A Single-Center Case Series from Spain. *Am. J. Transplant.* **2020**, *20*, 1849–1858. [CrossRef]
23. Godoy, H.L.; Guerra, C.M.; Viegas, R.F.; Dinis, R.Z.; Branco, J.N.; Neto, V.A.; Almeida, D.R. Infections in Heart Transplant Recipients in Brazil: The Challenge of Chagas' Disease. *J. Heart Lung Transplant.* **2010**, *29*, 286–290. [CrossRef] [PubMed]
24. Inga, L.A.C.; Olivera, M.J. Reactivation of Chagas Disease in a Heart Transplant Patient Infected by Sylvatic Trypanosoma Cruzi Discrete Typing Unit I. *Rev. Soc. Bras. Med. Trop.* **2019**, *52*, e20180512. [CrossRef] [PubMed]
25. Leemans, S.; Maillart, E.; Van Noten, H.; Oliveira Dos Santos, L.; Leahu, L.M.; Kamgang, P.; Gallerani, A.; Clevenbergh, P. Cytomegalovirus Haemorrhagic Colitis Complicating COVID-19 in an Immunocompetent Critically Ill Patient: A Case Report. *Clin. Case Rep.* **2020**. [CrossRef]
26. Romanelli, A.; Mascolo, S. Immunosuppression Drug-Related and Clinical Manifestation of Coronavirus Disease 2019: A Therapeutical Hypothesis. *Am. J. Transplant.* **2020**, *20*, 1947–1948. [CrossRef] [PubMed]
27. Cavagna, L.; Seminari, E.; Zanframundo, G.; Gregorini, M.; Di Matteo, A.; Rampino, T.; Montecucco, C.; Pelenghi, S.; Cattadori, B.; Pattonieri, E.F.; et al. Calcineurin Inhibitor-Based Immunosuppression and COVID-19: Results from a Multidisciplinary Cohort of Patients in Northern Italy. *Microorganisms* **2020**, *8*, 977. [CrossRef] [PubMed]
28. D'Antiga, L. Coronaviruses and Immunosuppressed Patients: The Facts During the Third Epidemic. *Liver Transplant.* **2020**, *26*, 832–834. [CrossRef]
29. Liang, W.; Guan, W.; Chen, R.; Wang, W.; Li, J.; Xu, K.; Li, C.; Ai, Q.; Lu, W.; Liang, H.; et al. Cancer Patients in SARS-CoV-2 Infection: A Nationwide Analysis in China. *Lancet Oncol.* **2020**, *21*, 335–337. [CrossRef]
30. Li, X.; Xu, S.; Yu, M.; Wang, K.; Tao, Y.; Zhou, Y.; Shi, J.; Zhou, M.; Wu, B.; Yang, Z.; et al. Risk Factors for Severity and Mortality in Adult COVID-19 Inpatients in Wuhan. *J. Allergy Clin. Immunol.* **2020**, *146*, 110–118. [CrossRef] [PubMed]
31. Jin, S.X.; Juthani, V.V. Acute Corneal Endothelial Graft Rejection with Coinciding COVID-19 Infection. *Cornea* **2021**, *40*, 123–124. [CrossRef] [PubMed]
32. Neurath, M.F. COVID-19 and Immunomodulation in IBD. *Gut* **2020**, *69*, 1335–1342. [CrossRef] [PubMed]
33. Zaidel, E.J.; Forsyth, C.J.; Novick, G.; Marcus, R.; Ribeiro, A.L.P.; Pinazo, M.J.; Morillo, C.A.; Echeverría, L.E.; Shikanai-Yasuda, M.A.; Buekens, P.; et al. COVID-19: Implications for People with Chagas Disease. *Glob. Heart* **2020**, *15*, 69. [CrossRef] [PubMed]

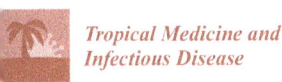

Article

SARS-CoV-2 Seroprevalence Post-First Wave among Primary Care Physicians in Catania (Italy)

Caterina Ledda [1,*], Flavia Carrasi [1], Maria Teresa Longombardo [2], Gianluca Paravizzini [2] and Venerando Rapisarda [1]

1. Occupational Medicine, Department of Clinical and Experimental Medicine, University of Catania, 95100 Catania, Italy; L98002367@studium.unict.it (F.C.); vrapisarda@unict.it (V.R.)
2. Clinical Laboratories "Girlando and Paravizzini", 95100 Catania, Italy; m.longombardo@girlandoeparavizzini.com (M.T.L.); gianluca@paravizzini.net (G.P.)
* Correspondence: cledda@unict.it; Tel./Fax: +39-095-3782049

Abstract: Family physicians or pediatricians and general practitioners (GPs) work in non-hospital settings. GPs usually visit many patients, frequently at their homes, with low potential, if any, to control the work setting. Particularly during the initial phases of the COVID-19 outbreak, they were not informed about the occurrence of SARS-CoV-2-infected patients, with inadequate information regarding the risk, a lack of suitable protective measures and, in some cases, deficient or poor accessibility to personal protective equipment (PPE). During the first wave of COVID-19, primary care physicians were on the front line and isolated the first cases of the disease. The present study aims to estimate the seroprevalence of SARS-CoV-2 in a cohort of 133 GPs working in Catania (Italy) after the first wave of COVID-19. Serological analysis revealed a low seroprevalence (3%) among GPs. The low seroprevalence highlighted in the results can be attributed to correct management of patients by GPs in the first wave. It is now hoped that mass vaccination, combined with appropriate behavior and use of PPE, can help further reduce the risk of COVID-19 disease.

Keywords: COVID-19; healthcare worker; healthcare personnel; SARS-CoV-2; general practitioners; medical doctor

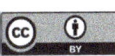

1. Introduction

The novel coronavirus (SARS-CoV-2), the causative agent of Corona Virus Disease-2019 (COVID-19), is the most severe global public health emergency of the twenty-first century [1].

The disease, which appeared in Wuhan, China, in December 2019, quickly spread across continents and was declared a pandemic by the World Health Organization (WHO) on 11 March 2020 [2].

At 5 February 2021, SARS-CoV-2 has infected over 104,000,000 persons and caused over 2,200,000 deaths globally [2].

Current information suggests that, in community settings, person-to-person transmission most commonly occurs via the respiratory droplets of the infected individual (through coughing, sneezing, talking, etc.), close interaction with the infected person, or self-delivery of the microorganism to the eyes, nose, or mouth via SARS-CoV-2 contaminated hands [3].

In health care scenarios, in addition to respiratory droplet-borne or contact-borne transmission, airborne transmission can also occur via aerosol-generating operations [3].

SARS-CoV-2 is highly transmissible, and health care workers (HCWs) have been occupied with the important risk of providing care to supposed or confirmed COVID-19 cases. Some reports have shown that numerous HCWs have contracted COVID-19 in health care settings globally [4–8].

The WHO, the Center for Disease Control and Prevention (CDC), and the European Centre for Disease Prevention and Control (ECDC) issued procedures for COVID-19 management that endorse safety protocols for HCWs, such as using appropriate personal protective equipment (PPE).

Nevertheless, because the suggested infection control protections have not been adequate to prevent the spread of the SARS-CoV-2 infection among HCWs, unrecognized risk factors may contribute to the transmission of viruses in hospitals [4–8].

However, not all healthcare is provided in a hospital setting. In particular, family physicians or pediatricians and general practitioners (GPs) work in a setting away from the hospital.

GPs usually visit numerous patients, frequently at their homes, with low potential, if any, to control the work setting. Particularly during the initial phases of the COVID-19 outbreak, GPs were not informed of the occurrence of SARS-CoV-2-infected patients, with inadequate information about the risk, a lack of suitable protective measures and, in some cases, deficient or poor accessibility to PPE [9].

Modenese and Gobba reported that 44% of the COVID-19 related deaths among Italian physicians were GPs [10].

In Italy, the first wave started at the end of January 2020 and in March, the government implemented a series of restrictive measures. On March 5th, all schools and universities in Italy locked their buildings to scholars. From 8 March to 4 May, the population was forced to respect the lockdown.

In the province of Catania, 777 cases [11] of COVID-19 were reported until the end of June, that is, the period of the effect of the lockdown.

The present study aims to estimate the seroprevalence of SARS-CoV-2 in a cohort of GPs working in Catania (Italy) after the first wave of COVID-19.

2. Materials and Methods

In the province of Catania, there are approximately 1100 working GPs. From June to July 2020, GPs working in the province of Catania (Italy) were recruited in this study through contacts made via mail from a GP database obtained from the Medical Board.

The GPs who made themselves available to participate in the study were contacted by email and filled out an online form that included the registration of: personal and work data, number of patients with COVID-19, any previous diagnosis of COVID-19 through molecular swab, eventual close contact with cases of COVID-19, possible presence of symptoms of COVID-19 attributable to contact, presence of other pathologies.

Following the receipt of answers from the GPs, blood sampling sessions were organized, two at the University of Occupational Medicine, and four in the province. The collected serum was immediately taken to the laboratory and analyzed the same day.

Serological analysis was performed using The NovaLisa® SARS-CoV-2 IgG (NovaTec Immundiagnostics GmbH, Dietzenbach, Germany) ELISA method. The aim of the test was the qualitative detection of IgG antibodies to SARS-CoV-2 virus in human serum.

Informed consent was obtained from all GPs. The present study was approved by the ethics committee of Catania University Hospital (n. 54/2020).

Data were analyzed with the software SPSS 22.0 (SPSS Inc., Chicago, IL, USA) for Windows. Descriptive analyses were performed using frequency percentages and mean and standard deviation.

3. Results

An invitation email was sent to 170 GPs. A total of 133 elected to participate in the study (response rate: 78%). The characteristics of the participating GPs are detailed in Table 1.

As reported in Table 1, three GPs had a COVID-19 diagnosis. SARS-CoV-2 antibodies were detected in 4 of 133 (3%) of GPs, and 2 (2%) had a "borderline" result. Table 2 reports the seroprevalence results after ELISA analysis.

Table 1. Characteristics of participating general practitioners (GPs).

Variables	Results
Gender (Male; n, %)	62 (47%)
Age (Mean ± SD)	55.65 ± 11.24
Working seniority (Mean ± SD)	15.14 ± 13.62
Patients	994.44 ± 358.33
GPs with COVID-19 patients (n., %)	51 (38%)
GPs who had swabbed for SARS-CoV-2 RT detection (n., %)	21 (16%)
GPs with COVID-19 diagnosis	3 (2%)
GPs with close contacts with cases of COVID-19 (n., %)	78 (59%)
Probable cases	21 (20%)
Presence of COVID-19 symptoms (n., %)	
Hyposmia * (n., %)	4 (3%)
Ageusia * (n., %)	2 (2%)
Fever > 37.5 °C * (n., %)	23 (23%)
Fatigue * (n., %)	65 (49%)
Muscle aches * (n., %)	52 (52%)
Sore throat * (n., %)	50 (50%)
Dry cough * (n., %)	48 (36%)
Nasal congestion * (n., %)	41 (31%)
Rhinorrhea * (n., %)	40 (30%)
Dyspnea * (n., %)	9 (7%)
Headache * (n., %)	53 (40%)
Abdominal pain * (n., %)	23 (17%)

* More than one answers was given.

Table 2. Seroprevalence of GPs.

Results	n. (%)
Negative	127 (95%)
Positive	4 (3%)
Borderline	2 (2%)

4. Discussion

The aim of this study was to assess the SARS-CoV-2 seroprevalence, after the first wave of the disease, among GPs working in Catania province (Italy). Probable cases, according to WHO criteria [12], were 21 (20%). Serological analysis revealed a low seroprevalence (3%) among GPs.

These low seroprevalence rates were found despite the treatment of 777 patients with COVID-19 infections during the first wave [11] period in which GPs worked with very few PPE available from the local health authority. Nevertheless, the degree of contagion was lower in GPs compared to HCWs in direct contact with COVID-19 patients in hospital settings. Other seroprevalence studies carried out among HCWs working in hospital report higher rates of prevalence: Belgium (12.6%) [13], Spain (11.2%) [14], Italy (14.4%) [15], Sweden (19.1%) [16], the United Kingdom (10.8–43.5%) [13,17], and the United States of America (7.6–13.7%) [18,19]. The differences in these rates may be due to differences in seroprevalence in the general population by May 2020: 8.0% in Belgium, 5.5% in Spain, 4.6% in Italy, 3.7% in Sweden, 5.1% in the United Kingdom, and only 0.85% in Germany [20].

A recent study on duration of SARS-CoV-2 antibody carried out by Lumley et al. [21] evidences that anti-spike IgG levels remained stably detected after a positive result in 94% of health care workers after 180 days, instead anti-nucleocapsid IgG levels rose to a peak at 24 and the mean estimated antibody half-life was 85 days. Ongoing longitudinal studies are required to track the long-term duration of antibody levels and their association with immunity to SARS-CoV-2 reinfection and evaluate these two IgG fractions for guide vaccination modalities.

To date, no seroprevalence studies have been carried out among GPs by other research groups.

Due to the type of work and the shortage of PPE, GPs contracted the virus at the beginning of the spread of SARS-CoV-2. Subsequently, distancing rules were also adopted within clinics, and overnight stays and contact were avoided unless requested. Thus, contagion was able to be reduced.

It is has been found that rigorous use of appropriate PPE by HCWs when providing direct care of all patients efficiently prevents COVID-19 transmission [22,23]. Moreover, a study carried out by Brehm underlines that mindfulness of COVID-19 is crucial even when suitable PPE is used.

Our results are in line with an investigation carried out by Arons [24], which proved that pre-symptomatic patients play a crucial role in the spread of SARS-CoV-2 associated with both community and healthcare facilities.

It is important to finalize strategies and procedures to prevent SARS-CoV-2 infection among GPs, for example, specific guidelines for GPs to safely guarantee care for patients during the spread of COVID-19. Another input could be the introduction of telemedicine procedures to reduce direct contact with patients [10,25–27].

In conclusion, the low seroprevalence highlighted in these results can be attributed to correct management of patients by GPs during the first wave. It is now hoped that mass vaccination, in combination with appropriate behavior and use of PPE, can help further reduce the risk of COVID-19 disease.

Author Contributions: Conceptualization, C.L. and V.R.; methodology, G.P.; validation, C.L., V.R. and M.T.L.; formal analysis C.L. and M.T.L.; investigation, C.L.; data curation, C.L. and F.C.; writing—original draft preparation, F.C.; writing—review and editing, C.L.; supervision, V.R. All authors have read and agreed to the published version of the manuscript.

Funding: This research received no external funding.

Institutional Review Board Statement: The study was conducted according to the guidelines of the Declaration of Helsinki, and approved by the Ethics Committee of Catania 1 (n. 54/2020).

Informed Consent Statement: Informed consent was obtained from all subjects involved in the study.

Data Availability Statement: Data available on request due to privacy restrictions.

Conflicts of Interest: The authors declare no conflict of interest.

References

1. Vella, F.; Senia, P.; Ceccarelli, M.; Vitale, E.; Maltezou, H.; Taibi, R.; Lleshi, A.; Rullo, E.V.; Pellicano, G.F.; Rapisarda, V.; et al. Transmission mode associated with coronavirus disease 2019: A review. *Eur. Rev. Med. Pharmacol. Sci.* **2020**, *24*, 7889–7904.
2. Coronavirus Disease (COVID-2019) Situation Reports. Available online: https://www.who.int/emergencies/diseases/novel-coronavirus-2019/situation-reports (accessed on 5 February 2021).
3. Interim, U.S. Guidance for Risk Assessment and Work Restrictions for Healthcare Personnel with Potential Exposure to COVID-19. Available online: https://www.cdc.gov/coronavirus/2019-ncov/hcp/guidance-risk-assesment-hcp.html (accessed on 9 January 2021).
4. Xiang, Y.; Jin, Y.; Wang, Y.; Zhang, Q.; Zhang, L.; Cheung, T. Tribute to health workers in china: A group of respectable population during the outbreak of the COVID-19. *Int. J. Biol. Sci.* **2020**, *16*, 1739–1740. [CrossRef]
5. Chou, R.; Dana, T.; Buckley, D.I.; Selph, S.; Fu, R.; Totten, A.M. Update alert: Epidemiology of and risk factors for coronavirus infection in health care workers. *Ann. Intern. Med.* **2020**, *173*, W46–W47. [CrossRef]
6. Reusken, C.B.; Buiting, A.; Bleeker-Rovers, C.; Diederen, B.; Hooiveld, M.; Friesema, I.; Koopmans, M.; Kortbeek, T.; Lutgens, S.P.M.; Meijer, A.; et al. Rapid assessment of regional SARS-CoV-2 community transmission through a convenience sample of healthcare workers, the netherlands, march 2020. *Eurosurveillance* **2020**, *25*, 2000334. [CrossRef]
7. Heinzerling, A.; Stuckey, M.J.; Scheuer, T.; Xu, K.; Perkins, K.M.; Resseger, H.; Magill, S.; Verani, J.R.; Jain, S.; Acosta, M.; et al. Transmission of COVID-19 to health care personnel during exposures to a hospitalized patient-solano county, california, february 2020. *Morb. Mortal. Wkly Rep.* **2020**, *69*, 472–476. [CrossRef] [PubMed]
8. Keeley, A.J.; Evans, C.; Colton, H.; Ankcorn, M.; Cope, A.; State, A.; Bennett, T.; Giri, P.; De Silva, T.I.; Raza, M. Roll-out of SARS-CoV-2 testing for healthcare workers at a large NHS foundation trust in the united kingdom, march 2020. *Eurosurveillance* **2020**, *25*, 000433. [CrossRef] [PubMed]

9. Kamerow, D. Covid-19: Don't forget the impact on US family physicians. *BMJ* **2020**, *368*, m1260. [CrossRef] [PubMed]
10. Modenese, A.; Gobba, F. Increased Risk of COVID-19-Related Deaths among General Practitioners in Italy. *Healthcare* **2020**, *8*, 155. [CrossRef] [PubMed]
11. Covid 19-Ripartizione dei Contagiati per Provincia-21/06/2020 ore 17. Available online: http://www.salute.gov.it/imgs/C_17_notizie_4922_1_file.pdf (accessed on 9 January 2021).
12. World Health Organization. *Global Surveillance for COVID-19 Caused by Human Infection with COVID-19 Virus: Interim guidance, 20 March 2020*; World Health Organization: Geneva, Switzerland, 2020. Available online: https://apps.who.int/iris/handle/10665/331506 (accessed on 5 February 2021).
13. Martin, C.; Montesinos, I.; Dauby, N.; Gilles, C.; Dahma, H.; Van Den Wijngaert, S.; De Wit, S.; Delforge, M.; Clumeck, N.; Vandenberg, O. Dynamics of SARS-CoV-2 RT-PCR positivity and seroprevalence among high-risk healthcare workers and hospital staff. *J. Hosp. Infect.* **2020**, *106*, 102–106. [CrossRef]
14. Garcia-Basteiro, A.L.; Moncunill, G.; Tortajada, M.; Vidal, M.; Guinovart, C.; Jiménez, A.; Santano, R.; Sanz, S.; Méndez, S.; Llupià, A.; et al. Seroprevalence of antibodies against SARS-CoV-2 among health care workers in a large spanish reference hospital. *Nat. Commun.* **2020**, *11*, 3500. [CrossRef]
15. Sotgiu, G.; Barassi, A.; Miozzo, M.; Saderi, L.; Piana, A.; Orfeo, N.; Colosio, C.; Felisati, G.; Davì, M.; Gerli, A.G.; et al. SARS-CoV-2 specific serological pattern in healthcare workers of an italian COVID-19 forefront hospital. *BMC Pulm. Med.* **2020**, *20*, 203. [CrossRef]
16. Rudberg, A.; Havervall, S.; Månberg, A.; Jernbom Falk, A.; Aguilera, K.; Ng, H.; Gabrielsson, L.; Salomonsson, A.-; Hanke, L.; Murrell, B.; et al. SARS-CoV-2 exposure, symptoms and seroprevalence in healthcare workers in sweden. *Nat. Commun.* **2020**, *11*, 5064. [CrossRef]
17. Houlihan, C.F.; Vora, N.; Byrne, T.; Lewer, D.; Kelly, G.; Heaney, J.; Gandhi, S.; Spyer, M.J.; Beale, R.; Cherepanov, P.; et al. Crick COVID-19 Consortium, SAFER Investigators. Pandemic peak SARS-CoV-2 infection and seroconversion rates in london frontline health-care workers. *Lancet* **2020**, *396*, e6–e7. [CrossRef]
18. Moscola, J.; Sembajwe, G.; Jarrett, M.; Farber, B.; Chang, T.; McGinn, T.; Davidson, K.W. Prevalence of SARS-CoV-2 antibodies in health care personnel in the New York city area. *JAMA* **2020**, *324*, 893–895. [CrossRef] [PubMed]
19. Stubblefield, W.; Talbot, H.; Feldstein, L. Seroprevalence of SARS-CoV-2 among frontline healthcare personnel during the first month of caring for COVID-19 patients-nashville, tennessee. *Clin. Infect. Dis.* **2020**, ciaa936. [CrossRef] [PubMed]
20. Flaxman, S.; Mishra, S.; Gandy, A.; Unwin, H.J.T.; Mellan, T.A.; Coupland, H.; Whittaker, C.; Zhu, H.; Berah, T.; Eaton, J.W.; et al. Imperial College COVID-19 Response Team. Estimating the effects of non-pharmaceutical interventions on COVID-19 in europe. *Nature* **2020**, *584*, 257–261. [CrossRef]
21. Sheila, F.L.; Jia, W.; Denise, O.; Nicole, E.S.; Philippa, C.M.; Alison, H.; Stephanie, B.H.; Brian, D.M.; Stuart, C.; Tim, J.; et al. Oxford University Hospitals Staff Testing Group, The duration, dynamics and determinants of SARS-CoV-2 antibody responses in individual healthcare workers. *Clin. Infect. Dis.* **2021**, ciab004. [CrossRef]
22. Wang, X.; Ferro, E.G.; Zhou, G.; Hashimoto, D.; Bhatt, D.L. Association between universal masking in a health care system and SARS-CoV-2 positivity among health care workers. *JAMA* **2020**, *324*, 703–704. [CrossRef]
23. Cirrincione, L.; Plescia, F.; Ledda, C.; Rapisarda, V.; Martorana, D.; Moldovan, R.E.; Theodoridou, K.; Cannizzaro, E. COVID-19 pandemic: Prevention and protection measures to be adopted at the workplace. *Sustainability* **2020**, *12*, 3603. [CrossRef]
24. Arons, M.M.; Hatfield, K.M.; Reddy, S.C.; Kimball, A.; James, A.; Jacobs, J.R.; Taylor, J.; Spicer, K.; Bardossy, A.C.; Oakley, L.P.; et al. Presymptomatic SARS-CoV-2 infections and transmission in a skilled nursing facility. *N. Engl. J. Med.* **2020**, *382*, 2081–2090. [CrossRef]
25. Rapporto ISS COVID-19 n. 12/2020—Indicazioni ad Interim per Servizi Assistenziali di Telemedicina Durante L'Emergenza Sanitaria COVID-19 (Italian National Institute of Health (ISS), COVID-19 Report n. 12/2020—Interim Indications for Telemedicine Assistance Services during the COVID-19 Health Emergency). Available online: https://www.iss.it/documents/20126/0/Rapporto+ISS+COVID-19+n.+12_2020+telemedicina.pdf/387420ca-0b5d-ab65-b60d-9fa426d2b2c7?t=1587107170414 (accessed on 9 January 2021).
26. Ramaci, T.; Barattucci, M.; Ledda, C.; Rapisarda, V. Social stigma during COVID-19 and its impact on HCWs outcomes. *Sustainability* **2020**, *12*, 3834. [CrossRef]
27. Marchesi, F.; Valente, M.; Riccò, M.; Rottoli, M.; Baldini, E.; Mecheri, F.; Bonilauri, S.; Boschi, S.; Bernante, P.; Sciannamea, A.; et al. Effects of bariatric surgery on COVID-19: A multicentric study from a high incidence area. *Obes Surg.* **2021**. [CrossRef]

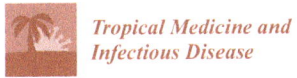

Review

Defusing COVID-19: Lessons Learned from a Century of Pandemics

Graciela Mujica [1,†], Zane Sternberg [1,†], Jamie Solis [1], Taylor Wand [1], Peter Carrasco [2,3], Andrés F. Henao-Martínez [4] and Carlos Franco-Paredes [4,5,*]

1. School of Medicine, University of Colorado, 13001 E 17th Pl, Aurora, CO 80045, USA; graciela.mujica@cuanschutz.edu (G.M.); zane.sternberg@cuanschutz.edu (Z.S.); Jamie.solis@cuanschutz.edu (J.S.); taylor.wand@cuanschutz.edu (T.W.)
2. International Association for Immunization Managers, Washington, DC 20037, USA; rcphs@aol.com
3. Department of Immunization and Vaccines, World Health Organization, 1202 Geneva, Switzerland
4. Department of Medicine, Division of Infectious Diseases, Anschutz Medical Center, University of Colorado, Aurora, CO 80045, USA; andres.henaomartinez@cuanschutz.edu
5. Hospital Infantil de México, Federico Gomez, México City 06720, Mexico
* Correspondence: carlos.franco-paredes@cuanschutz.edu
† These two authors contributed equally.

Received: 3 November 2020; Accepted: 26 November 2020; Published: 30 November 2020

Abstract: Amidst the COVID-19 global pandemic of 2020, identifying and applying lessons learned from previous influenza and coronavirus pandemics may offer important insight into its interruption. Herein, we conducted a review of the literature of the influenza pandemics of the 20th century; and of the coronavirus and influenza pandemics of the 21st century. Influenza and coronavirus pandemics are zoonoses that spread rapidly in consistent seasonal patterns during an initial wave of infection and subsequent waves of spread. For all of their differences in the state of available medical technologies, global population changes, and social and geopolitical factors surrounding each pandemic, there are remarkable similarities among them. While vaccination of high-risk groups is advocated as an instrumental mode of interrupting pandemics, non-pharmacological interventions including avoidance of mass gatherings, school closings, case isolation, contact tracing, and the implementation of infection prevention strategies in healthcare settings represent the cornerstone to halting transmission. In conjunction with lessons learned from previous pandemics, the public health response to the COVID-19 pandemic constitutes the basis for delineating best practices to confront future pandemics.

Keywords: pandemic; COVID-19; coronavirus; SARS-CoV-1; SARS-CoV-2; MERS; SARS; influenza

1. Introduction

Throughout the history of mankind, pandemics have consistently produced large-scale demographic, economic, and political disruptions [1,2]. Due to their unpredictable course, fear and anxiety amplify the overall impact of pandemics. Globally, we have experienced multiple waves of the spread of the coronavirus associated disease 2019 pandemic (COVID-19), which is caused by the novel coronavirus SARS-CoV-2 [3]. By November 2020, this pandemic has reached every corner of the planet, and similar to previous pandemics, it has caused substantial medical, economic, and social disruption leading to almost 58 million cases and more than one million deaths [4]. Modern-day experience with pandemics has combined a myriad of public health responses in an attempt to suppress these rapidly evolving pathogens during an era of increased globalization and international travel. While there is a large amount of uncertainty surrounding COVID-19, we have blueprints of similar widespread events that have occurred in the past, particularly the Black Death in the Middle Ages and many influenza pandemics [2]. Unfortunately, pandemics are becoming much more common compared to previous centuries, as shown by the proximity of the 2003 SARS pandemic, the influenza H1N1pdm2009, Chikungunya in 2014, Ebola from 2014–2015, and Zika in 2015. In this narrative review, we compare salient epidemiological aspects of the major influenza and coronavirus pandemics of the 20th and 21st century to identify potential patterns and lessons learned that may assist us in mitigating the impact of the current COVID-19 pandemic.

2. Emergence of the Third Coronavirus in the 21st Century

In November 2002, the severe acute respiratory syndrome (SARS) emerged in Southern China. This event marked the documented coronavirus emergence that spread through 20 countries, causing approximately 8000 cases and 800 deaths by producing viral pneumonia and respiratory failure (fatality rate of 9.5%). Traditional public health actions used to control the SARS pandemic included active case detection, isolation of cases, contact tracing with the isolation of cases, social distancing, and community quarantine. Since most of the transmission of SARS-CoV-1 occurred in healthcare settings, the implementation of effective infection prevention interventions resulted in the interruption of clusters of transmission by July 2003. Similarly, the human case of the Middle-East respiratory syndrome (MERS) appeared in Jordan in April 2012 and Saudi Arabia in September 2012, associated with important transmission in healthcare settings and a case-fatality rate of 34%. The COVID-19 pandemic has caused unprecedented medical, social, and economic turmoil that is only comparable to the 1918–1919 influenza pandemic and serves as a stark reminder of how pandemics have molded and marred the evolution and history of humanity [2]. The SARS-CoV-2 coronavirus has been circulating for more than 11 months since it was initially identified in China's Hubei province in December 2019 [3]. Some of the countries that were most heavily affected by the initial spread of COVID-19 are now seeing new waves of transmission with potentially catastrophic consequences in regions of the Northern Hemisphere entering the winter season [4].

The emergence of zoonotic infections capable of infecting humans has been a relatively common occurrence throughout history. The rate at which these infections cross the animal-human barrier has risen in the 21st century due to increased human-animal contact, habitat destruction, the industrial model of agriculture, and population growth [5]. The transmission has been facilitated by factors such as globalization and ease of travel. This context is important when examining the potential for SARS-CoV-2 to spread across multiple species and generate similar reservoirs. While SARS-CoV-1 and SARS-CoV-2 have proven animal origins, the prevailing theory is that both strains emerged in settings that allowed for a variety of animals to come into close contact with each other [6]. Evidence points to the fact that both coronaviruses were originally harbored in horseshoe bats; however, the identification of an intermediate host remains elusive [7,8]. There is evidence that SARS-CoV-1 is able to be spread to domestic cats, ferrets, and even macaque monkeys. With this knowledge and the growing evidence that SARS-CoV-2 could be highly transmissible to both cats and ferrets, the possible reservoirs for future spread are exponentially larger than was initially considered and across many continents [6,9,10].

The antigenic novelty of a pandemic virus or antigenic shift from a previous pandemic virus can profoundly influence pandemic severity across different regions, populations, and points in time. Indeed, an influenza pandemic arose when novel influenza A viruses containing a new hemagglutinin surface protein subtype present in viral strains derived from waterfowl or swine spread among immunologically naïve human populations. Furthermore, the underlying degree of immunological exposure can play an important role in the impact of a pandemic. This was exemplified during the H2N2 influenza pandemic of 1957, where genetic reassortment into the H3N2 strain was then responsible for the subsequent 1968 pandemic. The retained neuraminidase (N2) surface antigen in this recombination event conferred partial immunity to the pandemic in 1968–1969, particularly in the European and Asian countries that were heavily impacted by the pandemic in 1957 [11]. The partial immunity these areas gained in 1957 is thought to have contributed to the relatively mild first wave they experienced 10 years later. However, many of these areas were also impacted by an H3 antigenic shift that occurred mid-pandemic. This shift is thought to be a driver for the high number of deaths experienced during the second wave in Europe and Asia (70% of all deaths). This pattern was very different in North America, where 70% (USA) and 54% (Canada) of deaths occurred during the first, larger wave of the early fall, theorized to be partially due to the lack of partial immunity conferred from the 1957–1958 H2N2 pandemic [12]. In the case of SARS-CoV-2 infection, there is evidence that some cross-reactive immunity may be conferred by the long-term circulating coronaviruses associated with the common cold (CoV HKU1, CoV NL63, CoV OC43, and CoV 229E). While the degree of immunity conferred by coronaviruses is thought to be short-lived, it may affect the severity, age distribution, and geographic transmissibility of COVID-19 [13].

Mutations of the novel strain within the pandemic period can also influence which waves have the highest case fatality and affect differences in wave transmission patterns by country. An example of mutations occurring throughout multiple seasons of a pandemic took place during the 1918 H1N1 pandemic, where the first wave occurred quite early in June and July in Europe and North America. While there is fragmentary data on the sequence of the virus present in the first wave, we do know from samples that there were strains of the H1N1 virus present during the second wave. However, with the case of 1918–1919, there was conflicting evidence on the influence these H1N1 mutations had on mortality and transmissibility [14]. These mutations go both ways, as seen in the 2004 resurgence of SARS-CoV-1 in South Korea, where a mutation had occurred after the first wave/emergence of SARS. The mutation decreased the S2 protein to the ACE-2 receptor, resulting in decreased transmissibility, disease severity, and mortality compared to the original SARS-CoV-1 sequence [15].

Another inter-pandemic variable is cross-protection, or the number of people exposed who will have immunity in subsequent waves. The basic concept being the relative steps to herd immunity in each wave. In the 1918 influenza pandemic, both the US and British military bases exposed to the first wave provided a 35–94% protection against severe symptoms and 56–89% protection against death during the second wave [16–18]. This strategy was recently employed in Sweden, where lockdowns were minimized compared to most countries facing COVID-19 with the expectation that herd immunity would be reached faster to minimize further waves of transmission. It should be stated that this is not a realistic approach for many countries as it works best when a country has a certain age demographic (younger and healthier populations) and a healthcare system capable of handling a large number of cases.

During the COVID-19 pandemic, case isolation and tracing of contacts have given way to mitigation interventions attempting to reduce the number of hospitalization and fatalities. Indeed, the SARS-CoV-2 coronavirus has shown to be efficiently transmitted within households and in the community and with a significant amount of transmission occurring during the incubation period by presymptomatic individuals and by asymptomatic infections[2]. Timely quarantine of close contacts is important in preventing onward transmission during the incubation phase of the infection. In many countries, we have witnessed subsequent waves of community and household transmission leading to significant disruption, suffering, healthcare utilization, and a growing number of case-fatalities.

3. Seasonality of Pandemics

Multiple waves of infections are often a mainstay of pandemics (Table 1). It should be stated that when analyzing wave pattern projections for SARS-CoV-2, little data can be drawn from the other coronavirus pandemics. The 2003–2004 SARS-CoV-1 pandemic would appear as if it occurred in a single wave. However, the confinement of this virus and its limited spread to just over 8000 people make drawing parallels nearly impossible. The main thing noted in the seasonality of SARS-CoV-1 was that it appeared to spread rapidly in humans from March to June of 2003. Similarly, with MERS, this virus has had a much smaller total number of cases, was facilitated by camel to human transmission and arose in a very different environment than other pandemic viruses. The main trend seen with MERS seasonality was that between 2012–2017 the smallest number of cases were seen in July and tended to increase throughout the year, with 52.7% of all cases having occurred in April, May, and June of each year [19]. For these reasons, the discussion of seasonality and multiple waves will be limited to influenza pandemics. The timing of multiple pandemic waves is highly variable and unpredictable due to the large number of factors contributing to disease emergence and spread. Most pandemics have multiple waves peaking in non-summer months, with subsequent waves causing high levels of mortality and large variability between different regions around the globe. Although mechanisms leading to subsequent waves of infection and predicting future pandemic wave patterns are not well understood, there are a series of determinant variables we know to influence wave timing and severity. Discussed in more depth during this section, it would appear climate and environment is the major driver in seasonal timing of waves and lack of summer outbreaks. Viral (prior immunity, cross-wave immunity, mutation, etc.) and human determinants (changing population size, NPI employments, vaccines, and social changes) appear to be major drivers in the number of waves seen and help to determine the variations seen in different pandemics (Table 1).

Table 1. Comparison of influenza pandemics from late 19th to 21st century.

Virus Pandemic Years	Waves (Duration)	Timing	Most Severe Wave	Post-Pandemic Resurgences	Other facts
H3N8 Russian Flu 1889–1890	3 (3 years)	W1: 1889–1890 W2: 1890–1891 W3: 1892–1893	N/A	3 each separated by 3 years. Concurrent with seasonal flu	Gradually from Asia to North America, with peak wave timing spread over months.
H1N1 Spanish Flu 1918–1919	3 (9 months)	W1: Jun–Jul 1918 W2: Oct–Nov 1918 W3: Feb–Mar 1919	2	R1: Jan–Apr 1920 R2: Dec 20–May 21 R3: Dec 21–Apr 22	W1 mostly in the US and Europe. W2 and 3 similar timing globally
H2N2 Asian Flu 1957–1959	3 (15–18 months)	W1: Sep–Dec 1957 W2: Dec–Mar 1958 W3: Dec 58–Apr 59	2	-	Midst of Vietnam war with heavy annual travel of soldiers from Asia to United States
H3N2 Hong Kong 1968–1970	2 (12–18 months)	Based on global circ. W1: Jul 68 to Aug 69 W2: Sept 69–Sept 70	2	-	Travel based spread due to the Vietnam war. US and Canada W1 most severe. All other countries W2 had highest mortality
H1N1 Swine Flu 2009–2010	1 Epidemic 2 Pandemic (12 months)	E1: Jan–Mar 2009 W1: Mar–Aug 2009 W2: Aug 09–Jan 10	2 (Fall)	-	Following the 2008 economic crisis with overflow effects on the availability of international aid

Part of the variability of seasonality we have seen is also due to the fact that human society has been a moving target for each strain. For example, the 1889 pandemic had the first wave initiated in Europe during the end of spring in 1889 and did not peak in the United States until the beginning of 1889–1890. The lack of globalization and intercontinental travel may have influenced both the slow spread and its waves being annual [20]. This may have also been a factor as in 1889, the three resurgent spikes in strain infectivity were approximately spaced by 3 years. However, with the pandemic of 1918 and many of the pandemics since, the viral strains have had their resurgent waves follow a more annual pattern along with other seasonal flu viruses. With the exception of the severity of the 1918 H1N1 influenza pandemic, the gradual increase in travel and the global population has altered the homogeneity of waves around the world in subsequent pandemics. The SARS-CoV-2 first wave occurred within Asia, Europe, and North America within a 3-month period. For our current pandemic and future novel viruses that have a threshold transmissibility, the likelihood of global spread is elevated and is more likely to share simultaneous wave patterns than wave patterns described in influenza pandemics of the 20th and 21st centuries; and of the SARS pandemic.

The influence of seasonality has been one of the strongest and most consistent variables in wave timing and refractory periods. This is true for both seasonal pandemic influenza strains with decreased infectivity during periods with increased temperature and absolute humidity [21]. This can help to account for why most pandemic strains have shown a refractory period of decreased cases during the summer months. However, while these trends have also been seen with beta-coronaviruses, a recent study on the likelihood of SARS-CoV-2 entering into the seasonal flu community in the post-pandemic period has estimated that the influence of summer climate aspects may only decrease the likelihood of spread of SARS-CoV-2 by less than 20% [13,22–25]. While it is likely that environmental factors decrease the transmissibility of SARS-CoV-2, we are unable to say whether it occurs to the same degree as seen with influenza [22,26–28].

In 1968–1969, the H3N2 pandemic was the first time the United States engaged in wide-scale federal regulation of quarantine, social distancing, and personal protective equipment for both health care workers and civilians. All of these measures would have helped decrease the initial wave severity. Unfortunately, the lack of regulations allowed schools to commence following the winter break, which likely catalyzed the dual peaked first wave observed 2 months later [5]. This was by no means the only factor in the United States, as military bases and communal areas potentiated the chain of transmission. It appears that another wave of SARS-CoV-2 transmission in the United States correlates with school openings and, to some degree, to the political events and messaging prior to the elections of 3 November 2020.

4. Clinical Outcomes of the Different Pandemics

The pandemics discussed here span a period of over 100 years, during which advances in the biomedical and clinical landscape have improved our understanding of severe pandemic outcomes. One of the most common severe outcomes of most viral respiratory pandemics is acute respiratory distress syndrome (ARDS). Multiple mechanisms contribute to this syndrome's progression, such as the host's immunophenotype as well as their comorbidities [29,30]. As a result, ARDS severity and presentation can differ dramatically. Early COVID-19 studies report that 20–42% of hospitalized patients develop ARDS, subsequently some of these critically ill patients are then discharged home and expected to reintegrate into their communities. While improvements in ICU care will save many lives, many of these individuals will suffer from long-term sequelae dubbed "post-ICU syndrome" [31]. This includes reductions in their mental, cognitive, and psychological health, muscle weakness, decreased pulmonary function, and prolonged return to their activities of daily life. Health care systems must plan for the surge in post-ICU syndrome and its complications, especially for the most vulnerable groups in our community.

Secondary bacterial infections (SBI) are a well-studied severe outcome of influenza pandemics. Data indicate that, on average, between 11–35% of hospitalized patients with influenza have a bacterial co-infection, with this number being as high as 65% in immunocompromised individuals [32]. This outcome was also a likely cause of death during the 1918 influenza pandemic, prior to the advent of penicillin [33].

The role of SBIs in COVID-19 is less clear. Early reports suggested co-infections with respiratory pathogens were a rare occurrence, but recent studies have identified co-infections in up to 25.8% of hospitalized patients, with rates rising to 65% among ICU patients alone [34,35]. The majority of these were caused by viral pathogens, with bacterial and fungal infections being more common among severely ill patients [35]. Most of these studies do not provide data on the timing and development of SBIs, but the prolonged length of illness and high intubation rates may explain many of these cases. As in most pandemics, with the 2009 H1N1 pandemic being the exception, those above 65 years of age have represented one of the groups most at risk for severe outcomes, including ICU admission, mechanical ventilation, and death [3,9,36].

5. Mortality and Case Fatality of Pandemics

The ways in which we access mortality and case-fatality for each pandemic have changed drastically from 1918 to the present [37–45]. This should first be explained as direct comparisons are often difficult due to these differences in mortality parameters (Table 2). This table is by no means a definitive record of the infection and mortality rates brought about by these pandemics. These numbers are widely contested, many of the cases may not have been recorded, and the records that do exist vary greatly in coverage and reliability.

Table 2. Comparison of influenza and coronavirus pandemics of the 20th and 21st centuries.

Pandemic	Viral Strain	Total Infected (Globally)	Total Deaths (Globally)	Case Fatality Rate (%)	Basic Reproductive Number (R_0)	Reference for CFR Estimates
Spanish Flu (1918–1919)	aH1N1	300–450 million	20–50 million	CMR ~2.5% *	2.11–2.5	[37]
Asian Flu (1957)	aH2N2	500,000,000	700,000–1.5 million	0.02–0.05%	1.8	[43]
Hong Kong Flu (1968)	aH3N2	500,000,000	500,000–2.0 million	0.67%	1.28–1.58	[43]
Swine Flu (2009)	H1N1pdm	200,000,000	2185–284,000	1.09%	1.33–1.38	[28]
SARS (2003)	SARS-CoV-1	8098	774	9.6%	2.4	[44]
MERS (2012)	MERS-CoV	2499	858	34.4%	1.1–1.2	[44]
COVID-19 (2020)	SARS-CoV-2	58,480,000	1,385,000	2–3%	1.5–3.5	[45]

* Crude mortality rate (CMR) of ~2.5% calculated based on excess mortality observations, which may be misleading due to large geographic variations and gaps in data. Note that CMR should not be confused with Case Fatality Rate (CFR). Estimates of R_0 were based on analysis of mortality data from the fall wave in the United States and United Kingdom.

When looking at the earliest pandemic discussed here (1918–1919 H1N1), the lack of data from both the time period and chaotic environment of WWI limit wide analysis of mortality. Much of these data are taken from retrospective studies on individual communities, areas which took a more detailed recording of the deaths and probable causes than much of the world at this time, usually documented as "total deaths". These data are often extrapolated and overall estimates should be seen to have a very large range of error. This changed for both the 1957–1958 and 1968–1969 pandemics, where technology had progressed to the point of identifying the viral culprit during the pandemic and the implementation of better tracking and mortality data for non-pandemic years. In these cases, "excess mortality" for various age groups is the most common method. Usually using the Serfling Regression model, which compares deaths during the pandemic to pneumonia and influenza deaths in the preceding 5–10 year's seasonal flu mortality data. The most recent pandemics tend not to use "excess mortality" to the same degree. With the advent of PCR in the late 1980's allowing for confirmation of infection in patients and post-mortem viral detection in unknown cases, pandemics such as SARS-CoV-1 are often reported as total infections, total deaths, and age group share of total deaths (what percentage of all deaths can be attributed to each group) [23].

It is also important to state that the statistics of mortality may be somewhat skewed as there is little data for any pandemic on the number of infections and deaths for equatorial countries, with the majority of data coming out of Europe, North America, Australia, and a handful of countries in Asia. This has implications as there are differences in life expectancy and the average age of populations, thus the impact each pandemic may have had is different in different areas. For the most part, understanding how these viruses affected various age groups in Europe and North America, with data from China, Japan, and South Korea coming with more recent pandemics. This can be seen with SARS-CoV-1 where it appears that the CFR and percentage of total deaths in Mainland China are higher in the 60–79 age range (25.51% CFR and 36.15% of total deaths) than in the 80–93 age range (17.74% CFR and 3.21% of total deaths) [24]. While this data looks different than in other countries, which have age and age-dependent CFR directly correlated, it may be due to the younger demographics in China and the proportionally smaller 80–93 aged population having decreased exposure in metropolitan public spaces (Figure 1). There is also a certain degree of change that happens as models progress overtime. This was seen as recently as with the 2009 H1N1 pandemic where in the years following the pandemic, the CDC has estimated the global death toll may be closer to 280,000 deaths than the 2184 lab-confirmed deaths initially reported [25]. Knowing the implications of excess mortality definitions changing over time and the somewhat limited ability to extrapolate data from a limited geographical and economic subset to the world, let us discuss the general trends seen.

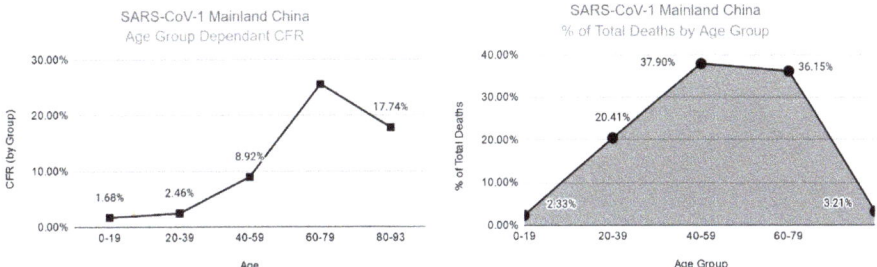

Figure 1. Age group dependent CFR (left column) as compared to % of total deaths for various age groups (right column) mortality (left column) for SARS-CoV-1 in Mainland China. Showing how CFR is much higher for advanced age while the majority of deaths occurred in younger populations exposed to the virus in both the community and hospitals [24].

For influenza, there tends to be a general trend that the two most heavily hit age groups are the very young and those over the age of 65, commonly referred to as the "U-shaped" distribution. This trend has been true for the most part for both seasonal and pandemic strains. There is, however, an exception for the H1N1 pandemics of both 1918 and 2009. In these two cases, there seems to be increased excess mortality for young adults not seen with other influenza (Figures 1 and 2). This is especially true for 1918, where a "W-shaped" excess mortality curve is seen. With a number of compounding factors, young adults (15–35 years of age) had a heightened death rate (per 100,000 population) [14].

The other atypical trend seen in 1918 was that when comparing death rates to pneumonia and influenza of 1913 to 1917, people over the age of 74 had negative excess mortality [26]. A similar trend was seen in 2009 with elevated mortality of those under the age of 20 [27,28]. In both these cases, there seems to be a trend where a H1N1 related strain had been circulating decades beforehand and then gone dormant for a few decades. This provided mortality protection for older generations and increased mortality for younger generations that were not exposed to the virus during their lifetime. The 1957 and 1968 pandemic both show a more typical influenza excess mortality curve where the two most affected groups are those under the age of 4–5 and those over the age of 65, as can be seen for 1957–1959 below (Figure 3). When looking at the changes from 1918 to 2009, one of the most consistent trends is that excess mortality for those over the age of 65 has remained quite high, while the excess mortality for young children has decreased with medical advances. Lastly, it is important to note that while excess mortality and the percentage of total deaths have decreased for young children, just like in 2009, these groups still maintain a large number of hospitalizations and a large total burden on the health care system.

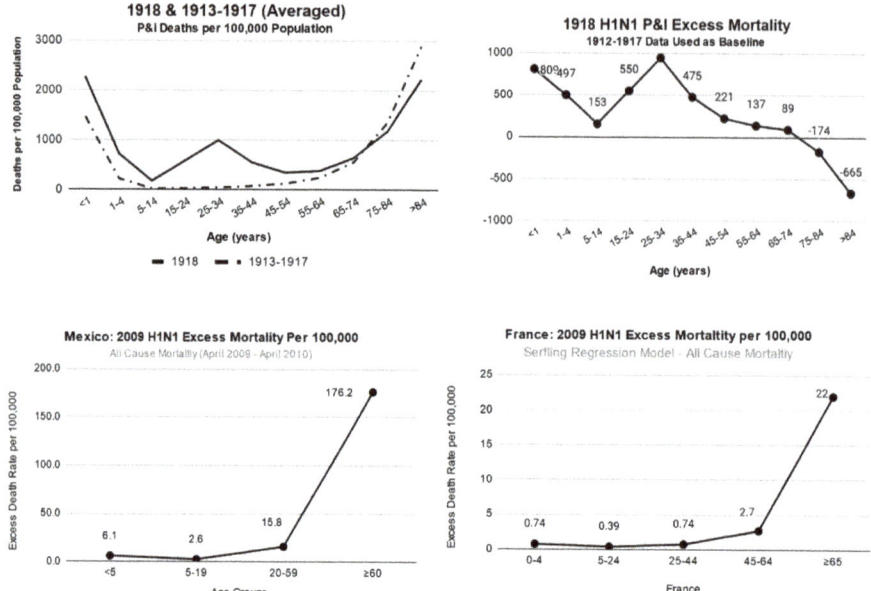

Figure 2. Mortality visualizations for H1N1 pandemics of both 1918–1919 and 2009. Averaged mortality (upper left) as compared to excess mortality (upper right) due to 1918 H1N1 pneumonia and influenza (P&I) pandemic. Excess death rates [5] are shown for the 2009 H1N1 pandemic for both the country of Mexico (lower left) [38] and France (lower right) [39].

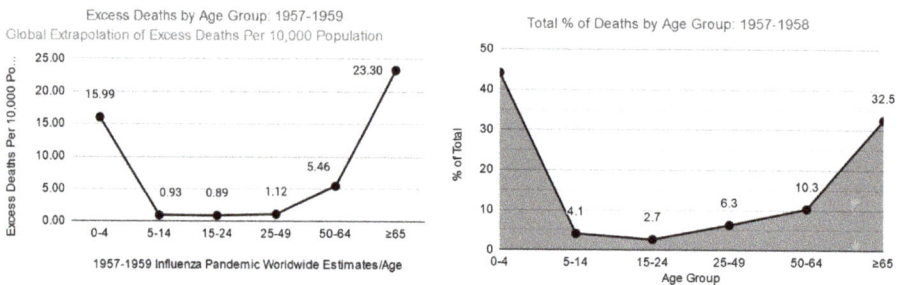

Figure 3. Excess deaths (right column) and total percentage of deaths (right column) due to 1957–1959 Influenza pandemic [40].

This is quite different from Coronavirus excess mortality and total deaths. For both seasonal and pandemic CoV strains, there is a consistent trend where increases in age and mortality are directly related. When analyzing SARS-CoV-1 and MERS-CoV, there are still cases of children and young adults having some deaths. As referenced in the "Clinical outcomes of different pandemics" section, the proportion of hospitalizations and deaths increases with each decade of life, somewhat stabilizing with those over the age of 65–75. This trend is seeming to be true for SARS-CoV-2 as well, even when looking at countries with different relative age group populations. What is also noticeable about the regional data available for SARS-CoV-2 is the changes to the total % of deaths depending upon the demographics of the area. When comparing the United States, Colorado, and New York City (Figure 4), it can be shown how demographic data can often skew how the total death share appears. This is most evident in New York City, where the population demographics are noticeably younger than for the United States as whole.

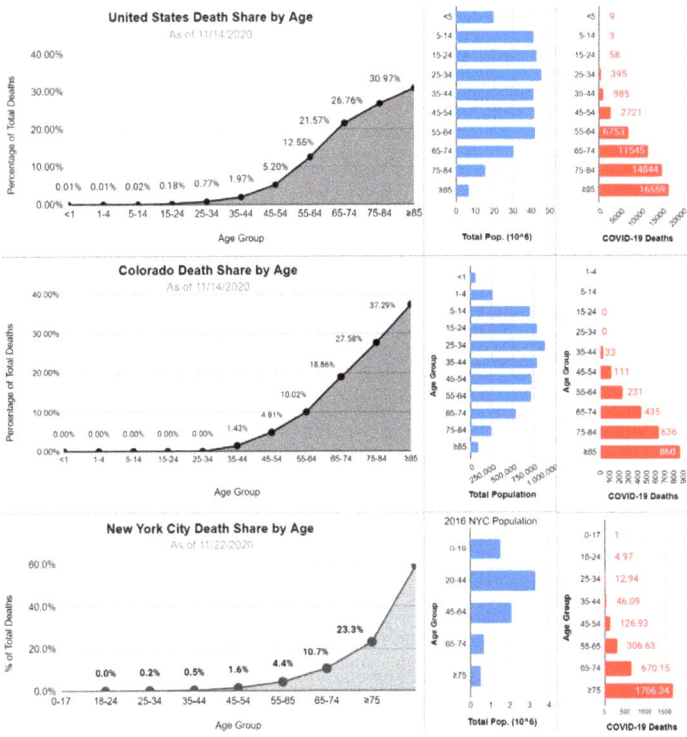

Figure 4. Deaths based on three regions for SARS-CoV-2, data included was last updated between 14 November–22 November 2020. The top row shows the percentage of total SARS-CoV-2 deaths (left column), regional demographics (middle column), and the total number of deaths (right column) for the United States, Colorado, and New York City. This serves to show how regional demographics can influence total death share data and can change noticeably throughout different regions. For the United States and Colorado, data were compiled from the CDC Provisional COVID-19 Data Sets [41]. For New York City, the city government's data set was used [42].

6. Conclusions

When comparing major influenza and coronavirus pandemics in recent history, it becomes clear that their similarities are not mere coincidences but seem to be somewhat inherent to how and why certain pathogens are easily transmitted from person to person and usually by multiple modes of transmission. In the past 100 years, all major pandemics have been caused by respiratory viruses that emerged during the winter season in the Northern Hemisphere during the second half of the normal flu season. They have all originated from a non-human source and most have exhibited the ability to cross from humans back into certain animal populations serving as the site for antigenic shifts or genetic recombination events. While there is no guarantee all future pandemics will follow these trends, understanding these animal to human transmission patterns may assist us in preparing for future emerging infections. Pandemics tend to occur in at least two consecutive waves of transmission. The impact of each wave depends on the underlying level of immunity of the population and community mitigation interventions. In every pandemic, there are specific age groups at risk of developing severe disease and dying. Most of these outcomes are the result of large pools of immunologically naïve populations, immunosenescence of the elderly, and a high prevalence of medical comorbidities. Among many influenza pandemics, school-age children were major drivers of household transmission. The COVID-19 pandemic has been associated with a high-attack rate among household contacts. Therefore, the prompt institution of mitigation interventions including non-pharmaceutical interventions such as social distancing, travel restrictions, interruption of mass gatherings, and community quarantine is critical to achieving at least a 50% reduction in transmission, which correlates with a basic reproductive number lower or equal to one ($R_0 \leq 1$).

The development of vaccines is a vital part of any pandemic response. However, in all cases starting with the great influenza pandemic of 1918–1919, the timeline for vaccine development, testing, approval, and production has been inadequate to have a substantial effect in mitigating the spread and impact of each pandemic. The first 2–3 waves are most likely to occur within 12–15 months of the virus originating and therefore it is crucial to focus on mitigating interventions targeting infection prevention strategies [12]. Indeed, it is important to allocate the bulk of our public health efforts to non-pharmacologic interventions and to the medical care of symptomatic cases to reduce fatalities until safe and efficacious vaccines are fully developed and distributed. Another important aspect to consider during a pandemic is maintaining adequate coverage levels of routine childhood vaccination in order to prevent the occurrence of outbreaks of vaccine-preventable diseases.

Given the degree of globalization and interconnectivity of modernity, pandemics remain as perennial threats for human societies. We can never be fully prepared for future pandemics. However, given that pandemics tend to disproportionately impact socially disadvantaged populations, there is an important urgency to continue addressing health inequities and structural social vulnerabilities that many people globally endure.

Author Contributions: G.M., Z.S., C.F.-P., J.S. drafted the initial manuscript and reviewed the literature. Edited and approved the last version. A.F.H.-M., P.C., T.W. reviewed the literature, edited, and approved the last version. All authors have read and agreed to the published version of the manuscript.

Funding: This research received no external funding.

Conflicts of Interest: The authors declare no conflict of interest.

References

1. McNeill, W.H.; McNeill, W. *Plagues and Peoples*; Anchor: New York, NY, USA, 1998.
2. Morens, D.M.; Daszak, P.; Markel, H.; Taubenberger, J.K. Pandemic COVID-19 Joins History's Pandemic Legion. *mBio* **2020**, *11*. [CrossRef] [PubMed]
3. World Health Organization. Report of the WHO-China Joint Mission on Coronavirus Disease 2019 (COVID-19). 2020. Available online: https://www.who.int/publications-detail/report-of-the-who-china-joint-mission-on-coronavirus-disease-2019-(covid-19) (accessed on 12 October 2020).
4. Johns Hopkins Coronavirus Resource Center. Available online: https://coronavirus.jhu.edu/map.html (accessed on 30 October 2020).
5. Mummert, A.; Weiss, H.; Long, L.-P.; Amigó, J.M.; Wan, X.-F. A Perspective on Multiple Waves of Influenza Pandemics. *PLoS ONE* **2013**, *8*, e60343. [CrossRef] [PubMed]
6. Groneberg, D.; Hilgenfeld, R.; Zabel, P. Molecular mechanisms of severe acute respiratory syndrome (SARS). *Respir. Res.* **2005**, *6*, 8. [CrossRef] [PubMed]
7. Li, R.; Pei, S.; Chen, B.; Song, Y.; Zhang, T.; Yang, W.; Shaman, J. Substantial undocumented infection facilitates the rapid dissemination of novel coronavirus (SARS-CoV-2). *Science* **2020**, *368*, 489–493. [CrossRef] [PubMed]
8. Wang, L.-F.; Shi, Z.; Zhang, S.; Field, H.; Daszak, P.; Eaton, B.T. Review of Bats and SARS. *Emerg. Infect. Dis.* **2006**, *12*, 1834–1840. [CrossRef]
9. World Health Organization. *Summary of Probable SARS Cases with Onset of Illness from 1 November 2002 to 31 July 2003*; World Health Organization: Geneva, Switzerland, 2013. Available online: https://www.who.int/csr/sars/country/table2004_04_21/en/ (accessed on 12 October 2020).
10. Shi, J.; Wen, Z.; Zhong, G.; Yang, H.; Wang, C.; Huang, B.; Liu, R.; He, X.; Shuai, L.; Sun, Z.; et al. Susceptibility of ferrets, cats, dogs, and other domesticated animals to SARS–coronavirus 2. *Science* **2020**, *368*, 1016–1020. [CrossRef]
11. Kilbourne, E.D. Influenza Pandemics of the 20th Century. *Emerg. Infect. Dis.* **2006**, *12*, 9–14. [CrossRef]

12. Viboud, C.; Grais, R.F.; Lafont, A.B.; Miller, M.A.; Simonsen, L. Multinational Influenza Seasonal Mortality Study Group: Multinational impact of the 1968 Hong Kong influenza pandemic: Evidence for a smoldering pandemic. *Int. J. Infect. Dis.* **2005**, *192*, 233–248. [CrossRef]
13. Ng, K.W.; Faulkner, N.; Cornish, G.H.; Rosa, A.; Harvey, R.; Hussain, S.; Ulferts, R.; Earl, C.; Wrobel, A.G.; Benton, D.J.; et al. Preexisting and de novo humoral immunity to SARS-CoV-2 in humans. *Science* **2020**, eabe1107. [CrossRef] [PubMed]
14. Morens, D.M.; Breman, J.G.; Calisher, C.H.; Doherty, P.C.; Hahn, B.H.; Keusch, G.T.; Kramer, L.D.; LeDuc, J.W.; Monath, T.P.; Taubenberger, J.K. The Origin of COVID-19 and Why It Matters. *Am. J. Trop. Med. Hyg.* **2020**, *103*, 955–959. [CrossRef] [PubMed]
15. Li, W.; Zhang, C.; Sui, J.; Kuhn, J.H.; Moore, M.J.; Luo, S.; Wong, S.-K.; Huang, I.-C.; Xu, K.; Vasilieva, N.; et al. Receptor and viral determinants of SARS-coronavirus adaptation to human ACE2. *EMBO J.* **2005**, *24*, 1634–1643. [CrossRef] [PubMed]
16. Barry, J.M.; Viboud, C.; Simonsen, L. Cross-Protection between Successive Waves of the 1918–1919 Influenza Pandemic: Epidemiological Evidence from US Army Camps and from Britain. *J. Infect. Dis.* **2008**, *198*, 1427–1434. [CrossRef] [PubMed]
17. Kawaoka, Y.; Krauss, S.; Webster, R.G. Avian-to-human transmission of the PB1 gene of influenza A viruses in the 1957 and 1968 pandemics. *J. Virol.* **1989**, *63*, 4603–4608. [CrossRef] [PubMed]
18. Ma, W.; Kahn, R.E.; Richt, J.A. The pig as a mixing vessel for influenza viruses: Human and veterinary implications. *J. Mol. Genet. Med.* **2009**, *3*, 158–166. [CrossRef]
19. Nassar, M.S.; Bakhrebah, M.A.; Meo, S.A.; Alsuabeyl, M.S.; Zaher, W.A. Global seasonal occurrence of middle east respiratory syndrome coronavirus (MERS-CoV) infection. *Eur. Rev. Med. Pharmacol. Sci.* **2018**, *22*, 3913–3918.
20. Taubenberger, J.K.; Morens, D.M. 1918 Influenza: The mother of all pandemics. *Rev. Biomed.* **2006**, *17*, 69–79. [CrossRef]
21. Shaman, J.; Pitzer, V.E.; Viboud, C.; Grenfell, B.T.; Lipsitch, M. Absolute humidity and the seasonal onset of influenza in the continental United States. *PLoS Biol.* **2010**, *8*, e1000316. [CrossRef]
22. Ilie, P.C.; Stefanescu, S.; Smith, L. The role of vitamin D in the prevention of coronavirus disease 2019 infection and mortality. *Aging Clin. Exp. Res.* **2020**, *32*, 1195–1198. [CrossRef]
23. Mackay, I. Real-time PCR in virology. *Nucleic Acids Res.* **2002**, *30*, 1292–1305. [CrossRef]
24. Jia, N.; Feng, D.; Fang, L.-Q.; Richardus, J.H.; Han, X.-N.; Cao, W.-C.; De Vlas, S.J. Case fatality of SARS in mainland China and associated risk factors. *Trop. Med. Int. Heal.* **2009**, *14*, 21–27. [CrossRef]
25. Simonsen, L.; Spreeuwenberg, P.; Lustig, R.; Taylor, R.J.; Fleming, D.M.; Kroneman, M.; Van Kerkhove, M.D.; Mounts, A.W.; Paget, W.J.; GLaMOR Collaborating Teams. Global Mortality Estimates for the 2009 Influenza Pandemic from the GLaMOR Project: A Modeling Study. *PLoS Med.* **2013**, *10*, e1001558. [CrossRef] [PubMed]
26. Luk, J.; Gross, P.; Thompson, W.W. Observations on Mortality during the 1918 Influenza Pandemic. *Clin. Infect. Dis.* **2001**, *33*, 1375–1378. [CrossRef]
27. Lemaitre, M.; Carrat, F. Comparative age distribution of influenza morbidity and mortality during seasonal influenza epidemics and the 2009 H1N1 pandemic. *BMC Infect. Dis.* **2010**, *10*, 162. [CrossRef] [PubMed]
28. Dawood, F.S.; Iuliano, A.D.; Reed, C.; Meltzer, M.I.; Shay, D.K.; Cheng, P.-Y.; Bandaranayake, D.; Breiman, R.F.; Brooks, W.A.; Buchy, P.; et al. Estimated global mortality associated with the first 12 months of 2009 pandemic influenza A H1N1 virus circulation: A modelling study. *Lancet Infect. Dis.* **2012**, *12*, 687–695. [CrossRef]
29. Matthay, M.A.; Hendrickson, C.M. Viral Pathogens and Acute Lung Injury: Investigations Inspired by the SARS Epidemic and the 2009 H1N1 Influenza Pandemic. *Semin. Respir. Crit. Care Med.* **2013**, *34*, 475–486. [CrossRef] [PubMed]
30. Herold, S.; Becker, C.; Ridge, K.M.; Budinger, G.S. Influenza virus-induced lung injury: Pathogenesis and implications for treatment. *Eur. Respir. J.* **2015**, *45*, 1463–1478. [CrossRef]
31. Sigurdsson, M.I.; Sigvaldason, K.; Gunnarsson, T.S.; Moller, A.; Sigurdsson, G.H. Acute respiratory distress syndrome: Nationwide changes in incidence, treatment and mortality over 23 years. *Acta Anaesthesiol. Scand.* **2013**, *57*, 37–45. [CrossRef]
32. Klein, E.Y.; Monteforte, B.; Gupta, A.; Jiang, W.; May, L.; Hsieh, Y.; Dugas, A. The frequency of influenza and bacterial coinfection: A systematic review and meta-analysis. *Influ. Respir. Viruses* **2016**, *10*, 394–403. [CrossRef]

33. Morens, D.M.; Taubenberger, J.K.; Fauci, A.S. Predominant Role of Bacterial Pneumonia as a Cause of Death in Pandemic Influenza: Implications for Pandemic Influenza Preparedness. *J. Infect. Dis.* **2008**, *198*, 962–970. [CrossRef]
34. Kim, D.; Quinn, J.; Pinsky, B.; Shah, N.H.; Brown, I. Rates of co-infection between SARS-CoV-2 and other respiratory pathogens. *JAMA* **2020**, *323*, 2085–2086. [CrossRef]
35. Zhang, G.; Hu, C.; Luo, L.; Fang, F.; Chen, Y.; Li, J.; Peng, Z.; Pan, H. Clinical features and short-term outcomes of 221 patients with COVID-19 in Wuhan, China. *J. Clin. Virol.* **2020**, *127*, 104364. [CrossRef] [PubMed]
36. Van Wijhe, M.; Ingholt, M.M.; Andreasen, V.; Simonsen, L. Loose Ends in the Epidemiology of the 1918 Pandemic: Explaining the Extreme Mortality Risk in Young Adults. *Am. J. Epidemiol.* **2018**, *187*, 2503–2510. [CrossRef] [PubMed]
37. Johnson, N.P.A.S.; Mueller, J. Updating the Accounts: Global Mortality of the 1918-1920 "Spanish" Influenza Pandemic. *Bull. Hist. Med.* **2002**, *76*, 105–115. [CrossRef] [PubMed]
38. Charu, V.; Chowell, G.; Mejia, L.S.P.; Echevarría-Zuno, S.; Borja-Aburto, V.H.; Simonsen, L.; Miller, M.A.; Viboud, C. Mortality Burden of the A/H1N1 Pandemic in Mexico: A Comparison of Deaths and Years of Life Lost to Seasonal Influenza. *Clin. Infect. Dis.* **2011**, *53*, 985–993. [CrossRef]
39. Lemaitre, M.; Carrat, F.; Rey, G.; Miller, M.; Simonsen, L.; Viboud, C. Mortality Burden of the 2009 A/H1N1 Influenza Pandemic in France: Comparison to Seasonal Influenza and the A/H3N2 Pandemic. *PLoS ONE* **2012**, *7*, e45051. [CrossRef]
40. Viboud, C.; Simonsen, L.; Fuentes, R.; Flores, J.; Miller, M.A.; Chowell, G. Global Mortality Impact of the 1957–1959 Influenza Pandemic. *J. Infect. Dis.* **2016**, *213*, 738–745. [CrossRef]
41. Provisional COVID-19 Death Counts by Sex, Age, and State |Data| Centers for Disease Control and Prevention. Available online: https://data.cdc.gov/NCHS/Provisional-COVID-19-Death-Counts-by-Sex-Age-and-S/9bhg-hcku (accessed on 22 November 2020).
42. COVID-19: Data Totals-NYC Health. Available online: https://www1.nyc.gov/site/doh/covid/covid-19-data-totals.page#rates (accessed on 22 November 2020).
43. Nickol, M.E.; Kindrachuk, J. A year of terror and a century of reflection: Perspectives on the great influenza pandemic of 1918–1919. *BMC Infect. Dis.* **2019**, *19*, 1–10. [CrossRef]
44. Gilbert, G.L. Commentary: SARS, MERS and COVID-19—new threats; old lessons. *Int. J. Epidemiol.* **2020**, *49*, 726–728. [CrossRef]
45. Mortality Analyses. Johns Hopkins Coronavirus Resource Center. Available online: https://coronavirus.jhu.edu/data/mortality (accessed on 22 November 2020).

Publisher's Note: MDPI stays neutral with regard to jurisdictional claims in published maps and institutional affiliations.

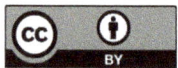

© 2020 by the authors. Licensee MDPI, Basel, Switzerland. This article is an open access article distributed under the terms and conditions of the Creative Commons Attribution (CC BY) license (http://creativecommons.org/licenses/by/4.0/).

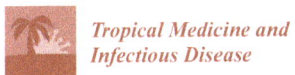 *Tropical Medicine and Infectious Disease*

Review

Efficacy and Safety of Lopinavir/Ritonavir for Treatment of COVID-19: A Systematic Review and Meta-Analysis

Saad Alhumaid [1,*], Abbas Al Mutair [2], Zainab Al Alawi [3], Naif Alhmeed [4], Abdul Rehman Zia Zaidi [5] and Mansour Tobaiqy [6]

1. Administration of Pharmaceutical Care, Ministry of Health, Al-Ahsa 31982, Saudi Arabia
2. Research Center, Almoosa Specialist Hospital, Al-Ahsa 31982, Saudi Arabia; abbas.almutair@almoosahospital.com.sa
3. Department of Pediatrics, College of Medicine, King Faisal University, Al-Ahsa 31982, Saudi Arabia; dr_z.alawi@hotmail.com
4. Administration of Supply and Shared Services, Ministry of Health, Riyadh 11461, Saudi Arabia; nalhmeed@moh.gov.sa
5. Research Center, Dr. Sulaiman Al Habib Medical Group, Riyadh 11461, Saudi Arabia; ar-zia@hotmail.com
6. Department of Pharmacology, College of Medicine, University of Jeddah, Jeddah 21442, Saudi Arabia; mtobaiqy@uj.edu.sa
* Correspondence: saalhumaid@moh.gov.sa; Tel.: +966-561-522-581

Received: 22 October 2020; Accepted: 26 November 2020; Published: 28 November 2020

Abstract: (Background) Lopinavir-ritonavir (LPV/RTV) is a human immunodeficiency virus (HIV) antiviral combination that has been considered for the treatment of COVID-19 disease. (Aim) This systematic review aimed to assess the efficacy and safety of LPV/RTV in COVID-19 patients in the published research. (Methods) A protocol was developed based on the Preferred Reporting Items for Systematic reviews and Meta-Analysis (PRISMA) statement. Articles were selected for review from 8 electronic databases. This review evaluated the effects of LPV/RTV alone or in combination with standard care ± interferons/antiviral treatments compared to other therapies, regarding duration of hospital stay, risk of progressing to invasive mechanical, time to virological cure and body temperature normalization, cough relief, radiological progression, mortality and safety. (Results) A consensus was reached to select 32 articles for full-text screening; only 14 articles comprising 9036 patients were included in this study; and eight of these were included for meta-analysis. Most of these studies did not report positive clinical outcomes with LPV/RTV treatment. In terms of virological cure, three studies reported less time in days to achieve a virological cure for LPV/RTV arm relative to no antiviral treatment (−0.81 day; 95% confidence interval (CI), −4.44 to 2.81; $p = 0.007$, $I^2 = 80\%$). However, the overall effect was not significant ($p = 0.66$). When comparing the LPV/RTV arm to umifenovir arm, a favorable affect was observed for umifenovir arm, but not statically significant ($p = 0.09$). In terms of time to body normalization and cough relief, no favorable effects of LPV/RTV versus umifenovir were observed. The largest trials (RECOVERY and SOLIDARITY) have shown that LPV/RTV failed to reduce mortality, initiation of invasive mechanical ventilation or hospitalization duration. Adverse events were reported most frequently for LPV/RTV ($n = 84$) relative to other antivirals and no antiviral treatments. (Conclusions) This review did not reveal any significant advantage in efficacy of LPV/RTV for the treatment of COVID-19 over standard care, no antivirals or other antiviral treatments. This result might not reflect the actual evidence.

Keywords: COVID-19; efficacy; safety; kaletra; lopinavir/ritonavir; meta-analysis

1. Introduction

Since the emergence of an unknown viral infection with its first cases in China in December 2019 and following the identification of this infection as 2019-new coronavirus disease (2019-nCoV, also known as COVID-19), caused by severe acute respiratory syndrome coronavirus 2 (SARS-CoV-2) [1], the world has worked to find effective therapeutics and vaccinations to treat hundreds of thousands of affected patients and to reduce the spread of this global pandemic [2].

As of 2 June 2020, there were 1104 registered clinical trials of COVID-19 therapeutics or vaccinations worldwide that either had ongoing or were recruiting patients; however, at that stage no drug or vaccine had officially been approved for COVID-19 [2,3]. These trials have produced mixed and conflicting results of positive or negative outcomes and inclusive evidence of efficacy or safety, that render the suspension of some trials inevitable, as in the hydroxychloroquine trials, which was suggested by the World Health Organization (WHO) in light of safety concerns [4]. This decision was reversed on 3 June 2020 [5], following a retraction of the research article by the Lancet as certain authors were not granted access to the underlying data [6]. As the pandemic evolves, the amount of evidence regarding the benefit of hydroxychloroquine in the treatment of COVID-19 patients has grown. A recent systematic review included 32 studies for a total 29,192 studied participants found treatment with hydroxychloroquine confers no benefit in terms of mortality in hospitalized patients with COVID-19 compared to standard care [7].

Lopinavir-ritonavir (LPV/RTV) is a protease inhibitor and nucleoside analog combination used for human immunodeficiency virus (HIV-1) and was also thought to be a potential treatment for COVID-19 [8], as its therapeutic value in the treatment of COVID-19 was assessed by in-vitro studies that claimed inhibition of several viral corona respiratory illnesses, including severe acute respiratory syndrome (SARS-CoV), and Middle East Respiratory Syndrome (MERS) [9–11]. Only recently, LPV/RTV therapy was hypothesized to be of no antiviral efficacy against SARS-CoV or MERS-CoV because the recommended dosages supplied to patients included in the published studies were subtherapeutic [12] and doses higher than 400 mg/100 mg twice daily are suggested [13].

Lopinavir (LPV) is an aspartic acid protease inhibitor of HIV, where inhibition of proteases enzymes is essential for the intervening of the viral infectious cycle. LPV is co-formulated with ritonavir (RTV) to boost the pharmacokinetic activity and half-life of LPV through the inhibition of cytochromes P450, providing adequate suppression of viral load and constant improvements in CD4+ cell counts, as demonstrated in randomized trials in naïve and experienced adult and child HIV patients [8].

There is conflicting evidence regarding the use of LPV/RTV for the treatment of COVID-19 patients; and evidence is currently scarce and of low quality. LPV/RTV is available as a single-tablet formulation (Kaletra®, North Chicago, IL, USA) in dosage strengths of 400/100 mg or 200/50 mg, and in clinical trials, this combination reduced rates of acute respiratory distress syndrome (ARDS) or death compared to supportive care or ribavirin alone in a matched cohort group during the early phase of viral acquisition [11].

LPV/RTV is being examined in several international clinical trials, including the RECOVERY trial and SOLIDARITY WHO trial [14], but did not gain authorization to be used emergently in the current pandemic in the USA by the Food and Drug Administration (FDA), which has approved only three pharmacologically different therapeutics for treatments of COVID-19, including antibiotic-hydroxychloroquine, immunotherapy-convalescent plasma therapy, and antiviral-remdesivir [2,14].

Among the clinical trials that did not find positive results for LPV/RTV, a study conducted by Bin Cao et al. published in the New England Journal of Medicine [15] revealed that treatment with LPV/RTV was not associated with clinical improvement beyond standard care or reduction in mortality rate at 28 days in hospitalized adult patients with severe COVID-19.

To date, LPV/RTV combination is available in some countries' therapeutics guidelines including USA [16], Saudi Arabia [17], and Ireland [18], which means that the medicine has tenable evidence of efficacy; however, considering that early negative and conflicting results have emerged [15], there is a need to assess the efficacy and safety of this COVID-19 treatment in a systematic manner.

2. Aim of the Study

This systematic review and meta-analysis aimed to assess the efficacy and safety of LPV/RTV in COVID-19 patients in published research.

3. Methods

This systematic review was conducted with reference to the basics of Cochrane Handbook for Systematic Reviews of Interventions [19], described as stated by the Preferred Reporting Items for Systematic reviews and Meta-Analysis (PRISMA) statement [20].

3.1. Search Strategy and Selection Criteria

A systematic review protocol was developed based on PRISMA-P and the PRISMA statement. Published articles from 1 December 2019, to 20 November 2020, were selected for review from 8 electronic databases (PubMed, CINAHL, Embase, medRxiv, Proquest, Wiley online library, Medline, and Nature).

The focus of the review was LPV/RTV treatment in COVID-19 patients. The primary outcome was the efficacy of LPV/RTV in COVID-19 patients. The secondary outcome was adverse events associated with its use.

3.2. Inclusion Criteria

Readily accessible peer-reviewed full articles, observational cohort studies, and clinical trials were included.

3.3. Participants

Patients with a positive SARS-CoV-2 reverse-transcription polymerase chain reaction (RT-PCR) test of any age were included.

3.4. Intervention

The interventions were LPV/RTV alone or in combination with standard care ± interferons/antiviral treatments compared to other therapies.

3.5. Objectives

A. Virological cure on day 7 after initiation of therapy (+ve to −ve polymerase chain reaction (PCR): non-detection of SARS-CoV-2 in nasopharyngeal swab).
B. Clinical cure (time to body temperature normalization and time to cough relief).
C. Radiological progression during drug treatment.
D. Mortality at 28 days and death during treatment at any time.
E. Safety and tolerability of lopinavir/ritonavir.

3.6. Comparisons

A. lopinavir/ritonavir vs. no antiviral therapy (conventional therapy)/control.
B. lopinavir/ritonavir in combination with other agents versus conventional therapy/control.

3.7. Searching Keywords

The search keywords included 2019-nCoV, 2019 novel coronavirus, COVID-19, coronavirus disease 2019, SARS-COV-2, lopinavir, ritonavir, combination, kaletra, treatment, efficacy, clinical trial, cohort, retrospective, and prospective.

3.8. Exclusion Criteria

Types of articles that were excluded included duplicate articles, editorials, reviews, case reports, and letters to editors.

Any research articles that did not include data on lopinavir/ritonavir use, did not include control patients' group, or reported combined use of lopinavir/ritonavir with other antiviral medications were also excluded. Given the lack of clear benefit and potential for toxicity of hydroxychloroquine [21], studies with evidence on the benefit of LPV/RTV in combination with hydroxychloroquine use in hospitalized COVID-19 patients were excluded in our review.

3.9. Data Extraction and Analysis

Two reviewers (SA and MT) independently screened the titles with abstracts using the selection criteria. For relevant articles, full texts were obtained for further evaluation. Disagreements between the two reviewers after full text screening were reconciled via consensus by a third reviewer (AA) [22].

Inclusions and exclusions were recorded following PRISMA guidelines presented in the form of a PRISMA flow diagram and detailed reasons recorded for exclusion. Articles were categorized as clinical trials or cohort studies. The following data were extracted from the selected studies: authors; publication year; study location; study design and setting; sample size, age, and gender; details of study intervention and control therapies in addition to data on adverse events and treatment outcomes; time from symptom onset to treatment initiation; assessment of study risk of bias; and remarks on notable findings.

3.10. Risk of Biased Evaluation of Included Studies

The quality assessment of the studies was undertaken based on the revised Cochrane risk of bias tool (RoB 2.0) for randomized controlled studies [23]. The Risk of bias in non-randomized studies—of interventions (ROBINS-I) tool was used to assess non-randomized interventional studies [24], and the Newcastle Ottawa Scale for observational cohort studies [25]. Critical appraisal checklists appropriate to each study design were applied and checked by a third team member.

Three investigators (SA, MT, and AA) separately evaluated the possibility of bias using these tools. Publication bias was not evaluated by funnel plot as there were only three studies that were included in the meta-analysis part of the study.

3.11. Assessment of Heterogeneity

Statistical heterogeneity was evaluated using the χ^2 test and I^2 statistics [19]. An I^2 value of 0 to <40% was not considered as significant, 30% to 60% was regarded as moderate heterogeneity, 50% to 90% was considered substantial heterogeneity, and 75% to 100% was considered significant heterogeneity.

3.12. Statistical Analysis

Because all of the data were continuous and dichotomous data, either odds ratio (OR) or mean difference were used for estimating the point estimate, along with a 95% confidence interval (CI). In the absence of significant clinical heterogeneity, the meta-analysis using the Mantel Hazel method or inverse variance method for dichotomous data and continuous data were performed, respectively. Employing a conservative approach, a random effects model was used, which produces wider CIs than a fixed effect model. Review Manager (Version 5.3, Oxford, UK; The Cochrane Collaboration, 2014) was used to conduct all statistical analyses and generate forest plots.

4. Results

A total of 8 literature databases were screened and 76 non-duplicate articles were identified, which were evaluated for possible inclusion using titles and abstracts. Out of these, 32 articles were selected for full-text screening and finally, 14 articles (total participants = 9036) were included in the systematic review, and eight articles were included in the meta-analysis; 18 articles were excluded following full-text screening (reasons: review = 5, study with no relative data = 6, LPV/RTV use data not available = 2, no control patients in the study = 1, combined LPV/RTV use with other antiviral therapies/other medications data = 2, no extractable data = 2). The PRISMA chart for the studies included is displayed in Figure 1. The details of the included studies are depicted in Table 1. Among these, two articles were in preprint versions [26,27].

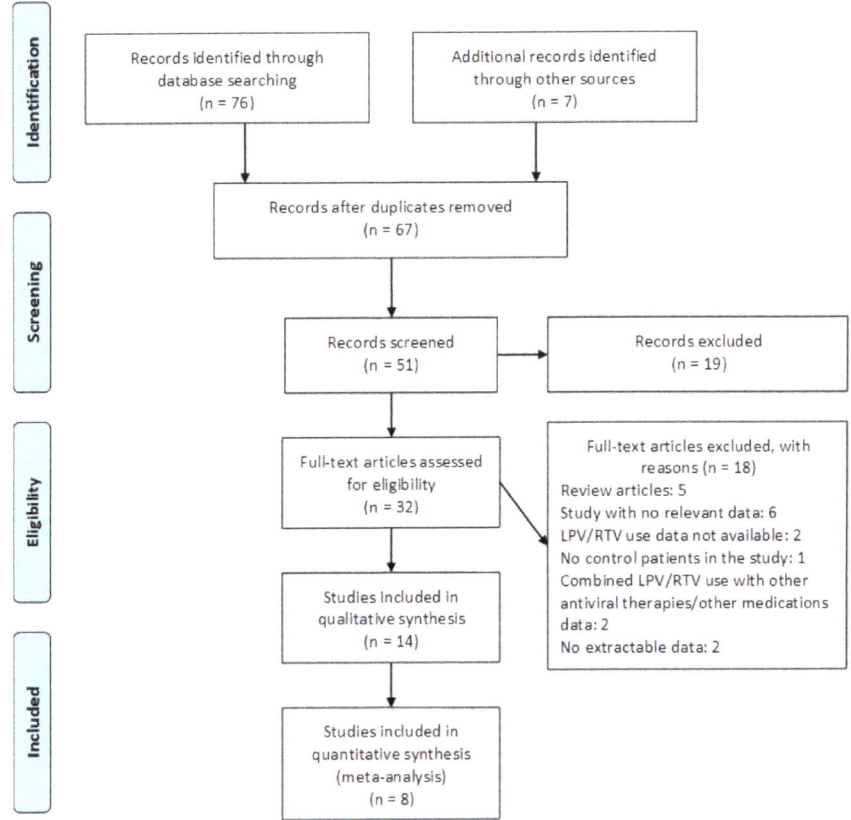

Figure 1. Preferred Reporting Items for Systematic reviews and Meta-Analysis (PRISMA) flow chart of the included studies. LPV/RTV, lopinavir/ritonavir.

Table 1. Data extracted from included papers ($n = 14$).

Author, Year [Reference] from, Study Location	Study Design and Setting	Age (Year)	Male, n (%)	Population	Intervention	Control	Time from Symptom Onset to Treatment Initiation	Outcome	AEs in LPV/RTV and Control Arm	Assessment of Study Risk of Bias (Tool Used; Finding)	Remark
Horby et al. 2020 [25]; United Kingdom	Randomized open-label controlled trial; multicenter	Mean (SD), 66.3 (15.9)	3077 (61.1)	Clinically suspected or laboratory confirmed SARS-CoV-2 infection cases of any age. Consistent characteristics across groups for age, sex, ethnicity, duration of symptoms before randomisation, amount of respiratory support at randomisation, and baseline predicted risk of death	1616 patients received: LPV/RTV (oral): 400 mg/100 mg twice daily for 10 days or until discharge, if sooner PLUS standard care * for 10 days or until discharge, if sooner	3424 patients received: Standard care alone * for 10 days or until discharge, if sooner	Not reported	Mortality at 28 days: 23% patients allocated to LPV/RTV and 22% patients allocated to usual care died within 28 days (RR 1.03, 95% CI 0.91–1.17; $p = 0.60$) Time until discharge alive from hospital: median 11 days [IQR 5 to >28] in both groups Patients discharged from hospital alive within 28 days: (RR 0.98, 95% CI 0.91–1.05; $p = 0.53$) Patients met the endpoint of invasive mechanical ventilation (RR 1.15, 95% CI 0.95–1.39; $p = 0.15$); or death (RR 1.04, 95% CI 0.93–1.16; $p = 0.54$)	In the LPV/RTV group, there was a serious case of elevated ALT that did not meet standard criteria for drug-induced liver injury. Detailed information on non-serious adverse reactions or reasons for stopping treatment were not collected	RoB 2, low risk of bias	LPV/RTV was not associated with reductions in 28-day mortality, duration of hospital stay, or risk of progressing to invasive mechanical ventilation or death Since preliminary results of RECOVERY trial were made public, WHO has halted the LPV/RTV monotherapy and the LPV/RTV plus IFN-b combination groups of the SOLIDARITY trial
Pan et al. 2020 [29]; Multi-country	Randomized open-label controlled trial; multicenter	<50 years: 36.5% 50–69 years: 7% 70+ years: 20.8%	1653 (59.6)	Hospitalized confirmed COVID-19 cases aged ≥18 years and not known to have received any study drug. Patient characteristics were well balanced between the two groups	1399 patients received: LPV/RTV (oral): 400 mg/100 mg twice daily for 10 days	1372 patients received: standard care *	Not reported	Death (with 95% CIs and numbers dead/randomized, LPV/RTV vs. its control) was: RR 1.00 (0.79–1.25, $p = 0.97$; 148/1399 vs. 146/1372). Initiation of ventilation: 124 (LPV/RTV) vs. 119 (control). Patients still hospitalized at day 7: 68% (LPV/RTV) vs. 59% (control)	No death was attributed to LPV/RTV due to renal or hepatic disease	RoB 2, low risk of bias	LPV/RTV did not reduce mortality (in unventilated patients or any other subgroup of entry characteristics), initiation of ventilation or hospitalization duration
Cai et al. 2020 [30]; China	Nonrandomized open-label controlled trial; single center	Median (IQR), 47 (35.7–61)	35 (43.8)	Confirmed COVID-19 cases aged 16–75 years. No significant differences between the baseline characteristics of the two arms. FPV treated patients were older (43 years) compared with LPV/RTV arm (49 years). All patients were moderate cases as defined by NHC [1]	45 patients received: FPV (oral): 1600 mg twice daily on Day 1 and 600 mg twice daily on days 2–14 PLUS IFN-α1b (aerosol inhalation): 5 million IUs twice daily	35 patients received: FPV (oral): 1600 mg twice daily on Day 1 and 600 mg twice daily on days 2–14 PLUS IFN-α1b (aerosol inhalation): 5 million IUs twice daily	Less than 7 days	Viral clearance: shorter viral clearance time in FPV arm (median (IQR), 4 (2.5–9) days versus 11 (8–13) days, $p < 0.001$) Chest CT changes: more imaging improvement rate in FPV arm (91.43% vs. 62.22%), $p = 0.004$	FPV arm patients had less AEs compared to the LPV/RTV group (11.43% vs. 55.56%) ($p < 0.001$). Two patients had diarrhea, one had a liver injury, and one had a poor diet in the FPV arm. There were five patients with diarrhea, five with vomiting, six with nausea, four with rash, three with liver injury, and two with chest tightness and palpitations in the LPV/RTV arm	ROBINS-I, moderate risk of bias	Two patients in the FPV group turned negative for viral RNA detection in nasopharyngeal swabs at days 18 and 21 For patients in the LPV/RTV group, the viral RNA detection all turned negative within 27 days

Table 1. Cont.

Author, Year [Reference] from, Study Location	Study Design and Setting	Age (Year)	Male, n (%)	Population	Intervention	Control	Time from Symptom Onset to Treatment Initiation	Outcome	AEs in LPV/RTV and Control Arm	Assessment of Study Risk of Bias (Tool Used; Finding)	Remark
Cao et al. 2020 [15]; China	Randomized open-label controlled trial; single center	Median (IQR), 58 (49–68)	120 (60.3)	Confirmed COVID-19, having a SaO$_2$ of 94% or less or a ratio of the PaO$_2$ to the FiO$_2$ of less than 300 mmHg. No important between-group differences in demographic characteristics, baseline laboratory test results, distribution of ordinal scale scores, or NEWS2 scores at enrollment	99 patients received: LPV/RTV (oral): 400/100 mg twice daily PLUS standard care * for 14 days	100 patients received: standard care * alone for 14 days	13 days (IQR, 11 to 16 days)	Time to clinical improvement: no difference in the time to clinical improvement for patients in the LPV/RTV group and the standard-care * group (HR for clinical improvement, 1.31; 95% CI, 0.95 to 1.80). Mortality at 28 days was similar in the two groups (19.2% vs. 25.0%; difference, −5.8 percentage points; 95% CI, −17.3 to 5.7). Percentages of patients with detectable viral RNA at various time points were similar. LPV/RTV led to a median time to clinical improvement that was shorter by 1 day than that observed with standard care * (HR, 1.39; 95% CI, 1.00 to 1.91)	GI AEs were more common in the LPV/RTV group, but serious AEs were more common in the standard care * group. LPV/RTV treatment was stopped early in 13.8% because of AEs	RoB 2, low risk of bias	Most patients were severely unwell and required urgent clinical attention. Systemic glucocorticoids were administered (33.0% in patients of LPV/RTV group and 35.7% in patients of standard-care * alone group)
Hung et al. 2020 [3]; Hong Kong	Randomized open-label trial; multicenter	Median (IQR), 52 (32–62)	68 (54)	Confirmed COVID-19 cases and aged at least 18 years, a NEWS2 of at least 1, and symptom duration of 14 days or less upon recruitment. Age, sex, and baseline demographics in each group were similar	41 patients received: LPV/RTV (oral): 400/100 mg twice daily (control group) for 14 days	86 patients received: LPV/RTV (oral): 400/100 mg twice daily PLUS Ribavirin (oral): 400 twice daily PLUS IFN-beta-1b (SC): three doses of 8 million IUs of interferon beta-1b on alternate days (combination group); for 14 days	5 days (IQR 3–7)	Combination group had a significantly shorter median time from start of study treatment to negative nasopharyngeal swab (7 days [IQR 5–11]) than the LPV/RTV group (12 days [8–15]; HR 4.37 [95% CI 1.86–10.24], $p = 0.0010$)	AEs included nausea and diarrhea with no difference between the two groups. One patient discontinued LPV/RTV because of biochemical hepatitis	RoB 2, some concerns risk of bias	No patients died during the study

Table 1. Cont.

Author, Year [Reference] from, Study Location	Study Design and Setting	Age (Year)	Male, n (%)	Population	Intervention	Control	Time from Symptom Onset to Treatment Initiation	Outcome	AEs in LPV/RTV and Control Arm	Assessment of Study Risk of Bias (Tool Used; Finding)	Remark
Li et al. 2020 [27]; China	Randomized blinded trial; single center	Mean (SD), 49.4 (14.7)	40 (46.5)	Mild/moderate confirmed COVID-19 cases aged 18–80 years Baseline characteristics of the three groups were comparable	34 patients received: LPV/RTV (oral): 200/50 mg twice daily for 7–14 days	35 patients received: Umifenovir (oral): 200 mg three times daily for 7–14 days OR 17 patients received no antiviral therapy (conventional)	3.5 days (IQR, 2 to 6 days)	Rate of positive-to-negative conversion of SARS-CoV-2 nucleic acid was similar between groups (all $p > 0.05$). There were no differences between groups in the rates of antipyresis, cough alleviation, or improvement of chest CT at day 7 or 14 (all $p > 0.05$). At day 7, 23.5% patients in the LPV/RTV group, 8.6% in the umifenovir group, and 11.8% in the control group showed a deterioration in clinical status from moderate to severe/critical ($p = 0.206$)	Overall, 35.3% of patients in the LPV/RTV group and 14.3% in the umifenovir group experienced AEs No apparent AEs occurred in the control group	RoB 2, high risk of bias	Study was blinded to participants, physicians, and radiologists who reviewed data but open label to clinicians who recruited patients and research staff All three groups were treated with Standard care * if in need
Lan et al. 2020 [26]; China	Retrospective; cohort; multicenter	Mean (SD), 55.8 (15.2)	37 (50.7)	Confirmed COVID-19 cases treated with LPV/RTV alone or combined with umifenovir Different age, sex, and baseline demographics in each group	34 patients received: LPV/RTV (oral): 400/100 mg twice daily for 14 days	39 patients received: LPV/RTV (oral): 400/100 mg twice daily PLUS Umifenovir (oral): 200 mg three times daily; at least for 3 days	Not reported	Treatment with LPV/RTV alone was not different from LPV/RTV combined with umifenovir in overall cure rate (92.3% and 97.1%, respectively) LPV/RTV combined with umifenovir led to a median time of hospital stay that was shorter by 1.5 days (12.5 days vs. 14 days) COVID-19 RNA clearance was 92.3% in LPV/RTV and 97.1% in combination therapies group Mean time of virus turning negative was 11.5 ± 9.0 days in combination group compared to 9.9 ± 7.5 in single therapy group	Not reported	NOS, 5	All eligible patients received standard care * if necessary

Table 1. Cont.

Author, Year [Reference] from, Study Location	Study Design and Setting	Age (Year)	Male, n (%)	Population	Intervention	Control	Time from Symptom Onset to Treatment Initiation	Outcome	AEs in LPV/RTV and Control Arm	Assessment of Study Risk of Bias (Tool Used; Finding)	Remark
Wen et al. 2020 [32]; China	Retrospective; cohort; single center	Mean (SD), 49.9 (16.1)	81 (45.5)	Confirmed COVID-19 cases aged ≥18 years with a hospital stay longer than 14 days. No statistically significant difference in baseline characteristics before treatment between patients in LPV/RTV group, umifenovir group, combination (LPV/RTV and umifenovir) group and conventional treatment (no antiviral therapy) group	59 patients received: LPV/RTV (oral): 200/50 mg twice daily for 7 days	36 patients received: Umifenovir (oral): 200 mg, three times daily for 7 days OR 25 patients received: Combined antiviral therapies (LPV/RTV AND umifenovir; same dosages for 7 days) OR 58 patients received no antiviral therapy (conventional group)	Not reported	Time for pharyngeal swab PCR to turn negative was (10.20 ± 3.49 days) in LPV/RTV group, (10.11 ± 4.68 days) in umifenovir group, (10.86 ± 4.74 days) in LPV/RTV plus umifenovir group, and (8.44 ± 3.51 days) in conventional group. No significant difference in the rate of nasopharyngeal swab new coronavirus nucleic acid conversion, clinical symptom improvement rate, and lung infection imaging improvement rate ($p > 0.05$). There was a statistically significant difference in the ratio of normal/mild to severely/critically severe on the 7th day in the four groups ($\chi^2 = 9.311, p = 0.017$): the combined group (24.0%), umifenovir group (16.7%), LPV/RTV group (5.4%), conventional treatment group (5.2%)	AEs in the three groups of patients using antiviral drugs was significantly higher than that in the conventional treatment group ($\chi^2 = 14.875, p = 0.002$)	NOS, 5	All three groups were treated with standard care * if in need
Jun et al. 2020 [33]; China	Retrospective; cohort; single center	Median (IQR), 48 (35–62)	69 (51.5)	Confirmed COVID-19 cases. No statistically significant differences in the demographic data, clinical manifestations, laboratory examinations, and chest CT examination of patients in the LPV/RTV group, umifenovir group, and control (no antiviral therapy) group (all $p > 0.05$)	52 patients received: LPV/RTV (oral): 200/50 mg twice daily for 5 days	34 patients received: Umifenovir (oral): 200 mg three times daily for 5 days OR 48 patients received no antiviral therapy (conventional group)	Not reported	Median time for the body temperature to return to normal in the umifenovir group and the LPV/RTV group was 6 days, and the conventional group was 4 days ($\chi^2 = 2.37, p = 0.31$). Median time of viral nucleic acid negative in respiratory tract specimens of the three groups was 7 days after treatment. Viral nucleic acid negative in the LPV/RTV group was 71.8% and 82.6% in the umifenovir group, the conventional group was 77.1% ($\chi^2 = 0.46, p = 0.79$). 42.3% patients in the LPV/RTV group, 35.3% patients in the umifenovir group, and 52.1% patients in the conventional group still had progressive imaging on the 7th day after treatment ($\chi^2 = 2.28, p = 0.30$)	17.3% in the LPV/RTV group had AEs, including nausea, diarrhea, and other GI symptoms; 8.8% in the umifenovir group had AEs, including diarrhea; 8.3% in the control group had AEs such as anorexia and diarrhea ($\chi^2 = 2.33, p = 0.33$)	NOS, 5	All patients received IFN α2b spray therapy and standard care *

Table 1. Cont.

Author, Year [Reference], Study Location	Study Design and Setting	Age (Year)	Male, n (%)	Population	Intervention	Control	Time from Symptom Onset to Treatment Initiation	Outcome	AEs in LPV/RTV and Control Arm	Assessment of Study Risk of Bias (Tool Used; Finding)	Remark
Yan et al. 2020 [34]; China	Retrospective; cohort; single center	Median (IQR), 52 (35–63)	54 (45)	Confirmed COVID-19 cases and had the available RNA viral data to estimate the duration of viral shedding	78 patients received: LPV/RTV (oral): 200/50 mg twice daily for 10 days or more	42 patients received no antiviral therapy (conventional group)	10 days (IQR 7–13)	Median duration of viral shedding was shorter in the LPV/RTV treatment group than that in no LPV/RTV treatment group (median, 22 days vs. 28.5 days, $p = 0.02$). Patients who started LPV/RTV treatment within 10 days from symptom onset had a shorter duration of SARS-CoV-2 RNA shedding than other patients who began after 10 days (median 19 days vs. 27.5 days, $p < 0.001$)	Not reported	NOS, 5	Many patients received and standard care * if in need
Yuan et al. 2020 [35]; China	Retrospective; cohort; single center	Median (range), 40 (1–78)	42 (45)	Confirmed COVID-19 cases of mild and/or moderate symptoms and critical conditions Significant different illness onset on the most common symptoms (fever, fatigue, and diarrhea)	46 patients received: LPV/RTV+ IFN-α (dosages, durations were not reported)	41 patients received: IFN-α + LPV/RTV PLUS Ribavirin; (dosages, durations were not reported)	Not reported	No significant difference in average LOS or PCR negative conversion times among different antivirus treatment groups. Correlation analysis indicated that the duration of hospital stay was significantly correlated with PCR negative conversion times in IFN-α + lopinavir/ritonavir + ribavirin group ($p = 0.0215$), as well as IFN-α + lopinavir/ritonavir group ($p = 0.012$). Average LOS and IFN treatment duration of moderate group was 14.12 (13.34–14.90) days and 14.24 (13.45–15.03) days, respectively, while those of the severe group took average 2.08 days and 1.44 days longer	Not reported	NOS, 6	Approximately 51% were aged ≤40 year, including 2 children under 3 year
Zhu et al. 2020 [36]; China	Retrospective; cohort; multicenter	Mean (SD), 39.8 (17.6)	26 (52)	Confirmed COVID-19 cases No significant difference in age and sex between the two groups	34 patients received: LPV/RTV (oral): 200/50 mg twice daily for 7 days	16 patients received: Umifenovir (oral): 200 mg three times daily (duration was not reported)	Not reported	No difference in fever duration between the two groups ($p = 0.61$). On day 14 after the admission, no viral load was detected in umifenovir group, but the viral load was found in 44.1% of patients treated with LPV/RTV. Patients in the umifenovir group had a shorter duration of positive RNA test compared to those in the LPV/RTV group ($p < 0.01$)	No apparent SEs were found in both groups	NOS, 6	All patients received and standard care * if in need

Table 1. Cont.

Author, Year [Reference] from, Study Location	Study Design and Setting	Age (Year)	Male, n (%)	Population	Intervention	Control	Time from Symptom Onset to Treatment Initiation	Outcome	AEs in LPV/RTV and Control Arm	Assessment of Study Risk of Bias (Tool Used; Finding)	Remark
Ye et al. 2020 [37]; China	Retrospective; cohort; single center	Range (5–68), of which 9 were <30 and 38 were >30	22 (46.8)	Confirmed COVID-19 cases treated with LPV/RTV or not during hospitalization. Different age, sex, and baseline demographics in each group	42 patients received: LPV/RTV (oral): 400/100 mg twice daily or 800/200 mg once daily PLUS Umifenovir (oral): 200 mg three times daily PLUS IFN-α1b (aerosol inhalation): 5 million IUs twice daily; (durations of use were not reported)	5 patients received: Umifenovir (oral): 200 mg three times daily PLUS IFN-α1b (aerosol inhalation): 5 million IUs twice daily; (durations of use were not reported)	Not reported	Patients in the LPV/RTV group returned to normal body temperature in a shorter time (test group: 4.8 ± 1.94 days vs. control group: 7.3 ± 1.53 days, $p = 0.0364$) Patients in the LPV/RTV group were able to turn negative in a shorter period of time (LPV/RTV group: 7.8 ± 3.09 days vs. control group: 12.0 ± 0.82 days, $p = 0.0219$)	Increased level of ALT enzyme in the LPV/RTV group	NOS, 5	All patients received and standard care * if in need
Deng et al. 2020 [38]; China	Retrospective; cohort; single center	Mean (SD), 44.6 (15.8)	17 (51.5)	Confirmed COVID-19 cases of adults (≥ 18 years) with laboratory-confirmed COVID-19 without invasive ventilation. Baseline clinical, laboratory, and chest CT characteristics were similar between groups	17 patients received: LPV/RTV (oral): 400/100 mg twice daily	16 patients received: LPV/RTV (oral): 400/100 mg twice daily PLUS Umifenovir (oral): 200 mg three times daily (until coronavirus is detected negative by RT-PCR for three times)	Not reported	SARS-CoV-2 could not be detected for 75% of patients' nasopharyngeal specimens in the combination group after 7 days, compared with 35% in the monotherapy group ($p < 0.05$). After 14 days, 94% in the combination group and 52.9% in the monotherapy group, respectively, SARS-CoV-2 could not be detected ($p < 0.05$) Chest CT scans were improving for 69% of patients in the combination group after seven days, compared with 29% in the monotherapy group ($p < 0.05$)	Elevated levels of bilirubin in patients (68.7%) Digestive upsets, such as mild diarrhea and nausea were reported in patients (43.7%)	NOS, 6	All patients received and standard care * if in need. Authors never stated which therapy group experienced AEs

Abbreviations: AEs, adverse events; ALT, alanine aminotransferase; CI, confidence interval; COVID-19, coronavirus disease 2019; CT, computed tomography; FiO2, fraction of inspired oxygen; FPV, favipiravir; GI, gastrointestinal; HR, hazard ratio; IFN, interferon; IQR, interquartile range; ITT, intention-to-treat; IUs, international units; LOS, length of hospital stay; LPV/RTV, lopinavir/ritonavir; NA, not applicable; NEWS2, National Early Warning Score 2; NHC, National Health Commission of China; NOS, Newcastle Ottawa Scale; PaO2, partial pressure of oxygen; RR, rate ratio; RoB 2, Version 2 of the Cochrane risk-of-bias tool for randomized trials; ROBINS-I, Risk of bias in non-randomized studies—of interventions; RT-PCR, real-time reverse transcription-polymerase chain reaction; SaO2, oxygen saturation; SARS-CoV-2, severe acute respiratory syndrome coronavirus 2; SCI, subcutaneous injection; SEs, side effects. * Standard care comprised, as necessary, supplemental oxygen, non-invasive and invasive ventilation, antibiotic agents, vasopressor support, renal replacement therapy, and extracorporeal membrane oxygenation (ECMO).

4.1. Comparison 1: Efficacy and Safety of Lopinavir-Ritonavir (LPV/RTV) versus No Antiviral Therapy (Conventional Therapy) or Control

A total of eight studies [26–29,32–34,36] reported on LPV/RTV versus no antiviral therapy (conventional therapy) or control ($n = 8405$) in terms of efficacy and safety.

4.1.1. Virological Cure on Day 7 Post-Initiation of Therapy (+ve to −ve PCR: Non-Detection of Severe Acute Respiratory Syndrome Coronavirus 2 (SARS-CoV-2) in Nasopharyngeal Swab)

LPV/RTV Versus No Antiviral Therapy (Conventional Cure): Virologic Cure at Day 7 Post-Initiation of Therapy

Three studies reported on virological cure ($n = 171$ in LPV/RTV alone arm vs. $n = 117$ in conventional arm) on day 7 [27,32,34]. Significant mean difference was observed between the two arms in terms of virological cure (mean difference = −0.81 day; 95% CI, −4.44 to 2.81; $p = 0.007$, $I^2 = 80\%$; Figure 2).

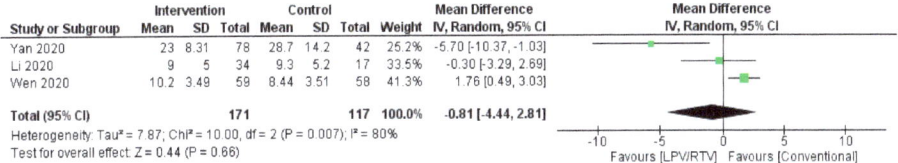

Figure 2. Time from +ve to −ve PCR (days) (LPV/RTV vs no antiviral treatment or conventional). CI, confidence interval; df, degrees of freedom; lopinavir/ritonavir (LPV/RTV).

LPV/RTV vs. Umifenovir: Virologic Cure at Day 7 Post-Initiation of Therapy

Three studies reported on virological cure ($n = 127$ in LPV/RTV alone arm vs. $n = 87$ in umifenovir arm) on day 7 [27,32,36]. No significant mean difference was observed between the two arms in terms of virological cure (mean difference = 0.95 day; 95% CI, −1.11 to 3.01; $p = 0.09$, $I^2 = 58\%$; Figure 3).

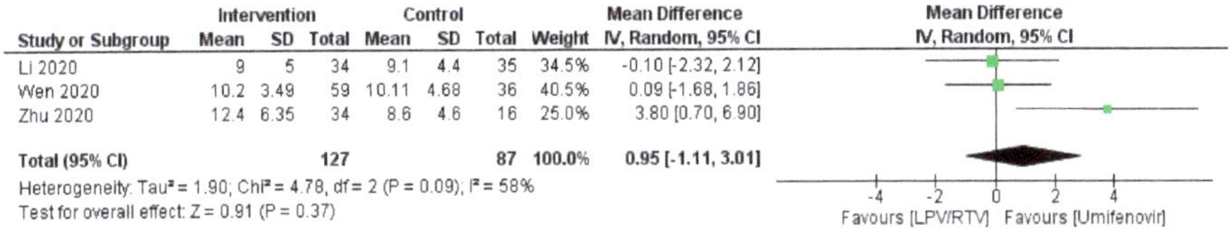

Figure 3. Time from +ve to −ve PCR (days) (LPV/RTV vs. umifenovir). CI, confidence interval; df, degrees of freedom; LPV/RTV, lopinavir/ritonavir.

LPV/RTV vs. Umifenovir Plus Lopinavir/Ritonavir: Virologic Cure at Day 7 Post-Initiation of Therapy

Two studies reported on virological cure ($n = 93$ in LPV/RTV alone arm vs. $n = 75$ in umifenovir plus LPV/RTV arm) on day 7 [26,32]. No significant mean difference was observed between the two arms in terms of virological cure (mean difference = −0.83 day; 95% CI, −2.45 to 0.78; $p = 0.66$, $I^2 = 0\%$; Figure 4).

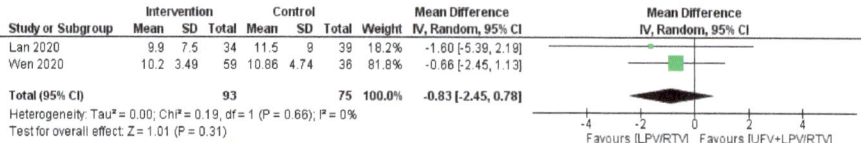

Figure 4. Time from +ve to−ve PCR (days) (LPV/RTV vs LPV/RTV plus umifenovir combination). CI, confidence interval; df, degrees of freedom; LPV/RTV, lopinavir/ritonavir; UFV, umifenovir.

4.1.2. Clinical Cure (Time to Body Temperature Normalization and Time to Cough Relief)

Time to Body Temperature Normalization

1. LPV/RTV vs. Umifenovir

Two studies reported on time to temperature normalization ($n = 93$ in LPV/RTV alone arm vs. $n = 71$ in umifenovir arm) [27,32]. No significant association was observed between the two arms in terms of temperature normalization (OR = 0.87 day; 95% CI, 0.42 to 1.78; $p = 0.61$, $I^2 = 0\%$; Figure 5).

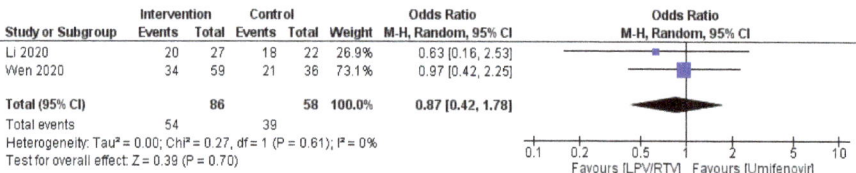

Figure 5. Time to body temperature normalization (days) (LPV/RTV vs umifenovir). CI, confidence interval; df, degrees of freedom; LPV/RTV, lopinavir/ritonavir.

2. LPV/RTV versus No Antiviral Therapy (Conventional)

Two studies reported on time to temperature normalization ($n = 93$ in LPV/RTV alone arm vs. $n = 75$ in conventional arm) [27,32]. No significant association was observed between the two arms in terms of temperature normalization (OR = 0.99 day; 95% CI, 0.49 to 1.99, $p = 0.35$, $I^2 = 0\%$; Figure 6).

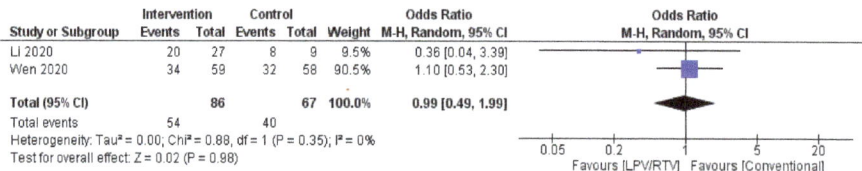

Figure 6. Time to body temperature normalization (days) (LPV/RTV vs. no antiviral treatment or conventional). CI, confidence interval; df, degrees of freedom; LPV/RTV, lopinavir/ritonavir.

Duration of Cough

1. LPV/RTV Versus Umifenovir: Rate of Cough Alleviation after 7 Days of Therapy

Two studies reported on cough alleviation ($n = 93$ in LPV/RTV alone arm vs. $n = 71$ in umifenovir arm) [27,32]. LPV/RTV alone arm had a significant lower number of cough days by 0.62 (95% CI 0.06 to 6.53, $p = 0.02$; $I^2 = 81\%$; Figure 7).

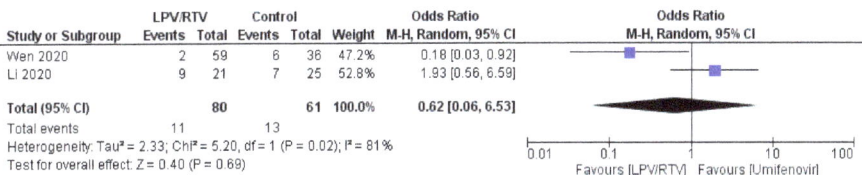

Figure 7. Rate of cough alleviation after 7 days of treatment (LPV/RTV vs. umifenovir). CI, confidence interval; df, degrees of freedom; LPV/RTV, lopinavir/ritonavir.

2. LPV/RTV vs. No Antiviral Therapy (Conventional): Rate of Cough Alleviation after 7 Days of Therapy

Two studies reported on cough alleviation ($n = 93$ in LPV/RTV alone arm vs. $n = 75$ in conventional arm) [27,32]. No significant association was observed between the two arms in terms of cough alleviation (OR = 0.87 day; 95% CI, 0.10 to 7.16; $p = 0.08$, $I^2 = 67\%$; Figure 8).

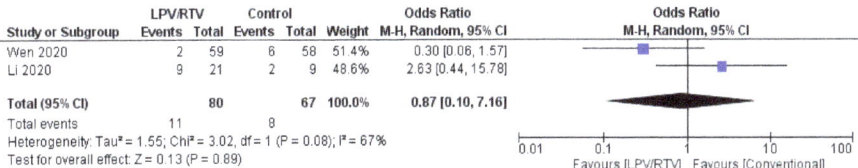

Figure 8. Rate of cough alleviation after 7 days of treatment (LPV/RTV vs. no antiviral treatment or conventional). CI, confidence interval; df, degrees of freedom; LPV/RTV, lopinavir/ritonavir.

4.1.3. Radiological Progression during Drug Treatment

Rate of Improvement on Chest Computed Tomography (CT) after 7 Days of Treatment

1. LPV/RTV vs. Umifenovir

In terms of CT evidence for radiological progression of pneumonia/lung damage ($n = 59$ in the LPV/RTV arm vs. $n = 71$ in the umifenovir arm), treatment with LPV/RTV resulted in no significant decrease in the radiological progression (OR = 0.80; 95% CI, 0.42 to 1.54; $p = 0.59$, $I^2 = 81\%$; Figure 9) [27,32].

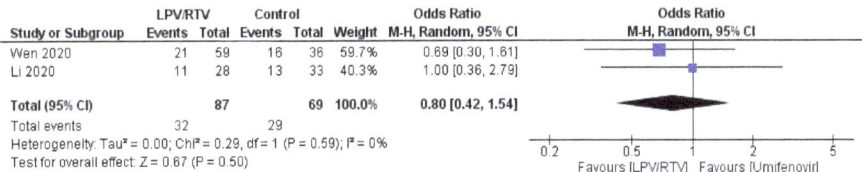

Figure 9. Rate of improvement on chest CT after 7 days of treatment (LPV/RTV vs. umifenovir). CI, confidence interval; df, degrees of freedom; LPV/RTV, lopinavir/ritonavir.

2. LPV/RTV vs. No Antiviral Therapy (Conventional)

In terms of CT evidence for radiological progression of pneumonia/lung damage ($n = 71$ in the LPV/RTV arm vs. $n = 75$ in conventional arm), treatment with LPV/RTV resulted in no significant decrease in the radiological progression (OR = 0.69; 95% CI, 0.36 to 1.31; $p = 0.42$, $I^2 = 0\%$; Figure 10) [27,32].

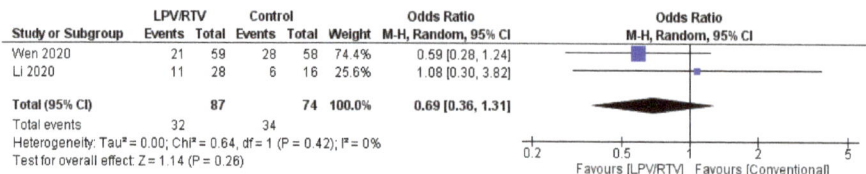

Figure 10. Rate of improvement on chest CT after 7 days of treatment (LPV/RTV vs. no antiviral treatment or conventional). CI, confidence interval; df, degrees of freedom; LPV/RTV, lopinavir/ritonavir.

4.1.4. Mortality at 28 Days and Death during Treatment at Any Time

Mortality at 28 Days

1. LPV/RTV vs. Standard of Care

Two trials reported on mortality at 28 days (n = 1715 in LPV/RTV plus standard of care arm vs. n = 3524 in standard of care arm) [15,28]. No significant association was observed between the two arms in terms of mortality at 28 days (OR = 1.00; 95% CI, 0.79 to 1.26; p = 0.28, I^2 = 15%; Figure 11).

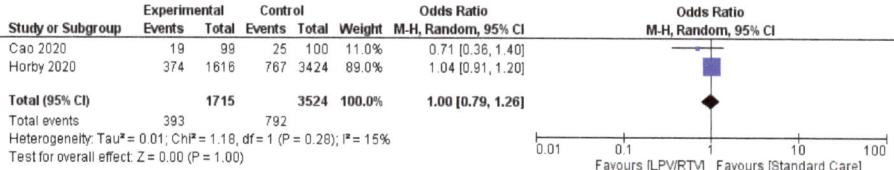

Figure 11. Rate of mortality at 28 days (LPV/RTV plus standard of care vs. standard of care alone). CI, confidence interval; df, degrees of freedom; LPV/RTV, lopinavir/ritonavir.

Death during Treatment at Any Time

1. LPV/RTV vs. Standard of Care

Two large trials reported on death during treatment at any time (n = 3015 in LPV/RTV plus standard of care arm vs. n = 4796 in standard of care arm) [28,29]. No significant association was observed between the two arms in terms of death during treatment at any time (OR = 1.03; 95% CI, 0.93 to 1.14; p = 0.78, I^2 = 0%; Figure 12).

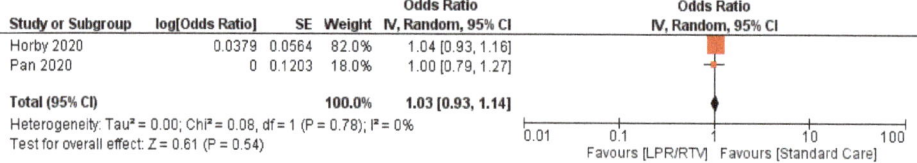

Figure 12. Rate of mortality at 28 days (LPV/RTV plus standard of care vs. standard of care alone). CI, confidence interval; df, degrees of freedom; LPV/RTV, lopinavir/ritonavir.

4.1.5. Safety and Tolerability

Rate of Adverse Events of Treatment: LPV/RTV vs. Umifenovir

A greater number of adverse events were reported in the LPV/RTV arms (n = 45) compared to the umifenovir groups (n = 14) (OR = 2.66; 95% CI, 1.36 to 5.19; p = 0.44, I^2 = 0%; Figure 13) [27,32,33].

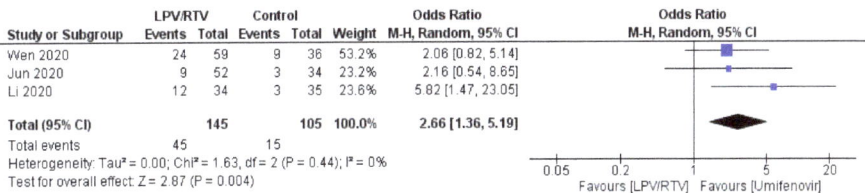

Figure 13. Rate of adverse events of treatment (LPV/RTV vs. umifenovir). CI, confidence interval; df, degrees of freedom; LPV/RTV, lopinavir/ritonavir.

Rate of Adverse Events of Treatment: LPV/RTV vs. No Antiviral Treatment (Conventional)

A greater number of adverse events were reported in the LPV/RTV arms ($n = 45$) compared to the no antiviral treatment or conventional arms ($n = 10$) (OR = 4.6; 95% CI, 1.91 to 11.07; $p = 0.29$, $I^2 = 18\%$; Figure 14) [27,32,33].

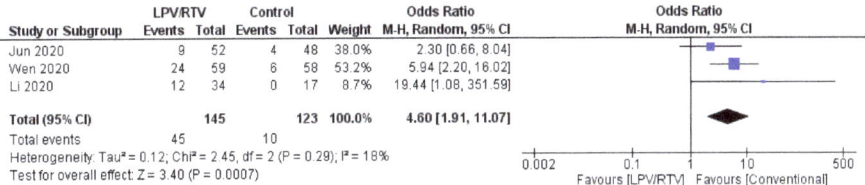

Figure 14. Rate of adverse events of treatment (LPV/RTV vs. no antiviral treatment or conventional). CI, confidence interval; df, degrees of freedom; LPV/RTV, lopinavir/ritonavir.

4.2. Comparison 2: Efficacy and Safety of LPV/RTV along in Combination with Other Agents versus No Antiviral Therapy (Conventional Therapy) or Control

A total of four studies evaluated the efficacy of LPV/RTV plus interferon (IFN) [30,31,35,37] and three studies [30,31,37] evaluated the safety of the combination. Other studies evaluated the efficacy of LPV/RTV plus standard care [15,28], ribavirin [31], or umifenovir [26,32,37], and evaluated the safety of these combinations.

In terms of the efficacy of the combination in patients with COVID-19, LPV/RTV plus IFN combination in addition to ribavirin was safe and superior to LPV/RTV alone by shortening the median time from the start of study treatment to negative nasopharyngeal swab (7 days [IQR 5–11]) compared to the LPV/RTV arm (12 days [IQR 8–15]; hazard ratio 4.37 [95% CI 1.86–10.24], $p = 0.001$) [31]. Additionally, combination treatment with LPV/RTV plus IFN and umifenovir had a more evident therapeutic effect in a shorter time by normalizing body temperature (4.8 ± 1.94 days vs. 7.3 ± 1.53 days, $p = 0.03$) and turning PCRs negative (7.8 ± 3.09 days vs. 12.0 ± 0.82 days, $p = 0.02$) compared to the umifenovir plus IFN arm with no evident toxic and side effects [37]. However, the use of LPV/RTV plus IFN combination resulted in fewer therapeutic responses on COVID-19 in terms of viral clearance [median (interquartile range, IQR), 4 (2.5–9) d versus 11 (8–13) d, $p < 0.001$] and chest CT changes (91.43% vs. 62.22%), $p = 0.004$] compared to the favipiravir plus IFN combination. Favipiravir arm patients had fewer adverse events (AEs) compared to the LPV/RTV arm (11.43% vs. 55.56%) ($p < 0.001$) [30]. Additionally, no significant difference in average PCR negative conversion times among IFN plus LPV/RTV or IFN plus LPV/RTV plus ribavirin treatment arms [35]. In another cohort study, more patients turned SARS-CoV-2 PCR negative in the LPV/RTV plus umifenovir combination group compared to the LPV/RTV monotherapy group (after 7 days: 75% vs. 35% of patients were PCR negative in the combination therapy and monotherapy, respectively, $p < 0.05$; and after 14 days: 94% vs. 52.9% of patients were PCR negative in the combination therapy and monotherapy, respectively, $p < 0.05$) [38]. Moreover, chest CT scans were improving for 69% of patients in the combination group after seven days, compared with 29% in the monotherapy group ($p < 0.05$) [38].

The combination of LPV/RTV, in addition to standard care, or standard care alone exhibited no difference in the time to clinical improvement (hazard ratio for clinical improvement, 1.31; 95% CI, 0.95 to 1.80) with similar 28-day mortality (19.2% vs. 25.0%; difference, −5.8 percentage points; 95% CI, −17.3 to 5.7) [15]. In another recent large study, LPV/RTV combined with standard care was not associated with reductions in 28-day mortality, duration of hospital stay, or risk of progressing to invasive mechanical ventilation or death [28].

5. Discussion

This systematic review included 14 articles relating to the efficacy and safety of LPV/RTV in COVID-19 patients, with a total of 9036 patients included, and only eight articles, that comprised 8438 patients had findings on the efficacy and safety of LPV/RTV alone or in combination with standard care ± interferons/antiviral treatments compared to other therapies in the treatment of COVID-19, were deemed legible for quantitative synthesis (meta-analysis) [26–29,32–34,36].

In terms of virological cure, three studies reported less time in days for LPV/RTV arm ($n = 171$) compared with no antiviral therapy (conventional) ($n = 117$); however, the overall effect was not significant (mean difference = −0.81 day; 95% CI, −4.44 to 2.81; $p = 0.66$), similarly the virological cure for LPV/RTV alone ($n = 127$) versus the umifenovir arm ($n = 87$) ($p = 0.37$), or LPV/RTV versus umifenovir plus LPV/RTV ($p = 0.31$) [26,27,32–34,36].

Two studies reported no significant effect on time to temperature normalization for LPV/RTV arm ($n = 93$) versus umifenovir arm ($n = 71$) (OR = 0.87 day; 95% CI, 0.42 to 1.78; $p = 0.70$, $I^2 = 0\%$); or alleviation of cough duration ($p = 0.69$) [27,32]. The total number of cough days was found to be lower in the LPV/RTV arm compared with the umifenovir arm or no antiviral therapy (conventional) arm after 7 days of treatment; however, the overall effect was found to be not significant [27,32]. Although a favorable therapeutic effect for umifenovir was observed in a small cohort study when the drug was combined with LPV/RTV treatment in ($n = 16$) COVID-19 patients rather than LPV/RTV alone ($n = 17$) [38]; it should be noted that the treatment of LPV/RTV alone groups ($n = 127$) versus umifenovir plus LPV/RTV groups ($n = 69$) did not reveal any significant mean difference between the two groups in terms of virological cure at day seven [26,32,37]. In another study that involved 81 COVID-19 patients, the umifenovir treatment group had a longer hospital stay than patients in the control group (13 days (IQR 9–17) vs. 11 days (IQR 9–14), $p = 0.04$) [39]. Of note, umifenovir, which is branded as Arbidol®, has a wide antiviral activity against RNA and DNA viruses, is licensed in Russia and China for the treatment and prophylaxis of influenza and recommended for treatment of MERS-CoV, was investigated in SARS-CoV, and is currently being trialed in COVID-19 patients [40].

In terms of CT evidence for radiological progression of pneumonia/lung damage, fewer patients exhibited radiological progression in the LPV/RTV arm compared with the umifenovir arm or no antiviral therapy (conventional) arm after 7 days of treatment, this effect was not significant ($p = 0.59$), and similarly, with LPV/RTV ($n = 71$) versus no antiviral therapy [27,32].

It is worth mentioning that initiating therapy earlier is known to be more effective [41], since systemic hyperinflammation rather than viral pathogenicity dominates later stages of SARS-CoV-2 infection. Although patients in five of the studies [15,27,30,31,34] included in our review were administered LPV/RTV early in the infection (median of <7 days); LPV/RTV therapy was not found to be totally effective.

In terms of safety, this study found greater adverse events reported in the LPV/RTV arm versus no antiviral treatment (conventional) or umifenovir, respectively. Adverse events associated with LPV/RTV alone or in combination with other medicines were reported in COVID-19 patients, and were typically gastrointestinal (GIT) in nature, including nausea, vomiting, and diarrhea [32]; nevertheless, serious GIT adverse drug reactions such as acute gastritis and GIT bleeding and acute kidney injury ($n = 3$) were also reported [32]. It was reported that most ADRs associated with LPV/RTV in combined groups of medicines are resolved within three days of drug initiation [30].

To address the efficacy and safety of LPV/RTV combined with other drugs in patients with COVID-9, LPV/RTV plus IFN combination in addition to ribavirin was found to be superior and safer than LPV/RTV alone by shortening the time to negative nasopharyngeal swab compared to the LPV/RTV arm alone [31]. Additionally, a combined treatment regimen of LPV/RTV plus IFN and umifenovir resulted in a shorter time by normalizing body temperature and turning PCRs negative compared to the umifenovir plus IFN arm with reasonable safety profile [37]. However, the use of LPV/RTV plus IFN combination resulted in less therapeutic responses on COVID-19 in terms of viral clearance and chest CT changes compared to the favipiravir plus IFN combination. Favipiravir arm patients had fewer AEs than patients in the LPV/RTV arm [30]. Additionally, there was no significant difference in average PCR negative conversion times among IFN plus LPV/RTV or IFN plus LPV/RTV plus ribavirin treatment arms [35]. The combination of LPV/RTV, in addition to standard care, or standard care alone revealed no difference in the time to clinical improvement, duration of hospitalization, initiation of invasive mechanical ventilation and death [15,28,29]. A serious case of elevated alanine aminotransferase (ALT) was reported [28], GI AEs were more common in the LPV/RTV group and treatment was stopped early in 13.8% because of AEs [15].

In a recent systematic review that included 41 studies which considered therapeutics for COVID-19, LPV/RTV was found to be the third therapy associated with positive outcomes (54.9%) with less negative outcomes (12.3%) compared to systemic corticosteroids (21.3%), remdesivir (16.9%), moxifloxacin (13.4%) and oseltamivir (12.5%) [2]; however, further controlled studies were needed to draw a valid conclusion. Antiviral ineffectiveness of LPV/RTV against SARS-CoV-2 in the studies included in our review was justified by the necessity to give the drug at a daily amount higher than 800 mg/200 mg; as an in vitro analysis identified antiviral activity of LPV/RTV against SARS-CoV-2 with a half-maximal effective concentration (EC_{50}) of 16.4 µg/mL [42]. However, there is a potential to intoxicate the patient, because high doses of LPV/RTV may lead to delayed ventricular repolarisation (QT prolongation) [7]. Thus, it might be logical to argue that there is a need to determine the effective and safe dose of LPV/RTV against the SARS-CoV-2 virus for better clinical benefit [13].

It is important to consider drug concentrations at the site of infection, and currently, the lack of robust lung penetration data is an important gap that exists for many agents being considered for repurposing. In the case of LPV/RTV, lung penetration is complex and not well understood; however, typically it is the plasma-free fraction that is available to penetrate into tissues. Therefore, given its potency, lung penetration of LPV/RTV would have to be high to provide concentrations in the therapeutic range [43]. The antiviral activity in vivo is estimated by calculating the ratio of unbound drug concentrations achieved in the lung at the administered dose to the in vitro EC50 (R_{LTEC}) [44]. Even though the majority of the observed total LPV/RTV plasma concentrations in COVID-19 patients were above the published EC50 for SARS-CoV-2 [42], boosted LPV/RTV is unlikely to attain sufficient effective levels in the lung to inhibit the virus. Indeed, the largest trials of RECOVERY [28] and SOLIDARITY [29] found LPV/RTV had little or no effect on overall mortality, initiation of ventilation and duration of hospital stay in hospitalized patients.

There is uncertainty about the optimal approach to treat hospitalized COVID-19 patients. Management approaches are based on limited data and evolves rapidly as clinical data emerge. For patients with non-severe disease, care is primarily supportive, with close monitoring for disease progression. Remdesivir is suggested in hospitalized patients with severe disease (i.e., they have hypoxia) but who are not yet on oxygen [45,46]. For patients who are receiving supplemental oxygen (including those who are on high-flow oxygen and noninvasive ventilation), low-dose dexamethasone and, if available, remdesivir is/are suggested [47,48]. However, the optimal role of remdesivir remains uncertain, and some guidelines panels (including the WHO) suggest not using it in hospitalized patients because there is no clear evidence that it improves patient-important outcomes for hospitalized patients (e.g., mortality, need for mechanical ventilation). In general, use of LPV/RTV for treatment of SARS-CoV-2 in hospitalized patients is not suggested as several trials have failed to prove efficacy [15,28,29]. Evidence as to whether LPV/RTV is beneficial in outpatients with mild or moderate severity COVID-19 infection is lacking; therefore, use of LPV/RTV is suggested in outpatients only in the context of a clinical trial.

Vaccines to prevent COVID-19 infection are considered the most promising approach for controlling the pandemic. COVID-19 vaccine development is occurring at an unprecedented pace. Several different platforms are being utilized to develop COVID-19 vaccines such as: inactivated virus or live-attenuated virus platforms (traditional methods); recombinant proteins and vector vaccines (newer methods); and RNA and DNA vaccines (methods never previously employed in a licensed vaccine) [49]. Several vaccine candidates have demonstrated immunogenicity without major safety concerns in early-phase human trials [50]. Two mRNA vaccine candidates have also been reported to have approximately 95% vaccine efficacy [51,52]. AstraZeneca's Oxford coronavirus vaccine is 70% effective on average, data shows, with no safety concerns [53]. Importantly, the AstraZeneca vaccine can be distributed and administered within existing healthcare systems, as it can be stored, transported and handled in normal refrigerated conditions for at least six months, the company said. The vaccine will also be cheaper than rival coronavirus vaccines from makers Pfizer and Moderna [53].

Since disease resulting from SARS-CoV infection is driven by both virus and host immune response factors, depending on the stage of the disease progression, early initiation of antiviral therapy, and/or holistic combination therapies will likely be needed to diminish virus replication, immunopathology, and/or promote repair and restoration of pulmonary homeostasis [54]. Until sufficient evidence is available, the WHO has warned against physicians and medical associations recommending or administering unproven treatments to patients with SARS-CoV-2 or people self-medicating with them.

The key limitations of this study were the limited number of clinical studies investigating the efficacy and safety of LPV/RTV in combination with a limited number of participants. Another limitation is the inability to perform any type of meta-analysis specifically for the results of efficacy and safety of using LPV/RTV in combination with other agents versus no antiviral therapy (conventional therapy) or control because of the large methodological differences. Despite these limitations, this systematic review provided valuable insight into the efficacy, safety, and clinical outcomes of LPV/RTV alone or with other antiviral medications.

6. Conclusions

The small number of studies included in this systematic review and meta-analysis study did not reveal any statistically significant advantage in the efficacy of LPV/RTV in COVID-19 patients, over no antiviral or other antiviral treatments. In terms of safety, this study found a greater number of adverse events reported in LPV/RTV arm versus no antiviral treatment (conventional) or umifenovir arms, respectively. There is a general understanding of the need to conduct large randomized clinical trials to determine the efficacy and safety of LPV/RTV in the treatment of COVID-19. Ideally, these studies should be double-blinded and conducted in a wide range of settings.

Author Contributions: M.T. conceived the study and, together with S.A. and A.A.M. designed and performed the study. The statistical analysis was performed by S.A. and the manuscript was written and reviewed by S.A., M.T., A.A.M., Z.A.A., N.A. and A.R.Z.Z. All authors have read and agreed to the published version of the manuscript.

Funding: This research received no external funding.

Acknowledgments: We would like to thank sauthors and their colleagues who contributed to the availability of evidence needed to compile this article. We would also like to thank the reviewers for very useful comments and suggestions for improving the paper.

Conflicts of Interest: The authors declare no conflict of interest.

Abbreviations

COVID-19	coronavirus disease 2019
SARS-CoV-2	severe acute respiratory syndrome coronavirus 2
MERS-CoV	Middle East respiratory syndrome coronavirus
LPV/RTV	lopinavir/ritonavir
PRISMA	Preferred Reporting Items for Systematic reviews and Meta-Analysis
RoB 2	Version 2 of the Cochrane risk-of-bias tool for randomized trials
ROBINS-I	Risk of bias in non-randomized studies—of interventions
RT-PCR	real-time reverse transcription-polymerase chain reaction

References

1. Yang, W.; Cao, Q.; Qin, L.; Wang, X.; Cheng, Z.; Pan, A.; Dai, J.; Sun, Q.; Zhao, F.; Qu, J. Clinical characteristics and imaging manifestations of the 2019 novel coronavirus disease (COVID-19): A multi-center study in Wenzhou city, Zhejiang, China. *J. Infect.* **2020**, *80*, 388–393. [CrossRef] [PubMed]
2. Tobaigy, M.; Qashqary, S.; Al-Dahery, A.; Mujallad, A.; Hershan, M.; Kamal, N. Therapeutic management of patients with COVID-19: A systematic review. *Infect. Prev. Pract.* **2020**, *2*, 100061. [CrossRef]
3. Statista. *Number of Coronavirus (COVID-19) Clinical Trials for Drugs and Vaccines Worldwide as of November 12, 2020, by Type*; Statista: Hamburg, Germany, 2020; Available online: https://www.statista.com/statistics/1119086/coronavirus-drug-trials-by-type-worldwide/?utm_campaign=Cureus%20U%20-%20Gastroenterology&utm_medium=email&utm_source=marketing_mailer (accessed on 26 November 2020).
4. Mehra, M.R.; Desai, S.S.; Ruschitzka, F.; Patel, A.N. Hydroxychloroquine or chloroquine with or without a macrolide for treatment of COVID-19: A multinational registry analysis. *Lancet* **2020**. [CrossRef]
5. Mehra, M.R.; Ruschitzka, F.; Patel, A.N. Retraction—Hydroxychloroquine or chloroquine with or without a macrolide for treatment of COVID-19: A multinational registry analysis. *Lancet* **2020**. [CrossRef]
6. *Coronavirus Updates: Trials to Resume of Anti-Viral Touted by Trump*; BBC News: London, UK, 2020.
7. Cortegiani, A.; Ippolito, M.; Ingoglia, G.; Iozzo, P.; Giarratano, A.; Einav, S.; Update, I. A systematic review on the efficacy and safety of chloroquine/hydroxychloroquine for COVID-19. *J. Crit. Care* **2020**, *59*, 176–190. [CrossRef]
8. Cvetkovic, R.S.; Goa, K.L. Lopinavir/ritonavir. *Drugs* **2003**, *63*, 769–802. [CrossRef]
9. Alhumaid, S.; Tobaiqy, M.; Albagshi, M.; Alrubaya, A.; Algharib, F.; Aldera, A.; Alali, J. MERS-CoV transmitted from animal-to-human vs MERSCoV transmitted from human-to-human: Comparison of virulence and therapeutic outcomes in a Saudi hospital. *Trop. J. Pharm. Res.* **2018**, *17*, 1155–1164. [CrossRef]
10. Chan, J.F.-W.; Yao, Y.; Yeung, M.-L.; Deng, W.; Bao, L.; Jia, L.; Li, F.; Xiao, C.; Gao, H.; Yu, P. Treatment with lopinavir/ritonavir or interferon-β1b improves outcome of MERS-CoV infection in a nonhuman primate model of common marmoset. *J. Infect. Dis.* **2015**, *212*, 1904–1913. [CrossRef]
11. Chan, K.; Lai, S.; Chu, C.; Tsui, E.; Tam, C.; Wong, M.; Tse, M.; Que, T.; Peiris, J.; Sung, J. Treatment of severe acute respiratory syndrome with lopinavir/ritonavir: A multicentre retrospective matched cohort study. *Hong Kong Med. J.* **2003**, *9*, 399–406.
12. Smolders, E.J.; Te Brake, L.H.; Burger, D.M. SARS-CoV-2 and HIV protease inhibitors: Why lopinavir/ritonavir will not work for COVID-19 infection. *Antivir. Ther.* **2020**. [CrossRef]
13. Schoergenhofer, C.; Jilma, B.; Stimpfl, T.; Karolyi, M.; Zoufaly, A. Pharmacokinetics of Lopinavir and Ritonavir in Patients Hospitalized With Coronavirus Disease 2019 (COVID-19). *Ann. Intern. Med.* **2020**, *173*, 670–672. [CrossRef] [PubMed]
14. Alhazzani, W.; Møller, M.H.; Arabi, Y.M.; Loeb, M.; Gong, M.N.; Fan, E.; Oczkowski, S.; Levy, M.M.; Derde, L.; Dzierba, A. Surviving Sepsis Campaign: Guidelines on the management of critically ill adults with Coronavirus Disease 2019 (COVID-19). *Intensiv. Care Med.* **2020**, *46*, 854–887. [CrossRef] [PubMed]
15. Cao, B.; Wang, Y.; Wen, D.; Liu, W.; Wang, J.; Fan, G.; Ruan, L.; Song, B.; Cai, Y.; Wei, M. A trial of lopinavir–ritonavir in adults hospitalized with severe Covid-19. *N. Engl. J. Med.* **2020**, *382*, 1787–1799. [CrossRef] [PubMed]
16. Massachusetts General Hospital. *Massachusetts General Hospital COVID-19 Treatment Guidance*; Massachusetts General Hospital: Boston, MA, USA, 2020.

17. MoH. *Coronavirus Disease 19 (COVID-19) Guidelines, Saudi Arabia*; MoH: Riyadh, Saudi Arabia, 2020.
18. HPSC. *Interim Public Health, Infection Prevention & Control Guidelines on the Prevention and Management of COVID-19 Cases and Outbreaks in Residential Care Facilities in Ireland*; HPSC: Dublin, Ireland, 2020.
19. Higgins, J.P.T.; Thomas, J.; Chandler, J.; Cumpston, M.; Li, T.; Page, M.J.; Welch, V.A. *Cochrane Handbook for Systematic Reviews of Interventions*; John Wiley & Sons: Chichester, UK, 2020.
20. Shamseer, L.; Moher, D.; Clarke, M.; Ghersi, D.; Liberati, A.; Petticrew, M.; Shekelle, P.; Stewart, L.A. Preferred reporting items for systematic review and meta-analysis protocols (PRISMA-P) 2015: Elaboration and explanation. *BMJ* **2015**, *349*. [CrossRef]
21. USFDA. *Coronavirus (COVID-19) Update: FDA Revokes Emergency Use Authorization for Chloroquine and Hydroxychloroquine*; USFDA: Montgomery, MD, USA, 2020.
22. Wang, Z.; Nayfeh, T.; Tetzlaff, J.; O'Blenis, P.; Murad, M.H. Error rates of human reviewers during abstract screening in systematic reviews. *PLoS ONE* **2020**, *15*, e0227742. [CrossRef]
23. Sterne, J.A.; Savović, J.; Page, M.J.; Elbers, R.G.; Blencowe, N.S.; Boutron, I.; Cates, C.J.; Cheng, H.-Y.; Corbett, M.S.; Eldridge, S.M. RoB 2: A revised tool for assessing risk of bias in randomised trials. *BMJ* **2019**, *366*. [CrossRef]
24. Sterne, J.A.; Hernán, M.A.; Reeves, B.C.; Savović, J.; Berkman, N.D.; Viswanathan, M.; Henry, D.; Altman, D.G.; Ansari, M.T.; Boutron, I. ROBINS-I: A tool for assessing risk of bias in non-randomised studies of interventions. *BMJ* **2016**, *355*. [CrossRef]
25. Wells, G.A.; Shea, B.; O'Connell, D.; Peterson, J.; Welch, V.; Losos, M.; Tugwell, P. *Ottawa Hospital Research Institute: The Newcastle-Ottawa Scale (NOS) for Assessing the Quality of Nonrandomised Studies in Meta-Analyses*; Ottawa Hospital Research Institute: Ottawa, ON, Canada, 2020.
26. Lan, X.; Shao, C.; Zeng, X.; Wu, Z.; Xu, Y. Lopinavir-ritonavir alone or combined with arbidol in the treatment of 73 hospitalized patients with COVID-19: A pilot retrospective study. *MedRxiv* **2020**. [CrossRef]
27. Li, Y.; Xie, Z.; Lin, W.; Cai, W.; Wen, C.; Guan, Y.; Mo, X.; Wang, J.; Wang, Y.; Peng, P. Efficacy and safety of lopinavir/ritonavir or arbidol in adult patients with mild/moderate COVID-19: An exploratory randomized controlled trial. *Med* **2020**. [CrossRef]
28. Horby, P.W.; Mafham, M.; Bell, J.L.; Linsell, L.; Staplin, N.; Emberson, J.; Palfreeman, A.; Raw, J.; Elmahi, E.; Prudon, B. Lopinavir–ritonavir in patients admitted to hospital with COVID-19 (RECOVERY): A randomised, controlled, open-label, platform trial. *Lancet* **2020**, *396*, 1345–1352. [CrossRef]
29. Pan, H.; Peto, R.; Karim, Q.A.; Alejandria, M.; Restrepo, A.M.H.; García, C.H.; Kieny, M.P.; Malekzadeh, R.; Murthy, S.; Preziosi, M.-P. Repurposed antiviral drugs for COVID-19; interim WHO SOLIDARITY trial results. *MedRxiv* **2020**. [CrossRef]
30. Cai, Q.; Yang, M.; Liu, D.; Chen, J.; Shu, D.; Xia, J.; Liao, X.; Gu, Y.; Cai, Q.; Yang, Y. Experimental treatment with favipiravir for COVID-19: An open-label control study. *Engineering* **2020**. [CrossRef] [PubMed]
31. Hung, I.F.-N.; Lung, K.-C.; Tso, E.Y.-K.; Liu, R.; Chung, T.W.-H.; Chu, M.-Y.; Ng, Y.-Y.; Lo, J.; Chan, J.; Tam, A.R. Triple combination of interferon beta-1b, lopinavir–ritonavir, and ribavirin in the treatment of patients admitted to hospital with COVID-19: An open-label, randomised, phase 2 trial. *Lancet* **2020**, *395*, 1695–1704. [CrossRef]
32. Wen, C.; Xie, Z.; Li, Y.; Deng, X.; Chen, X.; Cao, Y.; Ou, X.; Lin, W.; Li, F.; Cai, W. Real-world efficacy and safety of lopinavir/ritonavir and arbidol in treating with COVID-19: An observational cohort study. *Zhonghua Nei Ke Za Zhi* **2020**, *59*, E012. [PubMed]
33. Jun, C.; Yun, L.; Xiuhong, X.; Ping, L.; Feng, L.; Tao, L.; Shang, Z.; Mei, W.; Yinzhong, S.; Hongzhou, L. Efficacies of lopinavir/ritonavir and abidol in the treatment of novel coronavirus pneumonia. *Chin. J. Infect. Dis.* **2020**, *12*, E008.
34. Yan, D.; Liu, X.-Y.; Zhu, Y.-N.; Huang, L.; Dan, B.-T.; Zhang, G.-J.; Gao, Y.-H. Factors associated with prolonged viral shedding and impact of Lopinavir/Ritonavir treatment in hospitalised non-critically ill patients with SARS-CoV-2 infection. *Eur. Respir. J.* **2020**. [CrossRef] [PubMed]
35. Yuan, J.; Zou, R.; Zeng, L.; Kou, S.; Lan, J.; Li, X.; Liang, Y.; Ding, X.; Tan, G.; Tang, S. The correlation between viral clearance and biochemical outcomes of 94 COVID-19 infected discharged patients. *Inflamm. Res.* **2020**, *69*, 599–606. [CrossRef]
36. Zhu, Z.; Lu, Z.; Xu, T.; Chen, C.; Yang, G.; Zha, T.; Lu, J.; Xue, Y. Arbidol monotherapy is superior to lopinavir/ritonavir in treating COVID-19. *J. Infect.* **2020**, *81*, e21–e23. [CrossRef]

37. Ye, X.; Luo, Y.; Xia, S.; Sun, Q.; Ding, J.; Zhou, Y.; Chen, W.; Wang, X.; Zhang, W.; Du, W. Clinical efficacy of lopinavir/ritonavir in the treatment of Coronavirus disease 2019. *Eur. Rev. Med. Pharm. Sci.* **2020**, *24*, 3390–3396.
38. Deng, L.; Li, C.; Zeng, Q.; Liu, X.; Li, X.; Zhang, H.; Hong, Z.; Xia, J. Arbidol combined with LPV/r versus LPV/r alone against Corona Virus Disease 2019: A retrospective cohort study. *J. Infect.* **2020**, *81*, e1–e5. [CrossRef]
39. Lian, N.; Xie, H.; Lin, S.; Huang, J.; Zhao, J.; Lin, Q. Umifenovir treatment is not associated with improved outcomes in patients with coronavirus disease 2019: A retrospective study. *Clin. Microbiol. Infect.* **2020**, *26*, 917–921. [CrossRef] [PubMed]
40. Haviernik, J.; Štefánik, M.; Fojtíková, M.; Kali, S.; Tordo, N.; Rudolf, I.; Hubálek, Z.; Eyer, L.; Ruzek, D. Arbidol (Umifenovir): A broad-spectrum antiviral drug that inhibits medically important arthropod-borne flaviviruses. *Viruses* **2018**, *10*, 184. [CrossRef] [PubMed]
41. Klement-Frutos, E.; Burrel, S.; Peytavin, G.; Marot, S.; Lê, M.P.; Godefroy, N.; Calvez, V.; Marcelin, A.-G.; Caumes, E.; Pourcher, V. Early administration of ritonavir-boosted lopinavir could prevent severe COVID-19. *J. Infect.* **2020**. [CrossRef] [PubMed]
42. Choy, K.-T.; Wong, A.Y.-L.; Kaewpreedee, P.; Sia, S.-F.; Chen, D.; Hui, K.P.Y.; Chu, D.K.W.; Chan, M.C.W.; Cheung, P.P.-H.; Huang, X. Remdesivir, lopinavir, emetine, and homoharringtonine inhibit SARS-CoV-2 replication in vitro. *Antivir. Res.* **2020**, 104786. [CrossRef]
43. Smith, P.F.; Dodds, M.; Bentley, D.; Yeo, K.; Rayner, C. Dosing will be a key success factor in repurposing antivirals for COVID-19. *Br. J. Clin. Pharmacol.* **2020**. [CrossRef]
44. Fan, J.; Zhang, X.; Liu, J.; Yang, Y.; Zheng, N.; Liu, Q.; Bergman, K.; Reynolds, K.; Huang, S.-M.; Zhu, H. Connecting hydroxychloroquine in vitro antiviral activity to in vivo concentration for prediction of antiviral effect: A critical step in treating COVID-19 patients. *Clin. Infect. Dis.* **2020**. [CrossRef]
45. Lamontagne, F.; Agoritsas, T.; Macdonald, H.; Leo, Y.-S.; Diaz, J.; Agarwal, A.; Appiah, J.A.; Arabi, Y.; Blumberg, L.; Calfee, C.S. A living WHO guideline on drugs for covid-19. *BMJ* **2020**, *370*. [CrossRef]
46. World Health Organization. *Therapeutics and COVID-19: Living Guideline*; WHO: Geneva, Switzerland, 2020.
47. National Institutes of Health. *Coronavirus Disease 2019 (COVID-19) Treatment Guidelines*; NIH: Bethesda, MD, USA, 2020.
48. Infectious Diseases Society of America. *Guidelines on the Treatment and Management of Patients with COVID-19*; IDSA: Arlington, VA, USA, 2020.
49. WHO. *Draft Landscape of COVID-19 Candidate Vaccines*; WHO: Geneva, Switzerland, 2020.
50. Krammer, F. SARS-CoV-2 vaccines in development. *Nature* **2020**, *586*, 516–527. [CrossRef]
51. Moderna, Inc. *Moderna's COVID-19 Vaccine Candidate Meets Its Primary Efficacy Endpoint in the First Interim Analysis of the Phase 3 COVE Study*; Moderna, Inc.: Cambridge, MA, USA, 2020.
52. BioNTech, P.A. *Pfizer and BioNTech Conclude Phase 3 Study of COVID-19 Vaccine Candidate, Meeting All Primary Efficacy Endpoints*; BioNTech SE: Mainz, Germany, 2020.
53. Halasz, S.; Fox, K.; Cassidy, A. *AstraZeneca's Oxford Coronavirus Vaccine is 70% Effective on Average, Data Shows, with No Safety Concerns*; CNN: Atlanta, GA, USA, 2020.
54. Sheahan, T.P.; Sims, A.C.; Leist, S.R.; Schäfer, A.; Won, J.; Brown, A.J.; Montgomery, S.A.; Hogg, A.; Babusis, D.; Clarke, M.O. Comparative therapeutic efficacy of remdesivir and combination lopinavir, ritonavir, and interferon beta against MERS-CoV. *Nat. Commun.* **2020**, *11*, 222. [CrossRef]

Publisher's Note: MDPI stays neutral with regard to jurisdictional claims in published maps and institutional affiliations.

© 2020 by the authors. Licensee MDPI, Basel, Switzerland. This article is an open access article distributed under the terms and conditions of the Creative Commons Attribution (CC BY) license (http://creativecommons.org/licenses/by/4.0/).

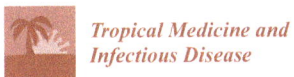

Brief Report

COVID-19-Induced Thrombosis in Patients without Gastrointestinal Symptoms and Elevated Fecal Calprotectin: Hypothesis Regarding Mechanism of Intestinal Damage Associated with COVID-19

Mauro Giuffrè [1,2,*], Stefano Di Bella [1], Gianluca Sambataro [3], Verena Zerbato [4], Marco Cavallaro [5], Alessandro Agostino Occhipinti [6], Andrea Palermo [7], Anna Crescenzi [8], Fabio Monica [9], Roberto Luzzati [1] and Lory Saveria Crocè [1,2]

1. Department of Medical, Surgical and Health Sciences, University of Trieste, 34151 Trieste, Italy; stefano932@gmail.com (S.D.B.); roberto.luzzati@asuits.sanita.fvg.it (R.L.); lcroce@units.it (L.S.C.)
2. Italian Liver Foundation, 34149 Basovizza, Trieste, Italy
3. University Hospital "Policlinico-Vittorio Emanuele", Department of Clinical and Experimental Medicine, University of Catania, 95100 Catania, Italy; dottorsambataro@gmail.com
4. Infectious Diseases Department, Udine University, 33100 Udine, Italy; verena.zerbato@gmail.com
5. Department of Radiology, Trieste University Hospital, 34139 Trieste, Italy; mrc.cavallaro@virgilio.it
6. Emergency Department, Trieste University Hospital, 34139 Trieste, Italy; alexander82@tiscali.it
7. Unit of Endocrinology and Diabetes, Campus Bio-Medico University, 00128 Rome, Italy; a.palermo@unicampus.it
8. Section of Pathology, Campus Bio-Medico University, 00128 Rome, Italy; a.crescenzi@unicampus.it
9. Department of Gastroenterology, Trieste University Hospital, 34139 Trieste, Italy; fabio.monica@asuits.sanita.fvg.it
* Correspondence: gff.mauro@gmail.com

Received: 6 August 2020; Accepted: 12 September 2020; Published: 16 September 2020

Abstract: Background: Patients with coronavirus infectious disease 2019 (COVID-19) and gastrointestinal symptoms showed increased values of fecal calprotectin (FC). Additionally, bowel abnormalities were a common finding during abdominal imaging of individuals with COVID-19 despite being asymptomatic. The current pilot study aims at evaluating FC concentrations in patients without gastrointestinal symptoms. Methods: we enrolled 25 consecutive inpatients with COVID-19 pneumonia, who were admitted without gastrointestinal symptoms and a previous history of inflammatory bowel disease. Results: At admission, 21 patients showed increased FC with median values of 116 (87.5; 243.5) mg/kg despite absent gastrointestinal symptoms. We found a strong positive correlation between FC and D-Dimer (r = 0.745, $p < 0.0001$). Two patients developed bowel perforation. Conclusion: our findings may change the current understanding of COVID-19 intestinal-related disease pathogenesis, shedding new light on the potential role of thrombosis and the consequent hypoxic intestinal damage.

Keywords: fecal calprotectin; COVID-19; SARS-CoV-2; bowel perforation; D-Dimer; thrombosis; ischemia

---

1. Main Text

At the time of writing this letter, the principal cause of mortality in patients with severe acute respiratory syndrome coronavirus 2 (SARS-CoV-2) infection is respiratory failure with exudative diffuse alveolar damage and massive capillary congestion often accompanied by microthrombi or, in lower percentages, by generalized thrombotic microangiopathy, as reported by post-mortem examinations [1]. With coronavirus infectious disease 2019 (COVID-19) being conceived as a solely respiratory disease [2,3], the scientific community initially assumed that the lungs represented the preferred and initial site of viral proliferation, as well as its primary source for shedding and transmission.

2. Gastrointestinal Manifestations of COVID-19

Recent findings indicated that SARS-CoV-2 could bind to gastrointestinal cells via specific receptors (such as the angiotensin converting enzyme-2 (ACE2) receptor and the transmembrane serine protease 2) [4], whose interaction is supposed to promote local inflammation by massive cytokine and chemokine release [5]. Additionally, an autoptic study on the small intestine of two COVID-19 patients showed endotheliitis of the submucosa vessels and evidence of direct viral infection of endothelial cells [6].

Regarding the clinical presentation, gastrointestinal symptoms are present in up to 28% of patients with COVID-19 [7–9], and fecal SARS-CoV-2-RNA was detected in approximately 50% of positive individuals [8–10]. Recently, Effenberger et al. [5] proposed the role of fecal calprotectin (FC) as a marker of intestinal inflammation in COVID-19 patients who developed gastrointestinal (GI) symptoms. In particular, the authors detected significantly higher FC values in patients with acute diarrhea if compared to patients without diarrhea or with ceased diarrhea (>48 h). In this pilot study, we aimed to externally validate the results of Effenberger et al. [5] by determining the actual absence of significant FC concentrations in patients who did not present gastrointestinal symptoms and without previous history of inflammatory bowel disease (IBD).

3. Materials and Methods

We performed a prospective observational cross-sectional study by enrolling 25 consecutive COVID-19 inpatients from May 2020 to June 2020, who were admitted without gastrointestinal symptoms and a previous history of IBD.

SARS-CoV-2 detection in nasopharyngeal swabs was determined by PCR (LightMix®-Modular-Wuhan CoV-RdRP and E genes). FC concentration was determined by the DiaSorin-LIAISON®-Calprotectin according to the manufacturer's specification (normal range <50 mg/kg). Both tests were performed at admission. Potential infective causes for FC increase were investigated through canonical stool analysis for common bacteria, viral and parasitic pathogens.

Data were displayed as median (Quartile 1; Quartile 3). We explored the correlation between continuous variables via Spearman's correlation coefficient, considering a statistically significant two-tailed p-value < 0.05.

4. Results

From the 25 original patients, 21 (84%) showed increased FC, with median values of 116 (87.5; 243.5) mg/kg despite being asymptomatic for GI symptoms, and a median D-Dimer of 1.32 (0.82; 2) mg/L (normal value < 0.5 mg/L). Their clinical characteristics, possible risk factors, and biochemical parameters are reported in Table 1. We did not detect any significant correlation between FC and the C reactive protein (CRP), white blood cell count (WBC), platelet count, ferritin, lactate dehydrogenase (LDH) or albumin. However, we found a strong positive correlation between FC and D-Dimer ($r = 0.745, p < 0.0001$).

Table 1. Patients' Characteristics and Laboratory Parameters. Continuous Variables are Reported as the Median (Quartile1; Quartile3). CRP: C Reactive Protein; LDH: Lactate Dehydrogenase.

Characteristics	Patients with Abnormal Fecal Calprotectin N = 21	Patients without Abnormal Calprotectin N = 4
Age, years	78.3 (69; 81.5)	76 (70; 84)
Gender, Male	15 (71.4%)	3 (75%)
BMI (kg/m^2)	24 (21; 27)	25 (20; 26)
Hearth Diseases	10 (47.6%)	2 (50%)
Hypertension	7 (33.3%)	2 (50%)
Previous ACE-Inhibitors	5 (23.8%)	2 (50%)
Active Smokers	7 (33.3%)	1 (25%)
Antibiotic Therapy	5 (23.8%)	1 (25%)
Heparin Therapy	13 (61.9%)	2 (50%)
White Blood Cell Count	6530 (4050; 7350)	6110 (4350; 8365)
Platelets (10^9/L)	205 (141;357)	189 (153; 265)
PCR (mg/dL)	31 (24; 91)	40 (8; 115)
LDH (U/L)	290 (195; 381)	250 (190; 300)
Ferritin (µg/L)	645 (520; 1210)	550 (420; 610)
Fecal Calprotectin (mg/kg)	116 (87.5; 243.5)	
D-Dimer (mg/LFEU)	1.32 (0.82; 2)	0.87 (0.5; 1.23)

4.1. Intestinal Perforation

Two of the enrolled patients developed intestinal perforation. They were admitted to the emergency department for high-grade fever, cough and dyspnea. Both resulted positive to SARS-CoV-2 in nasopharyngeal swabs, and according to their comorbidities, they were admitted to the hospital.

The first patient, a 68-year-old female with an FC of 216 mg/kg, WBC of 17,940 cells/mm^3, CRP of 94 mg/L and D-Dimer of 1.28 mg/LFEU developed severe abdominal pain 20 days after hospital admission. The contrast-enhanced abdominal computed tomography (CT) showed rectal wall and sigmoid colon thickening surrounded by extraluminal free air; a small-sized fluid collection and a smoothly thickened peritoneum were noted. The patient was treated conservatively.

The second patient, an 84-year-old female with an FC of 290 mg/kg, WBC of 5990 cells/mm^3, CRP of 290 mg/dL and D-Dimer of 2.1 mg/LFEU developed severe abdominal pain the day after admission and septic shock. The contrast-enhanced abdominal CT showed rectal wall thickening, with free air organized circumferentially around the mesorectum, suggestive for retroperitoneal perforation; an inflammatory stranding of perivisceral fat tissue was also identified. The patient died the next day.

4.2. A Hypothesis on the Role of Thrombosis

In contrast to Effenberger et al. [5], we detected an increase in FC concentration in 88.2% of patients without GI symptoms. Besides, our findings also represent the first report of a significant positive correlation between FC and D-Dimer. This particular discovery may change our current understanding of COVID-19 intestinal-disease pathogenesis, shedding new light on the potential role of thrombosis and the consequent hypoxic intestinal damage. Indeed, FC is mainly expressed by neutrophils [11], whose functions are severely affected by intestinal ischemia [12]. The two patients that developed bowel perforation showed on the CT rectal and sigmoid colon wall thickening. In non-COVID-19 patients, left flexure and sigmoid colon segments have the highest risk of ischemic colitis, while distal rectum is usually spared due to its dual blood supply; at variance, in COVID-19 patients colon/rectal thickening was previously reported in seven cases [13] in agreement with our data, supporting a relationship between intestinal damage and COVID-19 infection. Notably, D-Dimer was found to increase in up to 47% of patients with COVID-19 at hospital admission [14], which resulted in higher mortality rates despite not presenting pulmonary embolism or deep vein thrombosis. Was the gut being responsible for these patients' death? Unfortunately, this question has no definitive answer, but according to a recent study, bowel abnormalities were a common finding (31%) during abdominal imaging of individuals with COVID-19. Patients who underwent laparotomy often showed histological ischemia due to small vessel thrombosis [13].

That being said, our data should be taken with caution due to the relatively small sample size and the possible limitations related to selection bias. While waiting for the additional validation, and data on gut histopathology (autoptic reports or in vivo endoscopic biopsies) in COVID-19 patients, we firmly believe that the correlation between FC and D-Dimer may yield the secrets behind the COVID-19 Pandora's box.

Author Contributions: S.D.B., G.S., V.Z., M.C., A.A.O., A.P., A.C., F.M., R.L. and L.S.C. wrote the manuscript. M.G., S.D.B., V.Z., F.C., R.L., M.C., A.A.O. and L.S.C. were involved in patient care and contributed to the preparation of the manuscript. G.S., V.Z., A.P. and A.C., given their expertise in the field, were involved in the discussion of the gut damage etiology. All authors have read and agreed to the published version of the manuscript.

Funding: The authors did not receive funding for the current work.

Conflicts of Interest: The authors declare no conflict of interest.

Ethics Approval: The study protocol was approved by the institutional ethics commission (Comitato Etico Unico Regionale, CEUR) with the following number 2020-OS-072.

References

1. Menter, T.; Haslbauer, J.; Nienhold, R.; Savic, S.; Hopfer, H.; Deigendesch, N.; Frank, S.; Turek, D.; Willi, N.; Pargger, H.; et al. Post-mortem examination of COVID19 patients reveals diffuse alveolar damage with severe capillary congestion and variegated findings of lungs and other organs suggesting vascular dysfunction. *Histopathology* **2020**. [CrossRef] [PubMed]
2. Sambataro, G.; Giuffrè, M.; Sambataro, D.; Palermo, A.; Vignigni, G.; Cesareo, R.; Crimi, N.; Torrisi, S.; Vancheri, C.; Malatino, L.; et al. The Model for Early COvid-19 Recognition (MECOR) Score: A Proof-of-Concept for a Simple and Low-Cost Tool to Recognize a Possible Viral Etiology in Community-Acquired Pneumonia Patients during COVID-19 Outbreak. *Diagnostics* **2020**, *10*, 619. [CrossRef] [PubMed]
3. Cabas, P.; Di Bella, S.; Giuffrè, M.; Rizzo, M.; Trombetta, C.; Luzzati, R.; Antonello, R.M.; Parenzan, K.; Liguori, G. Community pharmacists' exposure to COVID-19. *Res. Soc. Adm. Pharm.* **2020**. [CrossRef] [PubMed]
4. Hoffmann, M.; Kleine-Weber, H.; Schroeder, S.; Krüger, N.; Herrler, T.; Erichsen, S.; Schiergens, T.S.; Herrler, G.; Wu, N.-H.; Nitsche, A.; et al. SARS-CoV-2 Cell Entry Depends on ACE2 and TMPRSS2 and Is Blocked by a Clinically Proven Protease Inhibitor. *Cell* **2020**, *181*, 271–280. [CrossRef] [PubMed]
5. Effenberger, M.; Grabherr, F.; Mayr, L.; Schwaerzler, J.; Nairz, M.; Seifert, M.; Hilbe, R.; Seiwald, S.; Scholl-Buergi, S.; Fritsche, G.; et al. Faecal calprotectin indicates intestinal inflammation in COVID-19. *Gut* **2020**, *69*. [CrossRef] [PubMed]
6. Varga, Z.; Flammer, A.J.; Steiger, P.; Haberecker, M.; Andermatt, R.; Zinkernagel, A.S.; Mehra, M.R.; Schuepbach, R.A.; Ruschitzka, F.; Moch, H. Endothelial cell infection and endotheliitis in COVID-19. *Lancet* **2020**, *395*, 1417–1418. [CrossRef]
7. Liang, W.; Feng, Z.; Rao, S.; Xiao, C.; Xue, X.; Lin, Z.; Zhang, Q.; Qi, W. Diarrhoea may be underestimated: A missing link in 2019 novel coronavirus. *Gut* **2020**, *69*, 1141–1143. [CrossRef] [PubMed]
8. Xiao, F.; Tang, M.; Zheng, X.; Liu, Y.; Li, X.; Shan, H. Evidence for Gastrointestinal Infection of SARS-CoV-2. *Gastroenterology* **2020**, *158*, 1831–1833. [CrossRef] [PubMed]
9. Lin, L.; Jiang, X.; Zhang, Z.; Huang, S.; Zhang, Z.; Fang, Z.; Gu, Z.; Gao, L.; Shi, H.; Mai, L.; et al. Gastrointestinal symptoms of 95 cases with SARS-CoV-2 infection. *Gut* **2020**, *69*, 997–1001. [CrossRef] [PubMed]

10. Pan, Y.; Zhang, D.; Yang, P.; Poon, L.L.M.; Wang, Q. Viral load of SARS-CoV-2 in clinical samples. *Lancet Infect. Dis.* **2020**, *20*, 411–412. [CrossRef]
11. Magro, F.; Lopes, J.; Borralho, P.; Lopes, S.; Coelho, R.; Cotter, J.; De Castro, F.D.; De Sousa, H.T.; Salgado, M.; Andrade, P.; et al. Comparison of different histological indexes in the assessment of UC activity and their accuracy regarding endoscopic outcomes and faecal calprotectin levels. *Gut* **2018**, *68*, 594–603. [CrossRef] [PubMed]
12. Tahir, M.; Arshid, S.; Fontes, B.; Castro, M.S.; Luz, I.S.; Botelho, K.L.R.; Sidoli, S.; Schwämmle, V.; Roepstorff, P.; Fontes, W. Analysis of the Effect of Intestinal Ischemia and Reperfusion on the Rat Neutrophils Proteome. *Front. Mol. Biosci.* **2018**, *5*, 89. [CrossRef] [PubMed]
13. Bhayana, R.; Som, A.; Li, M.; Carey, D.; Anderson, M.A.; Blake, M.A.; Catalano, O.A.; Gee, M.S.; Hahn, P.F.; Harisinghani, M.; et al. Abdominal Imaging Findings in COVID-19: Preliminary Observations. *Radiology* **2020**, 201908. [CrossRef] [PubMed]
14. Zhang, L.; Yan, X.; Fan, Q.; Liu, H.; Liu, X.; Liu, Z.; Zhang, Z. D-dimer levels on admission to predict in-hospital mortality in patients with Covid-19. *J. Thromb. Haemost.* **2020**, *18*, 1324–1329. [CrossRef] [PubMed]

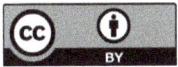

© 2020 by the authors. Licensee MDPI, Basel, Switzerland. This article is an open access article distributed under the terms and conditions of the Creative Commons Attribution (CC BY) license (http://creativecommons.org/licenses/by/4.0/).

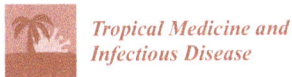 *Tropical Medicine and Infectious Disease*

Viewpoint

Malaria and COVID-19: Common and Different Findings

Francesco Di Gennaro [1], Claudia Marotta [1,*], Pietro Locantore [2], Damiano Pizzol [3] and Giovanni Putoto [1]

[1] Operational Research Unit, Doctors with Africa CUAMM, 35121 Padova, Italy; cicciodigennaro@yahoo.it (F.D.G.); g.putoto@cuamm.org (G.P.)
[2] Institute of Endocrinology, Università Cattolica del Sacro Cuore, 00168 Rome, Italy; pietro.locantore@icloud.com
[3] Italian Agency for Development Cooperation, Khartoum 79371, Sudan; damianopizzol8@gmail.com
* Correspondence: c.marotta@cuamm.org or claudia.marotta@gmail.com

Received: 31 July 2020; Accepted: 3 September 2020; Published: 6 September 2020

Abstract: Malaria and COVID-19 may have similar aspects and seem to have a strong potential for mutual influence. They have already caused millions of deaths, and the regions where malaria is endemic are at risk of further suffering from the consequences of COVID-19 due to mutual side effects, such as less access to treatment for patients with malaria due to the fear of access to healthcare centers leading to diagnostic delays and worse outcomes. Moreover, the similar and generic symptoms make it harder to achieve an immediate diagnosis. Healthcare systems and professionals will face a great challenge in the case of a COVID-19 and malaria syndemic. Here, we present an overview of common and different findings for both diseases with possible mutual influences of one on the other, especially in countries with limited resources.

Keywords: malaria; SARS-CoV-2; COVID-19; preparedness; Africa; emergency; pandemic

---

1. Background

On 11 March 2020, the WHO declared the outbreak of SARS-CoV-2 to be a pandemic infection. Just a few months earlier, pneumonia from a "new virus" was recorded in China; this ailment would later be identified as coronavirus disease 2019 (COVID-19) [1], a highly lethal viral disease with symptoms ranging from interstitial pneumonia to severe acute respiratory syndrome [2,3]. From February to July, around 12 million people were affected, with 500 thousand deaths occurring worldwide. While the figures related to COVID-19 seem to be slowly decreasing in Europe, with a seeming greater number of paucisymptomatic cases [4]; the epidemic is moving with greater force and aggression in Latin America (namely Mexico and Brazil), the United States of America, Asia (India), and Africa, where in the coming months the rainy season is expected along with the seasonal malaria epidemic.

Malaria—a parasitic disease caused by protozoan parasites of the genus *Plasmodium*, transmitted by mosquitoes of the genus *Anopheles*—is among the top ten causes of death in low-income countries and represents one of the great global health challenges. Although 100 countries worldwide have achieved disease elimination and are now malaria-free, around 300 million malaria cases and 500 thousand deaths still occurred worldwide in 2018, with sub-Saharan Africa bearing the greatest burden [5,6].

The association between COVID-19 and malaria epidemics can be devastating, especially in low- and middle-income countries (LMICs). Such countries are characterized by healthcare systems that are already fragile due to weak infrastructures, a scarcity of health workers, and limited financial resources. In this perspective, to avoid indirect short- and long-term effects of the COVID-19 pandemic [7] on malaria control programs and on healthcare systems of countries where the two diseases can coexist, preparedness is critical. For these reasons, in order to explore the current landscape and future outlook for a joint scenario of COVID-19 and malaria and the consequences thereof, here we provide an overview for physicians and public health authorities involved in the front line.

2. Epidemiology

2.1. Data

Quantifying the real number of SARS-CoV-2 cases is not easy since many different challenges are affecting surveillance systems over the world, from laboratory capacities to delay in case notification [8]. Although the mortality estimate is around 2%, different approaches to death cause monitoring and notification among different countries could affect this estimation [9]. What is for sure is that since the first case of SARS-CoV-2 infection identified in December 2019 in Wuhan—a commercial and university hub that is one of the ten most populous Chinese cities—the epidemic has spread all over the world very rapidly. On 13 January, the first confirmed case of COVID-19 outside China occurred in Thailand [10]. In a few weeks, the coronavirus epidemic had spread to 67 countries, from Italy to Iran, and a global pandemic was declared by the WHO on 11 March 2020 [11,12]. As of 17 August 2020, based on WHO reports, 21,689,832 confirmed cases and 770,273 deaths have been reported globally and are regionally distributed as follows: 6,540,222 cases and 420,753 deaths in the Americas, 1,119,579 cases and 25,633 deaths in Africa, 3,239,237 cases and 204,545 deaths in Europe, 5,606,2010 cases and 118,906 deaths in Asia, and 25,742 cases and 429 deaths in Oceania [4].

Meanwhile, malaria is still considered a huge killer, representing one of the biggest health challenges in the world, especially in contexts of poverty. According to the latest World Malaria Report, there were more than 200 million cases of malaria and almost 500 thousand deaths from malaria globally in 2018; although these figures represent a decrease from 2010, malaria is still one of the main causes of deaths in low-income countries [5]. The African region holds the sad record of having more than 90% of global malaria cases, followed by Southeast Asia and then the Eastern Mediterranean Region. Nineteen countries in sub-Saharan Africa and India share almost 85% of the global malaria burden. Six countries accounted for more than half of all malaria cases worldwide: Nigeria (25%); the Democratic Republic of the Congo (12%); Uganda (5%); and Cote d'Ivoire, Mozambique, and Niger (4% each) [5].

What emerged the global level is that at all countries are at a very high risk of COVID-19, while half of the world is at risk of malaria, with a greater risk for sub-Saharan Africa and Southeast Asia [5,13]. Although the extent of the COVID-19 epidemic is still relatively low in sub-Saharan Africa, an explosion of COVID-19 cases in Africa would be devastating given the severe impact this would have on healthcare systems that are already very weak [14].

Keeping in mind the reliability of data, the numbers of confirmed COVID-19 cases and deaths in the six countries with the biggest global burden of malaria, as of 17 August 2020, are as follows: 49,068 cases and 975 deaths in Nigeria, 9675 cases and 240 deaths in the Democratic Republic of the Congo, 1500 cases and 13 deaths in Uganda, 17,026 cases and 110 deaths in Cote d'Ivoire, 2855 cases and 19 deaths in Mozambique, and 1167 cases and 69 deaths in Niger [4].

To date, only a few clinical cases of malaria and COVID-19 co-infection [15,16] have been reported in the scientific literature, and wider studies are needed to improve knowledge on this topic.

2.2. Transmission and Prevention

The main route of transmission of SARS-CoV-2 is though respiratory droplets, with person-to-person contact by asymptomatic carriers also playing an important role. Accordingly, interhuman transmission can be prevented by (1) using face masks; (2) covering coughs and sneezes with tissues; (3) washing hands regularly with soap or disinfecting with sanitizers containing at least 60% alcohol; (4) avoiding contact with infected people; (5) maintaining a physical distance between people (1.5 m), and (6) refraining from touching eyes, nose, and mouth with unwashed hands [17].

The malaria parasite is mainly transmitted by female *Anopheles* mosquito bite, mainly between dusk and dawn. That is why prevention strategies are currently based on two complementary methods: chemoprophylaxis and protection against mosquito bites.

3. Clinical Manifestation and Diagnosis

The clinical diagnosis for both diseases is based on the patient's symptoms and findings upon physical examination (Table 1).

Table 1. Summary of the principal characteristics of COVID-19 and malaria.

	COVID–19	Malaria
Classification	Viral disease	Parasitic disease
Infectious agent	SARS-CoV-2	*Plasmodium falciparum, Plasmodium vivax, Plasmodium ovale, Plasmodium malariae, Plasmodium knowlesi*
Main symptoms	Fever, cough	Fever
Severe clinical disease manifestation	Acute respiratory distress syndrome, acute thromboembolic disease, pulmonary embolism	Confusion, coma, neurologic focal signs, severe anemia, acute respiratory distress syndrome, acute renal failure, pulmonary edema, seizure
Diagnostic tests	• Molecular tests (RT-PCR) on upper (nasopharyngeal/oropharyngeal swabs, nasal aspirate, nasal wash, or saliva) or lower respiratory tract (sputum or tracheal aspirate or bronchoalveolar lavage (BAL)) sample; • Antigen tests on upper or lower respiratory tract sample; • Antibody tests [enzyme-linked immunosorbent assays (ELISA), chemiluminescence assays (CLIA), and lateral flow assays (LFA)).	• Microscopic diagnosis on blood smear stained with Giemsa; • Antigen detection with RDTs using immunochromatographic methods; • Molecular diagnosis by PCR; • Serology, using either indirect immunofluorescence (IFA) or ELISA; • Drug resistance tests with in vitro tests or PCR molecular characterization.
Laboratory findings	Lymphopenia, increased prothrombin time (PT), increased lactate dehydrogenase (LDH), elevated C-reactive protein (CRP), elevated D-dimer, mildly elevated serum amylase, elevated alanine aminotransferase (ALT) and aspartate aminotransferase (AST)	Anemia, hypoglycemia, alterations in kidney function, hyperbilirubinemia, acid–base disturbances
Chest computed tomography (CT) scan	Ground-glass opacities, crazy-paving pattern	Not required for diagnosis
Transmission	Human-to-human; respiratory droplets	Mosquito vector
Age-group most affected by the severe form of the disease	Adult/Elderly	Children/Pregnancy
Defined treatment	No	Yes
Vaccine	Trials ongoing	Trials ongoing

Early symptoms of SARS-CoV-2 infection such as myalgia, fever, and fatigue could be confused with symptoms of malaria, leading to problems in early clinical diagnosis, especially where malaria is endemic. Different is the case of severe malaria (caused mainly by *Plasmodium falciparum*), where the predominance of neurological signs and symptoms such as confusion, coma, neurological focal signs, severe anemia, and respiratory difficulties can make us more inclined towards the diagnosis of malaria. Blood chemistry tests can also be confusing, as shown in Table 1; therefore, a laboratory test for both malaria and COVID-19 appears essential [18]. The gold standard for malaria diagnosis is the microscopic examination, which can detect the presence of the *Plasmodium*. However, it is an operator-dependent examination, and the sensitivity and specificity depend on the quality of the reagents, the microscope, and the experience of the technician. A useful alternative is provided by the rapid diagnostic tests (RDTs), which appear particularly useful when a reliable microscopic diagnosis is not available and also have the advantage of being a point-of-care method. Another method for diagnosing malaria is to search for parasite nucleic acids using polymerase chain reaction (PCR). Although this technique may be much more sensitive than smear microscopy, PCR results are often not available quickly enough and are therefore rarely used. However, PCR is useful for confirming the malarial parasite species after the diagnosis has been established by smear microscopy or rapid diagnostic tests (RDTs) [19,20].

On the other hand, for patients with suspected SARS-CoV-2 infection, in addition to clinical and/or radiological signs, the use of RT-PCR to detect SARS-CoV-2 nucleic acid in sputum or throat swabs and lower respiratory tract secretions appears essential for diagnosis [21]. Blood chemistry tests in patients with SARS-CoV-2 infection may show leukocytosis with leukopenia, increased liver function indices AST and ALT, elevated LDH, and especially high D-dimers that may indicate a concomitant pulmonary embolism [22]. Indeed, high levels of D-dimer and more severe lymphopenia have been associated with mortality. Chest computed tomography (CT) scans in COVID-19 patients show opacity of frosted glass with or without consolidating abnormalities, consistent with viral pneumonia. Furthermore, these lung lesions often appear to be bilateral and peripheral, and they involve the lower lobes more frequently. Less common findings include pleural thickening, pleural effusion, and lymphadenopathy [23,24]. Other authors presented the scientific community with controversial cases that had negative RT-PCR tests on oropharyngeal swabs despite the CT results being indicative of viral pneumonia and only subsequent positive nasopharyngeal swabs. This underlines how often there can be a divergence between the clinical and virological findings. In addition, IgA, IgM, and IgG serology tests are available to identify patients with recent or previous infection [25]. Malaria and COVID-19 share symptoms and geographic areas of disease spread. The use of laboratory investigations, and therefore the availability of adequate diagnostic capacity, as well as careful clinical surveillance and management of cases appear crucial in differential diagnosis. Furthermore, *Plasmodium* spp. and SARS-CoV-2 are similar in terms of incubation time. For SARS-CoV-2, an incubation period of 11.5 days has been calculated; for *Plasmodium* spp., the incubation period varies from 7 to 30 days in most cases, with a shorter period observed more frequently for *P. falciparum* and a longer one observed for *P. malaria* [5].

Medical and scientific attention should be paid to the potential of COVID-19/malaria co-infections. It would be recommended, especially in areas where malaria is endemic areas, and also because of the availability of malaria tests [26], to double-screen patients with suggestive symptoms for both COVID-19 and malaria. This could bring benefits in contrasting these two infectious diseases, reducing the death toll, and improving the outcome [5–25].

4. The Role of ACE 2 Receptor in *Plasmodium* spp. and SARS-CoV-2 Infection

Another interesting aspect of the correlation between SARS-CoV-2 and *Plasmodium* spp. can be seen by considering the angiotensin-converting enzyme receptor 2 (ACE2), since a genetic deletion or insertion polymorphism leads to a reduced expression of ACE2 by altering the concentration of ACE I and D alleles in both infections. This D/I polymorphism shows an important geographical variation [27] and would explain, although this is yet to be demonstrated, the variable prevalence of COVID-19 infections among the global distribution. In fact, SARS-CoV-2 uses the ACE2 receptor as a means of cell entry and requires the spike protein to be primed by cellular serine protease TMPRSS2 [28]. SARS-CoV-2 spike proteins bind to ACE2 receptors of numerous target cells, particularly the type II alveolar cells [29].

In SARS-CoV-2 patients, virus infection likely induces proinflammatory events through the activation of transcription nuclear factor (NF)-kB intracellular signaling pathway, leading to overexpression of cytokines and chemokines. In particular, an increased serum expression of interferon (IFN)-γ, interleukin (IL)-1β, IL-6, IL-12, IL-8, MCP-1, and IFN-γ inducible protein-10 has been demonstrated [30]. Similarly, in SARS-CoV-2 infection, increased serum concentrations of the proinflammatory molecules IL-1β, IFN-γ, IP-10, MCP-1, IL-4, and IL-10 has been demonstrated, with the higher levels being associated with more severe disease [31]. During severe infection, endothelial cell dysfunction induces hypercoagulability due to excessive thrombin generation and reduced fibrinolysis [32]. Moreover, virus-driven downregulation of ACE2 receptors may enhance the effects of angiotensin II, leading to increased thrombogenesis [33]. Some authors, in agreement with the role of ACE in lung infections caused by SARS-CoV-2 [4], have suggested how the ACE D/I genotype may influence the clinical course of the infection. Therefore, the ACE D/I polymorphism can play a role in the spread of COVID-19 and in the outcome of the infection, especially in European populations.

Similarly, for malaria, authors suggest a possible protective role in cerebral malaria due to the "D" allele of the ACE I/D polymorphism under both homozygous and heterozygous conditions [33]. In fact, studies reported how several ACE1 and ACE2 polymorphisms reduce erythrocyte invasion by *P. falciparum* [34], resulting in a "protective" effect influencing the development of the parasite and/or the host's susceptibility to the disease; this was also reported in children [35,36]. This aspect gains importance considering the great number of malaria deaths due to cerebral damage caused by *Plasmodium falciparum* [37] in sub-Saharan Africa.

In this scenario, more studies on the role of the D allele and other polymorphisms could help to better understand protective factors and develop intervention strategies. Matching data on prevalence of cerebral malaria, COVID-19, and this polymorphism could also be very interesting.

5. Relationship of SARS-CoV-2 Infection and *Plasmodium* spp. with Age

In LMICs, the average life expectancy at birth is low, and a huge burden of morbidity is still due to infectious diseases such as human immunodeficiency virus (HIV), malnutrition, tuberculosis, and malaria, with the coexistence of these conditions being a predictive risk factor of death [38,39].

For these reasons, even if it is currently believed that SARS-CoV-2 infection is less aggressive in children, some factors should be taken into account when considering this epidemic in a country with a high incidence of malaria. First of all, as for malaria, children, especially those under 5 years of age, are unfortunately the most affected age-group. Furthermore, economic and behavioral changes due to the COVID-19 pandemic could impact families' response to malaria and increase malaria morbidity and mortality in children. In fact, the cases of the young and elderly can be closely related. As adults and elderly are more susceptible to COVID-19, the fear of the contagion can cause them to be reluctant to visit healthcare facilities, even when they should bring their children with malaria-like symptoms to healthcare facilities. This could lead to a diagnostic delay and therefore a worse outcome. Especially in rural communities, which may have reduced attention, this will affect children with malaria, making an already vulnerable population even more vulnerable. In general, there could be a reduction in access to healthcare facilities due to the fear of contracting COVID-19 [40]. This could have a negative impact on pediatric care. As adults are increasingly implored adults to stay at home, they may hesitate to take their children to healthcare centers when needed, leading to diagnostic delay and the occurrence of more serious cases [19].

6. Antimalarials for Treatment of COVID-19

Although the therapeutic role of chloroquine (CQ) and hydroxychloroquine (HCQ) in COVID-19 infection is still not clear, several authors have underlined the antiviral and anti-inflammatory role of these molecules [41], since their action interferes with the ACE2 cell receptor and has activity against many proinflammatory cytokines (e.g., IL-1 and IL-6) [42]. The association of CQ or HCQ with an antibiotic such as azithromycin has been tested experimentally in the field with controversial results, but clinical trials are still ongoing [43–46] for an evidence-based utilization. However, it does not appear to have any role as a prophylactic in post-exposure prevention [47].

In the past, HCQ played a big role the treatment of malaria, even if the precise mechanism by which it exhibits activity against *Plasmodium* is still unknown. One hypothesis is that HCQ, like CQ, is a weak base and can exert its effect by concentrating on the acid vesicles of the parasite and inhibiting heme polymerization. However, the use of chloroquine in malaria has been suspended in most endemic areas due to resistance.

7. Possible Scenarios for COVID-19 in Countries with High Incidence of Malaria

There is great global concern surrounding the possible scenarios of the effects of the COVID-19 pandemic in Africa. It is prudent to assume that for a long time there will be a big gap between official data and the real situation of the COVID-19 pandemic. In part, the data on COVID-19 cases around the world are markedly unrepresentative due to the global scarcity of testing reagents, limited laboratory capabilities, and poor access to healthcare centers [4,48]. Whatever the scenario will be, what is known is that in emergencies, especially in epidemics, one of the most frequent risks is to neglect, suspend, postpone, or close essential prevention and treatment health services. In the end, the burden of avoidable morbidity and mortality from common pathologies causes more damage and creates more victims of the same epidemic; this particularly impacts mothers and children, making the already fragile part of the population even more vulnerable [48–50].

Moreover, in sub-Saharan Africa, there are no national healthcare systems capable of withstanding such a wave of patients suffering from acute respiratory failure as COVID-19 has caused in high-income countries. The number of intensive care beds is limited. To this end, the role of intermediate critical care facilities using frugal technology, already tested to be low-cost and effective in contexts with limited resources on other issues, could also be crucial with COVID-19 [51].

The Ebola lesson should be valued for the impact it had on malaria control measures, where a significant reduction in malaria diagnoses (but not deaths from malaria) was observed due to the perceived risk of Ebola contagion resulting in a lower number of people accessing healthcare centers [40,52]. In addition, during the Ebola outbreak, it was estimated that malaria cases in Guinea, Liberia, and Sierra Leone could increase to 1 million in 2014 following the disruption in the distribution of insecticide-treated bed nets (ITNs) [53]. The factors that contributed to that situation, i.e., the similarity of the first symptoms between the two diseases and the fear of contracting them in healthcare facilities, are very similar to what we could expect with COVID-19.

The impact of the epidemic on the health financing system as a whole should also be considered. A polarization of economic resources happened with Ebola, and this is also being observed with COVID-19. Therefore, in the next month, it could be possible to observe an important decrease in economic and human resources for malaria control programs, with a real risk of reducing prevention. This is turn may result in an increase in the numbers of cases, with a consequent increase in morbidity and mortality. The characteristics of COVID-19 and the previous experiences of the Ebola epidemic indicate the need for malaria-endemic countries to consider measures for preparation and prevention, focusing on not only the threat of COVID-19 but also the possible impact of other diseases, especially malaria [16].

In order to face these possible scenarios, COVID-19 preparedness and response in malaria-endemic countries should be focused on the following:

1. Local staff management, including protection, training, supervision, incentives, and rest shifts, should focus on all factors that together can help to ease the fear of contagion, diminish the anger over the death of colleagues, and contain strikes and protests;
2. Infection prevention and control measures should be applied for healthcare workers at the hospital and peripheral levels, making sure to institute appropriate low-technology measures such as washing hands with sodium hypochlorite, segregation of hospital waste, and proper application of the personal protective equipment;
3. Community engagement is crucial, as an effective communication campaign involving local leaders, indigenous associations, and media can compel the community to conform to the new behaviors (distancing, hand washing, stopping of traditional funeral rites, collaborating in contact tracing, etc.) and therefore in the end be able to retain trust in healthcare structures and operators;
4. Data management and operational research should not be neglected. It is of fundamental importance to monitor trends of routine health services use, maternal child health, TB, HIV, etc.

Operational research, especially when carried out with local and international partners, allows healthcare professionals to test ideas [54,55], check intuitions, and answer questions from different perspectives (e.g., epidemiology, organization of health services, and policies).

8. Conclusions

Malaria and COVID-19 may have similar aspects and seem to have a strong potential for mutual influence. They have already caused millions of deaths, and the regions where malaria is endemic regions are at risk of suffering from the consequences of COVID-19 due to mutual side effects, such as less access to treatment for patients with malaria due to the fear of access to healthcare centers leading to worse outcomes and diagnostic delays. Moreover, the similar and generic symptoms make it harder to achieve an immediate diagnosis. Healthcare systems and professionals will face a great challenge in case of a syndemic [56,57]. The role of young health professionals, well-motivated and trained in primary care, will also be essential [58] in countries with a high burden of malaria.

In patients with symptoms such as fever, fatigue, and headache, both malaria and COVID-19 tests should always be performed. According to recent WHO recommendations [59], in the case of challenges due to the COVID-19 pandemic (e.g., supply chain disruption for RDTs, health worker absenteeism, shortage of personal protective equipment) a malaria diagnosis should be considered for all fever cases in endemic countries. On the other hand, patients with COVID-19-related symptoms that negative for malaria must undergo isolation to exclude COVID-19 until repetition of the virological sample, thus reducing the potential risk of transmission.

Even though a COVID-19 outbreak may not occur in the malaria-endemic regions, the WHO has called for ministries of health and national malaria control programs to ensure that malaria control efforts are not disrupted while facing the COVID-19 response [59,60]. Preparedness is the key to tackling any public health crisis, and malaria-endemic countries need to be prepared for the challenges COVID-19 could pose. Finally, from a global perspective, it is necessary to increase and join efforts in order to develop an effective vaccine and it make available for everyone, as this would be the most effective preventive measure for both diseases.

Author Contributions: F.D.G. and C.M. conceived the idea; Methodology, F.D.G. and C.M.; Validation, F.D.G., C.M., P.L., D.P., G.P.; Formal writing—original draft preparation, F.D.G., C.M., Writing—review and editing, C.M., G.P., All authors reviewed the literature, drafted and critically revised the manuscript, and approved the final version before submission. All authors have read and agreed to the published version of the manuscript

Funding: This research received no external funding.

Conflicts of Interest: The authors declare no conflict of interest.

References

1. Lu, H.; Stratton, C.W.; Tang, Y. Outbreak of pneumonia of unknown etiology in Wuhan, China: The mystery and the miracle. *J. Med. Virol.* **2020**, *92*, 401–402. [CrossRef]
2. Coronaviridae Study Group of the International Committee on Taxonomy of Viruses; Gorbalenya, A.E. The species Severe acute respiratory syndrome-related coronavirus: Classifying 2019-nCoV and naming it SARS-CoV-2. *Nat. Microbiol.* **2020**, *5*, 536–544. [CrossRef] [PubMed]
3. Di Gennaro, F.; Pizzol, D.; Marotta, C.; Antunes, M.; Racalbuto, V.; Veronese, N.; Smith, L. Coronavirus Diseases (COVID-19) Current Status and Future Perspectives: A Narrative Review. *Int. J. Environ. Res. Public Health* **2020**, *17*, 2690. [CrossRef] [PubMed]
4. World Health Organization Coronavirus Disease (COVID-2019) Dashboard. Available online: https://covid19.who.int (accessed on 17 August 2020).
5. WHO. World Malaria Report 2019. World Health Organization. Available online: https://www.who.int/publications/i/item/9789241565721 (accessed on 16 July 2020).
6. Newby, G.; Bennett, A.; Larson, E.; Cotter, C.; Shretta, R.; A Phillips, A.; A Feachem, R.G. The path to eradication: A progress report on the malaria-eliminating countries. *Lancet* **2016**, *387*, 1775–1784. [CrossRef]

7. Haakenstad, A.; Harle, A.C.; Tsakalos, G.; E Micah, A.; Tao, T.; Anjomshoa, M.; Cohen, J.; Fullman, N.; Hay, S.I.; Mestrovic, T.; et al. Tracking spending on malaria by source in 106 countries, 2000-16: An economic modelling study. *Lancet Infect. Dis.* **2019**, *19*, 703–716. [CrossRef]
8. Lipsitch, M.; Swerdlow, D.L.; Finelli, L. Defining the Epidemiology of Covid-19—Studies Needed. *N. Engl. J. Med.* **2020**, *382*, 1194–1196. [CrossRef]
9. Lipsitch, M.; Donnelly, C.A.; Fraser, C.; Blake, I.M.; Cori, A.; Dorigatti, I.; Ferguson, N.M.; Garske, T.; Mills, H.L.; Riley, S.; et al. Potential Biases in Estimating Absolute and Relative Case-Fatality Risks during Outbreaks. *PLoS Negl. Trop. Dis.* **2015**, *9*, e0003846. [CrossRef]
10. World Health Organization Novel Coronavirus (2019-nCoV), Situation Report 1. Available online: https://www.who.int/docs/default-source/coronaviruse/situation-reports/20200121-sitrep-1-2019-ncov.pdf (accessed on 25 March 2020).
11. Di Castelnuovo, A.; Bonaccio, M.; Costanzo, S.; Gialluisi, A.; Antinori, A.; Berselli, N.; Blandi, L.; Bruno, R.; Cauda, R.; Guaraldi, G.; et al. Common cardiovascular risk factors and in-hospital mortality in 3,894 patients with COVID-19: Survival analysis and machine learning-based findings from the multicentre Italian CORIST Study. *Nutr. Metab. Cardiovasc. Dis.* **2020**. [CrossRef]
12. World Health Organization Coronavirus Disease. 2019 Situation Report. Available online: https://www.who.int/docs/default-source/coronaviruse/situation-reports/20200326-sitrep-66-covid-19.pdf?sfvrsn=9e5b8b48_2 (accessed on 20 July 2020).
13. Chiodini, J. COVID-19 and the impact on malaria. *Travel Med. Infect. Dis.* **2020**, *35*, 101758. [CrossRef]
14. Wang, J.; Xu, C.; Wong, Y.K.; He, Y.; A Adegnika, A.; Kremsner, P.G.; Agnandji, S.T.; A Sall, A.; Liang, Z.; Qiu, C.; et al. Preparedness is essential for malaria-endemic regions during the COVID-19 pandemic. *Lancet* **2020**, *395*, 1094–1096. [CrossRef]
15. Kishore, R.; Dhakad, S.; Arif, N.; Dar, L.; Mirdha, B.R.; Aggarwal, R.; Kabra, S.K. COVID-19: Possible Cause of Induction of Relapse of Plasmodium vivax Infection. *Indian J. Pediatr.* **2020**, 1–2. [CrossRef] [PubMed]
16. Zhu, M.; Zhu, Y.; Zhang, J.; Liu, W. A case of COVID-19 with Imported Falciparum Malaria Infection is Reported. *Front. Med.* **2020**, *21*, 1–9.
17. Centers for Disease Control and Prevention 2019 Novel Coronavirus, Wuhan, China. 2020. Available online: https://www.cdc.gov/coronavirus/2019-ncov/prevent-getting-sick/prevention.html (accessed on 16 August 2020).
18. Chanda-Kapata, P.; Kapata, N.; Zumla, A. COVID-19 and malaria: A symptom screening challenge for malaria endemic countries. *Int. J. Infect. Dis.* **2020**, *94*, 151–153. [CrossRef] [PubMed]
19. Nghochuzie, N.N.; Olwal, C.O.; Udoakang, A.J.; Amenga-Etego, L.N.-K.; Amambua-Ngwa, A. Pausing the Fight Against Malaria to Combat the COVID-19 Pandemic in Africa: Is the Future of Malaria Bleak? *Front. Microbiol.* **2020**, *11*. [CrossRef] [PubMed]
20. Di Gennaro, F.; Marotta, C.; Pizzol, D.; Chhaganlal, K.; Monno, L.; Putoto, G.; Saracino, A.; Casuccio, A.; Mazzucco, W. Prevalence and Predictors of Malaria in Human Immunodeficiency Virus Infected Patients in Beira, Mozambique. *Int. J. Environ. Res. Public Health* **2018**, *15*, 2032. [CrossRef] [PubMed]
21. Lippi, G.; Simundic, A.-M.; Plebani, M. Potential preanalytical and analytical vulnerabilities in the laboratory diagnosis of coronavirus disease 2019 (COVID-19). *Clin. Chem. Lab. Med.* **2020**, *58*, 1070–1076. [CrossRef] [PubMed]
22. Lagier, J.C.; Colson, P.; Dupont, H.T.; Salomon, J.; Doudier, B.; Aubry, C.; Gouriet, F.; Baron, S.; Dudouet, P.; Flores, R.; et al. Testing the repatriated for SARS-Cov2: Should laboratory-based quarantine replace traditional quarantine? *Travel Med. Infect. Dis.* **2020**, *34*, 101624. [CrossRef]
23. Ai, T.; Yang, Z.; Hou, H.; Zhan, C.; Chen, C.; Lv, W.; Tao, Q.; Sun, Z.; Xia, L. Correlation of Chest CT and RT-PCR Testing for Coronavirus Disease 2019 (COVID-19) in China: A Report of 1014 Cases. *Radiology* **2020**, *296*, E32–E40. [CrossRef]
24. Li, Y.; Xia, L. Coronavirus Disease 2019 (COVID-19): Role of Chest CT in Diagnosis and Management. *Am. J. Roentgenol.* **2020**, *214*, 1280–1286. [CrossRef]
25. Ling, Y.; Xu, S.-B.; Lin, Y.-X.; Tian, D.; Zhu, Z.-Q.; Dai, F.-H.; Wu, F.; Song, Z.-G.; Huang, W.; Chen, J.; et al. Persistence and clearance of viral RNA in 2019 novel coronavirus disease rehabilitation patients. *Chin. Med. J.* **2020**, *133*, 1039–1043. [CrossRef]
26. Landier, J.; Parker, D.M.; Thu, A.M.; Carrara, V.; Lwin, K.M.; Bonnington, C.A.; Pukrittayakamee, S.; Delmas, G.; Nosten, F. The role of early detection and treatment in malaria elimination. *Malar. J.* **2016**, *15*, 363. [CrossRef] [PubMed]

27. Saab, Y.B.; Gard, P.R.; Overall, A.D.J. The geographic distribution of the ACE II genotype: A novel finding. *Genet. Res.* **2007**, *89*, 259–267. [CrossRef] [PubMed]
28. Hoffmann, M.; Kleine-Weber, H.; Krüger, N.; Muller, M.; Drosten, C.; Pohlmann, S. The novel coronavirus 2019 (2019-nCoV) uses the SARS-coronavirus receptor ACE2 and the cellular protease TMPRSS2 for entry into target cells. *bioRxiv* **2020**. [CrossRef]
29. Zhao, Y.; Zhao, Z.; Wang, Y.; Zhou, Y.; Ma, Y.; Zou, W. Single-Cell RNA expression profiling of ACE2, the putative receptor of Wuhan 2019-nCoV. *BioRxiv* **2020**.
30. Wong, C.K.; Lam, C.W.K.; Wu, A.K.L.; Ip, W.K.; Lee, N.; Chan, I.H.S.; Lit, L.C.W.; Hui, D.S.C.; Chan, M.H.M.; Chung, S.S.C.; et al. Plasma inflammatory cytokines and chemokines in severe acute respiratory syndrome. *Clin. Exp. Immunol.* **2004**, *136*, 95–103. [CrossRef]
31. Huang, C.; Wang, Y.; Li, X.; Ren, L.; Zhao, J.; Hu, Y.; Znang, L.; Fan, G.; Xu, J.; Gu, X.; et al. Clinical features of patients infected with 2019 novel coronavirus in Wuhan, China. *Lancet* **2020**, *395*, 497–506. [CrossRef]
32. Liu, P.P.; Blet, A.; Smyth, D.; Li, H. The Science Underlying COVID-19: Implications for the Cardiovascular System. *Circulation* **2020**. [CrossRef]
33. Dhangadamajhi, G.; Mohapatra, B.N.; Kar, S.K.; Ranjit, M. Gene polymorphisms in angiotensin I converting enzyme (ACE I/D) and angiotensin II converting enzyme (ACE2 C→T) protect against cerebral malaria in Indian adults. *Infect. Genet. Evol.* **2010**, *10*, 337–341. [CrossRef]
34. Saraiva, V.B.; Silva, L.D.S.; Ferreira-DaSilva, C.T.; Da Silva-Filho, J.L.; Teixeira-Ferreira, A.; Perales, J.; Souza, M.C.; Henriques, M.D.G.M.O.; Caruso-Neves, C.; Pinheiro, A.A.S. Impairment of the Plasmodium falciparum Erythrocytic Cycle Induced by Angiotensin Peptides. *PLoS ONE* **2011**, *6*, e17174. [CrossRef]
35. Gallego-Delgado, J.; Rodriguez, A. Malaria and hypertension. Another co-evolutionary adaptation? Understanding SARS-CoV-2-mediated inflammatory responses: From mechanisms to potential therapeutic tools. *Front. Cell. Infect. Microbiol.* **2014**, *4*, 121.
36. Turner, L.; Lavstsen, T.; Berger, S.S.; Wang, C.W.; Petersen, J.E.V.; Avril, M.; Brazier, A.J.; Freeth, J.; Jespersen, J.S.; Nielsen, M.; et al. Severe malaria is associated with parasite binding to endothelial protein C receptor. *Nature* **2013**, *498*, 502–505. [CrossRef] [PubMed]
37. Rasti, N.; Wahlgren, M.; Chen, Q. Molecular aspects of malaria pathogenesis. *FEMS Immunol. Med. Microbiol.* **2004**, *41*, 9–26. [CrossRef] [PubMed]
38. Marotta, C.; Di Gennaro, F.; Pizzol, D.; Madeira, G.; Monno, L.; Saracino, A.; Putoto, G.; Casuccio, A.; Mazzucco, W. The At Risk Child Clinic (ARCC): 3 Years of Health Activities in Support of the Most Vulnerable Children in Beira, Mozambique. *Int. J. Environ. Res. Public Health* **2018**, *15*, 1350. [CrossRef] [PubMed]
39. Marotta, C.; Giaquinto, C.; Di Gennaro, F.; Chhaganlal, K.; Saracino, A.; Moiane, J.; Maringhini, G.; Pizzol, D.; Putoto, G.; Monno, L.; et al. Pathways of care for HIV infected children in Beira, Mozambique: Pre-post intervention study to assess impact of task shifting. *BMC Public Health* **2018**, *18*, 703. [CrossRef] [PubMed]
40. Quaglio, G.; Tognon, F.; Finos, L.; Bome, D.; Sesay, S.; Kebbie, A.; Di Gennaro, F.; Camara, B.S.; Marotta, C.; Pisani, V.; et al. Impact of Ebola outbreak on reproductive health services in a rural district of Sierra Leone: A prospective observational study. *BMJ Open* **2019**, *9*, e029093. [CrossRef]
41. Nicastri, E.; Petrosillo, N.; Bartoli, T.A.; Lepore, L.; Mondi, A.; Palmieri, F.; D'Offizi, G.; Marchioni, L.; Murachelli, S.; Ippolito, G.; et al. National Institute for the Infectious Diseases "L. Spallanzani" IRCCS. Recommendations for COVID-19 Clinical Management. *Infect. Dis. Rep.* **2020**, *12*. [CrossRef]
42. Yao, X.; Ye, F.; Zhang, M.; Cui, C.; Huang, B.; Niu, P.; Liu, X.; Zhao, L.; Dong, E.; Song, C.; et al. In Vitro Antiviral Activity and Projection of Optimized Dosing Design of Hydroxychloroquine for the Treatment of Severe Acute Respiratory Syndrome Coronavirus 2 (SARS-CoV-2). *Clin. Infect. Dis.* **2020**, *2*, 2. [CrossRef]
43. Cortegiani, A.; Ingoglia, G.; Ippolito, M.; Giarratano, A.; Einav, S. A systematic review on the efficacy and safety of chloroquine for the treatment of COVID-19. *J. Crit. Care* **2020**, *57*, 279–283. [CrossRef]
44. Geleris, J.; Sun, Y.; Platt, J.; Zucker, J.; Baldwin, M.; Hripcsak, G.; Labella, A.; Manson, D.K.; Kubin, C.; Barr, R.G.; et al. Observational Study of Hydroxychloroquine in Hospitalized Patients with Covid-19. *N. Engl. J. Med.* **2020**, *382*, 2411–2418. [CrossRef]
45. Liu, J.; Cao, R.; Xu, M.; Wang, X.; Zhang, H.; Hu, H.; Li, Y.; Hu, Z.; Zhong, W.; Wang, M. Hydroxychloroquine, a less toxic derivative of chloroquine, is effective in inhibiting SARS-CoV-2 infection in vitro. *Cell Discov.* **2020**, *6*, 1–4. [CrossRef]
46. Di Castelnuovo, A.; Costanzo, S.; Antinori, A.; Berselli, N.; Blandi, L.; Bruno, R.; Cauda, R.; Guaraldi, G.; Menicanti, L.; My, I.; et al. Use of hydroxychloroquine in hospitalised COVID-19 patients is associated with

reduced mortality: Findings from the observational multicentre Italian CORIST study. *Eur. J. Intern. Med.* **2020**. [CrossRef] [PubMed]
47. Boulware, D.R.; Pullen, M.F.; Bangdiwala, A.S.; Pastick, K.A.; Lofgren, S.M.; Okafor, E.C.; Skipper, C.P.; Nascene, A.A.; Nicol, M.R.; Abassi, M.; et al. A Randomized Trial of Hydroxychloroquine as Postexposure Prophylaxis for Covid-19. *N. Engl. J. Med.* **2020**, *383*, 517–525. [CrossRef] [PubMed]
48. Quaglio, G.; Preiser, W.; Putoto, G. COVID-19 in Africa. *Public Health* **2020**, *185*, 60. [CrossRef] [PubMed]
49. Di Gennaro, F.; Marotta, C.; Pisani, L.; Veronese, N.; Pisani, V.; Lippolis, V.; Pellizer, G.; Pizzol, D.; Tognon, F.; Bavaro, D.F.; et al. Maternal caesarean section infection (MACSI) in Sierra Leone: A case–control study. *Epidemiol. Infect.* **2020**, *148*, e40. [CrossRef]
50. Nkengasong, J.N.; Mankoula, W. Looming threat of COVID-19 infection in Africa: Act collectively, and fast. *Lancet* **2020**, *395*, 841–842. [CrossRef]
51. Marotta, C.; Di Gennaro, F.; Pisani, L.; Pisani, V.; Senesie, J.; Bah, S.; Koroma, M.M.; Caracciolo, C.; Putoto, G.; Amatucci, F.; et al. Cost-Utility of Intermediate Obstetric Critical Care in a Resource-Limited Setting: A Value-Based Analysis. *Annal. Glob. Health* **2020**, *86*, 1–8. [CrossRef]
52. Plucinski, M.M.; Guilavogui, T.; Sidikiba, S.; Diakité, N.; Diakité, S.; Dioubaté, M.; Bah, I.; Hennessee, I.; Butts, J.K.; Halsey, E.S.; et al. Effect of the Ebola-virus-disease epidemic on malaria case management in Guinea, 2014: A cross-sectional survey of health facilities. *Lancet Infect. Dis.* **2015**, *15*, 1017–1023. [CrossRef]
53. Walker, P.G.T.; White, M.T.; Griffin, J.T.; Reynolds, A.; Ferguson, N.M.; Ghani, A.C. Malaria morbidity and mortality in Ebola-affected countries caused by decreased health-care capacity, and the potential effect of mitigation strategies: A modelling analysis. *Lancet Infect. Dis.* **2015**, *15*, 825–832. [CrossRef]
54. Bobbio, F.; Di Gennaro, F.; Marotta, C.; Kok, J.; Akec, G.; Norbis, L.; Monno, L.; Saracino, A.; Mazzucco, W.; Lunardi, M. Focused ultrasound to diagnose HIV-associated tuberculosis (FASH) in the extremely resource-limited setting of South Sudan: A cross-sectional study. *BMJ Open* **2019**, *9*, e027179. [CrossRef]
55. Pizzol, D.; Di Gennaro, F.; Chhaganlal, K.D.; Fabrizio, C.; Monno, L.; Putoto, G.; Saracino, A. Prevalence of diabetes mellitus in newly diagnosed pulmonary tuberculosis in Beira, Mozambique. *Afr. Health Sci.* **2017**, *17*, 773–779. [CrossRef]
56. Gutman, J.R.; Lucchi, N.W.; Cantey, P.T.; Steinhardt, L.C.; Samuels, A.M.; Kamb, M.L.; Kapella, B.K.; McElroy, P.D.; Udhayakumar, V.; Lindblade, K.A. Malaria and Parasitic Neglected Tropical Diseases: Potential Syndemics with COVID-19? *Am. J. Trop. Med. Hyg.* **2020**, *103*, 572–577. [CrossRef] [PubMed]
57. Beshir, K.B.; Grignard, L.; Hajissa, K.; Mohammed, A.; Nurhussein, A.M.; Ishengoma, D.S.; Lubis, I.N.D.; Drakeley, C.; Sutherland, C.J. Emergence of Undetectable Malaria Parasites: A Threat under the Radar amid the COVID-19 Pandemic? *Am. J. Trop. Med. Hyg.* **2020**, *103*, 558–560. [CrossRef] [PubMed]
58. Mazzucco, W.; Marotta, C.; de Waure, C.; Marini, G.; Fasoletti, D.; Colicchio, A.; Luppi, D.; Pignatti, F.; Sessa, G.; Silenzi, A.; et al. Motivational aspects and level of satisfaction of Italian junior doctors with regard to knowledge and skills acquired attending specific general practice training courses. A national web survey. *Euro Mediterr. Biomed. J.* **2017**, *12*, 77–086. [CrossRef]
59. World Health Organization. Tailoring Malaria Interventions in the COVID-19 Response. 2020. Available online: https://www.who.int/malaria/publications/atoz/tailoring-malaria-interventions-covid-19.pdf?ua=1 (accessed on 17 August 2020).
60. Hogan, A.B.; Jewell, B.L.; Sherrard-Smith, E.; Vesga, J.F.; Watson, O.J.; Whittaker, C.; Hamlet, A.; A Smith, J.; Winskill, P.; Verity, R.; et al. Potential impact of the COVID-19 pandemic on HIV, tuberculosis, and malaria in low-income and middle-income countries: A modelling study. *Lancet Glob. Health* **2020**. [CrossRef]

© 2020 by the authors. Licensee MDPI, Basel, Switzerland. This article is an open access article distributed under the terms and conditions of the Creative Commons Attribution (CC BY) license (http://creativecommons.org/licenses/by/4.0/).

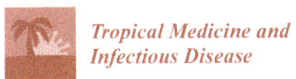

Viewpoint

Impact of the COVID-19 Pandemic on Tuberculosis Control: An Overview

Kefyalew Addis Alene [1,2,*], Kinley Wangdi [3] and Archie C A Clements [1,2]

[1] Faculty of Health Sciences, Curtin University, Bentley, WA 6102, Australia; archie.clements@curtin.edu.au
[2] Wesfarmers Centre of Vaccines and Infectious Diseases, Telethon Kids Institute, Perth, WA 6009, Australia
[3] Department of Global Health, Research School of Population Health, Australian National University, Canberra, ACT 2601, Australia; kinley.wangdi@anu.edu.au
* Correspondence: kefyalew.alene@curtin.edu.au; Tel.: +61-404-705-064

Received: 27 May 2020; Accepted: 21 July 2020; Published: 24 July 2020

Abstract: Throughout history, pandemics of viral infections such as HIV, Ebola and Influenza have disrupted health care systems, including the prevention and control of endemic diseases. Such disruption has resulted in an increased burden of endemic diseases in post-pandemic periods. The current coronavirus disease 2019 (COVID-19) pandemic could cause severe dysfunction in the prevention and control of tuberculosis (TB), the infectious disease that causes more deaths than any other, particularly in low- and middle-income countries where the burden of TB is high. The economic and health crisis created by the COVID-19 pandemic as well as the public health measures currently taken to stop the spread of the virus may have an impact on household TB transmission, treatment and diagnostic services, and TB prevention and control programs. Here, we provide an overview of the potential impact of COVID-19 on TB programs and disease burden, as well as possible strategies that could help to mitigate the impact.

Keywords: COVID-19; pandemic; endemic; tuberculosis; impact; control; overview

1. Historical Perspective

Tuberculosis (TB) is one of the oldest endemic diseases affecting humanity, but it remains a significant global public health problem today [1,2]. It is estimated that a quarter of the world's population has latent TB infection (a dormant form of TB) [3]. According to the World Health Organization (WHO) report, an estimated 10 million people develop active TB and more than one million people die due to TB each year [4].

The burden of TB has varied across human history. Major disruptions such as natural disasters, war and infectious disease pandemics have compromised TB programs and led to an increased burden of TB. For instance, during the First and Second World Wars, there were epidemics of TB in many European countries, which accounted for nearly one fourth of the total deaths during this period [5,6].

After World War II, following the discovery of TB medications, and improvements in the socioeconomic status of the population, TB was well controlled in high-income settings with TB burden decreasing dramatically [7]. However, when human immunodeficiency virus (HIV) emerged as a worldwide pandemic disease in the 1980s, TB re-emerged as an opportunistic infection and killed millions of people [8]. With the implementation of several TB prevention programmes and the introduction of anti-retroviral therapy (ART) for HIV, the mortality and morbidity of TB have decreased gradually over the last few decades [9].

More recently, the emergence of major viral disease outbreaks in several parts of the worlds has posed new challenges for global and national TB control efforts. For instance, the recent outbreak of Ebola in West Africa has severely compromised TB programs in the affected countries [10,11]. The outbreaks of Middle East respiratory syndrome coronavirus (MERS-CoV) complicated the control of TB in Saudi Arabia [12]. The direct and indirect effects of these viral outbreaks on TB programs have resulted in an increased burden of TB in the affected regions in subsequent years.

The United Nations Sustainable Development Goals (SDGs)include ending the TB epidemic by 2030, and the WHO set ambitious targets, including a 90% reduction in TB incidence and a 95% reduction in TB deaths compared with 2015, and no catastrophic costs due to TB, by 2035 [13]. Although progress continues to be made to achieve these ambitious targets, the current pandemic of coronavirus disease 2019 (COVID-19) could be a major challenge to achieving them.

Given the high levels of global disruption caused by the COVID-19 pandemic, it is critical to consider the potential impact on the control and prevention of common endemic diseases that might be even more devastating to human health than COVID-19 itself. The impact of COVID-19 on other diseases such as cancer and diabetes has been addressed in recent reviews [14,15]. However, there are no published reviews on the impacts of COVID-19 on TB. TB is the leading cause of death due to an infectious disease globally, and it is anticipated that people ill with both TB and COVID-19 may have poorer treatment outcomes. Most importantly, the public health response to COVID-19 to isolate people in their homes for extended periods could facilitate transmission of TB since close household contact, particularly in low-socioeconomic and overcrowded conditions, is a key risk factor for TB. Therefore, understanding the potential impacts of COVID-19 on TB is important for designing prevention strategies. Therefore, we review the potential impact of COVID-19 pandemics on the prevention and control of TB and provide possible strategies that could help to mitigate the impact.

2. The Coronavirus Disease 2019 (COVID-19) Pandemic and TB

The current pandemic of COVID-19 is a global health crisis, causing substantial disruptions to healthcare systems, including TB programs [16]. This section briefly summarizes the clinical features, epidemiological distribution, and transmission and prevention mechanisms of both COVID-19 and TB.

Clinical features: COVID-19 is a highly contagious acute viral disease, whereas TB is a chronic bacterial disease. Both COVID-19 and TB affect the respiratory system, primarily the lungs, and have similar symptoms such as cough, fever and breathing difficulty [17], although the severity and duration of the symptoms are varied. Up to 78% of patients with COVID-19 may be asymptomatic and recover spontaneously [18,19].

Epidemiology: TB has long been the leading cause of death due to an infectious disease globally, killing more than 1.5 million people, and with an estimated 10 million new cases in 2018 [20]. The COVID-19 pandemic has now become a public health crisis, and COVID-19 has overtaken TB as the infectious disease killing the most people per day [21]. According to the WHO, as of 8 July 2020, there were more than 11.7 million confirmed cases of COVID-19 and over 540,000 deaths globally. COVID-19 has affected at least 216 countries, areas and territories around the world. High-burden countries for TB have generally experienced a lower incidence of COVID-19 than countries in Europe and North America, although Russia, Brazil, China and India are amongst the top 20 countries for total numbers of cases and deaths due to COVID-19.

High-risk groups: Some population groups are at higher risk of developing severe COVID-19 complications [22]. In particular, a higher number of deaths have occurred in adults aged over 60 years [23], in particular men. Similarly, gender differences in TB burden have been reported worldwide, with men more likely to be affected by TB than women [24,25]. Patients with underlying chronic diseases such as hypertension, diabetes, lung cancer and chronic obstructive pulmonary disease are at a higher risk of COVID-19-related death and hospital admission, as well as poor outcomes for TB [17,22,26,27].

Transmission: While the exact route of transmission for COVID-19 and TB differ, the major mode of transmission for both diseases is through close contact with infected people [28,29]. For COVID-19, the source of infection can be both symptomatic and asymptomatic patients, while for TB the main source of infection is symptomatic patients with productive cough. The incubation period for TB (from infection to active TB) ranges from several months to two years [30], whereas the incubation period for COVID-19 is approximately 5 days [31].

Prevention: Various preventive measures have been taken at global, regional and national levels to reduce the risk of transmission of COVID-19 [32]. The common measures taken by countries to prevent the transmission of the disease include early case detection; prompt isolation of confirmed patients; contact tracing and quarantine of all contacts during the incubation period; social distancing; and communitywide containment, including closure of schools and public facilities, maintaining good hand hygiene through regular washing and use of sanitizers, and wearing of personal protective equipment [33,34]. Many countries have also undertaken strict measures, such as banning of public gatherings, complete lock-down of social and economic activities, and closure of borders to prevent importation of cases [35]. While some countries have been able to control transmission of the disease by implementing the aforementioned interventions, the number of new cases reported continues to rise in many countries at the current time [36]. While there are some vaccine trials under development, there is no evidence that any existing vaccine, including the Bacille Calmette-Guérin vaccine (BCG), protects people against infection with COVID-19 virus.

3. The Potential Impact of the COVID-19 Pandemic on Tuberculosis Control

COVID-19 could impact TB control in several ways, including increasing transmission of TB in the household, delaying the diagnosis and treatment of TB and increasing poor treatment outcomes and risks of developing drug-resistant TB. The direct and indirect effects of COVID-19 on national and global economies will have both short-term and long-term consequences for TB programs.

Impact of COVID-19 on household transmission of TB: One of the measures undertaken by countries to prevent the spread of COVID-19 is advising or requiring people to stay at home until the situation comes under control [33,34]. While this measure has several advantages in reducing the communitywide transmission of COVID-19, it may also facilitate household transmission of TB. Prolonged contact at household level is one of the risk factors that increases the transmission of TB [37]. A recent modelling study showed that a 3-month lockdown due to COVID-19 would cause an additional 1.65 million TB cases and 438,000 TB deaths in India over the next 5 years [38]. Another study conducted in Brazil showed that intensity of household exposure increased the risk of TB infection and disease among household members [37]. Previous studies have also shown that the prevalence of TB among children in household contact with adult patients is higher than in the general population [39,40], and the risk of household infection is significantly increased with prolonged household contact with sputum positive adults [39,41]. Since TB has a long incubation period, the impact of increased household transmission of TB is only likely to be observed in future years, when an increase in numbers of TB cases may be observed [42,43]. For instance, following the global pandemic of HIV, epidemics of TB were observed in several countries such as South Africa [44,45], which suggests that future public health vigilance is advisable.

Impact of COVID-19 on TB treatment and diagnostic services: Overwhelming of health care systems by COVID-19 cases is likely to impact on TB treatment and diagnostic services in several ways: (1) diversion of resources (including human and financial) away from routine services, to manage the pandemic; (2) health service and political leadership, the media and the public focusing on pandemic management and response with limited oversight and accountability of TB programmes; (3) health care personnel experiencing stress and anxiety, key predictors of errors and poor quality of care; (4) health care personnel being required to quarantine, or becoming ill or dying, and therefore not being available for routine services; and (5) stigma and fear of COVID-19 infection at health care facilities, discouraging people from visiting TB services. All of these factors will contribute to delays in the diagnosis and commencement of treatment. As untreated pulmonary TB is the main source of TB infection, late diagnosis and treatment of TB may increase the risk of transmission, especially the household transmission of TB as many people are currently at home. Late diagnosis and inappropriate treatment of TB can also increase the risk of poor treatment outcomes and development of drug-resistant

TB. Misdiagnosis and under-detection of TB are ongoing problems for TB programs [4]. It was estimated that globally 3 million TB cases were un-detected in 2018 [4]. This number is likely to increase due the current COVID-19 pandemic.

Impact of COVID-19 on the prevention and control of TB: Prevention and control strategies for TB have already been compromised due to the COVID-19 pandemic. Many fora for exchanging TB research and information, such as seminars, workshops and annual conferences, have not been conducted in 2020. For instance, the World Tuberculosis Day, which is celebrated on March 24 each year, to build public awareness about the prevention and control of TB and to raise funding to support TB control efforts, has been cancelled in several countries. Vaccination programs, including the BCG vaccination that has been given to prevent childhood TB, have been negatively affected by COVID-19 [46]. Furthermore, TB preventive therapy, which is often given to high-risk groups to prevent the progression of latent TB to active TB, may also be affected by COVID-19 [47].

The worldwide pandemic of COVID-19 may affect the global strategy of ending TB by 2035 in several ways. Many of the factors affecting diagnostic and testing services also affect prevention and control programmes. Shortages of resources, either directly due to diversion towards pandemic management or indirectly due to broader economic consequences of the pandemic and stretched national budgets, are likely to impact on routine public health programmes. Currently, the attention of the public, government, media and health professions is diverted to COVID-19. Prioritization of TB and other endemic diseases is likely to be less than pre-pandemic levels as a result.

Impact of COVID-19 on late reactivation of TB: The impact of COVID-19 on the health status of individuals, including on the functioning of the immune system [48,49], might be associated with a higher risk of developing active TB disease. Pneumonia and respiratory failure caused by COVID-19 might cause long-lasting damage to the respiratory system, particularly the lungs, which might increase the risk of TB [50]. Previous studies have shown that infections with viruses such as HIV and influenza play a role in the development of active TB disease, either directly after exposure to TB or through reactivation of latent TB infection [51–53].

Moreover, the COVID pandemic will severely damage global and national economies. The crisis will have a disproportionate impact on the poor, through job losses, loss of remittances, rising prices, and disruptions to services such as education and health care [54]. The World Bank estimates that the global extreme poverty rate could rise by 0.3 to 0.7 percentage points, to around 9 percent in 2020, and around 40 million to 60 million people will fall into extreme poverty in 2020 as a result of COVID-19. This will have a long-term impact on the burden of TB [55], because poverty is widely recognised as an important risk factor for being infected and developing active TB [55–57].

4. Possible Strategies to Mitigate the Impact of COVID-19 on TB Control

Several strategies can be implemented to mitigate the impact of COVID-19 on TB control (Table 1). For example, to limit household transmission of TB, basic infection prevention and control measures, recommended by the WHO for health care facilities and high-risk settings, can be implemented at home [58]. To avoid TB diagnosis and treatment delay due to COVID-19, use of virtual care and digital health technologies, decentralising TB treatment to community health workers, and supporting private health sectors and academic research institutions to provide TB testing and treatment might all be required.

Table 1. Possible strategies to mitigate the impact of COVID-19 on tuberculosis (TB) control.

Impact of COVID-19 on TB	Strategies to Mitigate the Impact of COVID-19 on TB Control
Increased household transmission of TB	<ul><li>Apply infection prevention and control measures (e.g., cough etiquette, personal protective equipment);</li><li>Consider using upper-room germicidal ultraviolet (GUV) where indicated;</li><li>Apply room ventilation (including natural, mixed-mode, mechanical ventilation, and recirculated air through high-efficiency particulate air (HEPA) filters);</li><li>Separate or isolate people with presumed or demonstrated infectious TB;</li><li>Provide TB preventive treatment for high-risk groups;</li><li>Initiate TB treatment early.</li></ul>
Delayed TB diagnosis and treatment services	<ul><li>Maintain supports to essential TB services during and after the COVID-19 pandemic;</li><li>Provide information to patients about COVID-19 and TB so they can protect themselves and continue their TB treatment;</li><li>Apply patient-centred delivery of TB prevention, diagnosis, treatment, and care services;</li><li>Decentralise TB treatment to community health workers and increase access to TB treatment for home-based TB care;</li><li>Provide adequate supply of TB medication to patients for safe storage at home;</li><li>Design mechanisms to deliver medicines and to collect specimens for follow-up testing at home;</li><li>Integrate TB and COVID-19 services for infection control, contact tracing, community-based care, surveillance and monitoring;</li><li>Provide short-term training for students and health professionals and recruit additional staff to work on TB programs;</li><li>Change policy if required and support private hospitals, and academic or research centres, to provide TB testing and treatment;</li><li>Use virtual care and digital health technologies (e.g., video observed therapy) for adherence support, early initiation of treatment, remote monitoring of TB patients, counselling, and follow-up consultations.</li></ul>
Affecting TB prevention and control strategies	<ul><li>Organize virtual conferences, seminars, workshops and fundraising;</li><li>Design strategies to deliver BCG and TB preventive therapy at home;</li><li>Create community awareness of the importance of TB services.</li></ul>
Reactivation of TB	<ul><li>Plan additional support and resources to reduce the burden of TB;</li><li>Conduct research to identify the impact of COVID-19 on reactivation of TB and to design interventions mitigating this problem.</li></ul>

5. Conclusions

The health and economic crisis created by the current COVID-19 pandemic, as well as the public health measures taken to stop the spread of the virus, could have a potential impact on TB prevention and control in many different ways. The proportion of the cumulative disease burden associated with the COVID-19 pandemic due to failures in endemic disease management might end up being greater than that directly caused by COVID-19 itself. It is essential that health systems attempt to maintain routine services for endemic infectious diseases to the highest level possible, recognizing that this may, through necessity, be lower than pre-pandemic levels. It is also essential that health systems have a plan for returning to full service levels as soon as possible, in particular for controlling major endemic diseases such as TB. Economic analyses of the impact of the pandemic should include indirect effects like disruption to routine services and subsequent burden of TB and other endemic infectious diseases. Public health vigilance is necessary to mitigate the impact of COVID-19 on TB prevention and control, with plans in place to manage any increases of TB burden in future years.

Author Contributions: K.A.A., A.C.A.C., and K.W. conceived the study; K.A.A. drafted the manuscript; A.C.A.C. and K.W. were involved in the critical revision of the manuscript. All authors have read and agreed to the published version of the manuscript.

Funding: This research received no specific grant from any funding agencies in the public, commercial or not-for-profit sectors.

Conflicts of Interest: The authors declare no conflict of interest.

References

1. Comas, I.; Coscolla, M.; Luo, T.; Borrell, S.; Holt, K.E.; Kato-Maeda, M.; Parkhill, J.; Malla, B.; Berg, S.; Thwaites, G.; et al. Out-of-Africa migration and Neolithic coexpansion of Mycobacterium tuberculosis with modern humans. *Nat. Genet.* **2013**, *45*, 1176–1182. [CrossRef] [PubMed]
2. Kyu, H.H.; Maddison, E.R.; Henry, N.J.; Mumford, J.E.; Barber, R.; Shields, C.; Brown, J.C.; Nguyen, G.; Carter, A.; Wolock, T.M.; et al. The global burden of tuberculosis: Results from the Global Burden of Disease Study 2015. *Lancet Infect. Dis.* **2018**, *18*, 261–284. [CrossRef]
3. Houben, R.M.; Dodd, P.J. The global burden of latent tuberculosis infection: A re-estimation using mathematical modelling. *PLoS Med.* **2016**, *13*, e1002152. [CrossRef] [PubMed]
4. WHO. *Global Tuberculosis Report 2019*; World Health Organization: Geneva, Switzerland, 2019.
5. Vynnycky, E.; Fine, P. Interpreting the decline in tuberculosis: The role of secular trends in effective contact. *Int. J. Epidemiol.* **1999**, *28*, 327–334. [CrossRef]
6. Glaziou, P.; Floyd, K.; Raviglione, M. Trends in Tuberculosis in the UK. *BMJ* **2018**. [CrossRef]
7. UN. *The Millennium Development Goals Report New York*; UN: New York, NY, USA, 2015.
8. Corbett, E.L.; Watt, C.J.; Walker, N.; Maher, D.; Williams, B.G.; Raviglione, M.C.; Dye, C. The growing burden of tuberculosis: Global trends and interactions with the HIV epidemic. *Arch. Intern. Med.* **2003**, *163*, 1009–1021. [CrossRef]
9. Edmonds, A.; Lusiama, J.; Napravnik, S.; Kitetele, F.; Van Rie, A.; Behets, F. Anti-retroviral therapy reduces incident tuberculosis in HIV-infected children. *Int. J. Epidemiol.* **2009**, *38*, 1612–1621. [CrossRef]
10. Zachariah, R.; Ortuno, N.; Hermans, V.; Desalegn, W.; Rust, S.; Reid, A.; Boeree, M.J.; Harries, A.D. Ebola, fragile health systems and tuberculosis care: A call for pre-emptive action and operational research. *Int. J. Tuberc. Lung Dis.* **2015**, *19*, 1271–1275. [CrossRef]
11. Ansumana, R.; Keitell, S.; Roberts, G.M.; Ntoumi, F.; Petersen, E.; Ippolito, G.; Zumla, A. Impact of infectious disease epidemics on tuberculosis diagnostic, management, and prevention services: Experiences and lessons from the 2014–2015 Ebola virus disease outbreak in West Africa. *Int. J. Infect. Dis.* **2017**, *56*, 101–104. [CrossRef]
12. Alfaraj, S.H.; Al-Tawfiq, J.A.; Altuwaijri, T.A.; Memish, Z.A. Middle East respiratory syndrome coronavirus and pulmonary tuberculosis coinfection: Implications for infection control. *Intervirology* **2017**, *60*, 53–55. [CrossRef]
13. Uplekar, M.; Weil, D.; Lonnroth, K.; Jaramillo, E.; Lienhardt, C.; Dias, H.M.; Falzon, D.; Floyd, K.; Gargioni, G.; Getahun, H.; et al. WHO's new end TB strategy. *Lancet* **2015**, *385*, 1799–1801. [CrossRef]
14. Hanna, T.P.; Evans, G.A.; Booth, C.M. Cancer, COVID-19 and the precautionary principle: Prioritizing treatment during a global pandemic. *Nat. Rev. Clin. Oncol.* **2020**, *17*, 268–270. [CrossRef] [PubMed]
15. Maddaloni, E.; Buzzetti, R. Covid-19 and diabetes mellitus: Unveiling the interaction of two pandemics. *Diabetes Metab. Res. Rev.* **2020**, e33213321. [CrossRef]
16. Hogan, A.B.; Jewell, B.L.; Sherrard-Smith, E.; Vesga, J.F.; Watson, O.J.; Whittaker, C.; Hamlet, A.; Smith, J.A.; Winskill, P.; Verity, R.; et al. Potential impact of the COVID-19 pandemic on HIV, tuberculosis, and malaria in low-income and middle-income countries: A modelling study. *Lancet Glob. Health* **2020**. [CrossRef]

17. Yang, J.; Zheng, Y.; Gou, X.; Pu, K.; Chen, Z.; Guo, Q.; Jia, R.; Wang, H.; Wang, Y.; Zhou, Y.; et al. Prevalence of comorbidities in the novel Wuhan coronavirus (COVID-19) infection: A systematic review and meta-analysis. *Int. J. Infect. Dis.* **2020**. [CrossRef]
18. Bai, Y.; Yao, L.; Wei, T.; Tian, F.; Jin, D.Y.; Chen, L.; Wang, M. Presumed asymptomatic carrier transmission of COVID-19. *JAMA* **2020**, *323*, 1406–1407. [CrossRef]
19. Day, M. Covid-19: Four fifths of cases are asymptomatic, China figures indicate. *BMJ* **2020**. [CrossRef]
20. Kyu, H.H.; Maddison, E.R.; Henry, N.J.; Ledesma, J.R.; Wiens, K.E.; Reiner, R., Jr.; Biehl, M.H.; Shields, C.; Osgood-Zimmerman, A.; Ross, J.M.; et al. Global, regional, and national burden of tuberculosis, 1990–2016: Results from the Global Burden of Diseases, Injuries, and Risk Factors 2016 Study. *Lancet Infect. Dis.* **2018**, *18*, 1329–1349. [CrossRef]
21. WHO. *Coronavirus Disease 2019 (COVID-19): Situation Report*; World Health Organization: Geneva, Switzerland, 2020.
22. Zhou, F.; Yu, T.; Du, R.; Fan, G.; Liu, Y.; Liu, Z.; Xiang, J.; Wang, Y.; Song, B.; Gu, X.; et al. Clinical course and risk factors for mortality of adult inpatients with COVID-19 in Wuhan, China: A retrospective cohort study. *Lancet* **2020**, *395*, 1054–1062. [CrossRef]
23. Wu, J.T.; Leung, K.; Bushman, M.; Kishore, N.; Niehus, R.; de Salazar, P.M.; Cowling, B.J.; Lipsitch, M.; Leung, G.M. Estimating clinical severity of COVID-19 from the transmission dynamics in Wuhan, China. *Nat. Med.* **2020**, *26*, 506–510. [CrossRef]
24. Horton, K.C.; MacPherson, P.; Houben, R.M.; White, R.G.; Corbett, E.L. Sex differences in tuberculosis burden and notifications in low-and middle-income countries: A systematic review and meta-analysis. *PLoS Med.* **2016**, *13*, e1002119. [CrossRef] [PubMed]
25. Horton, K.C.; White, R.G.; Houben, R.M. Systematic neglect of men as a key population in tuberculosis. *Tuberculosis* **2018**, *113*, 249–253. [CrossRef] [PubMed]
26. Xu, L.; Chen, G. Risk factors for severe corona virus disease 2019 (COVID-19) patients: A systematic review and meta analysis. *medRxiv* **2020**. [CrossRef]
27. Jeon, C.Y.; Murray, M.B. Diabetes mellitus increases the risk of active tuberculosis: A systematic review of 13 observational studies. *PLoS Med.* **2008**, *5*, e152.
28. Del Rio, C.; Malani, P.N. COVID-19—new insights on a rapidly changing epidemic. *JAMA* **2020**, *323*, 1339–1340. [CrossRef] [PubMed]
29. Morrison, J.; Pai, M.; Hopewell, P.C. Tuberculosis and latent tuberculosis infection in close contacts of people with pulmonary tuberculosis in low-income and middle-income countries: A systematic review and meta-analysis. *Lancet Infect. Dis.* **2008**, *8*, 359–368. [CrossRef]
30. Behr, M.A.; Edelstein, P.H.; Ramakrishnan, L. Revisiting the timetable of tuberculosis. *BMJ* **2018**, *362*, k2738. [CrossRef]
31. Lauer, S.A.; Grantz, K.H.; Bi, Q.; Jones, F.K.; Zheng, Q.; Meredith, H.R.; Azman, A.S.; Reich, N.G.; Lessler, J. The incubation period of coronavirus disease 2019 (COVID-19) from publicly reported confirmed cases: Estimation and application. *Ann. Intern. Med.* **2020**. [CrossRef]
32. Watkins, J. Preventing a covid-19 pandemic. *BMJ* **2020**. [CrossRef]
33. Anderson, R.M.; Heesterbeek, H.; Klinkenberg, D.; Hollingsworth, T.D. How will country-based mitigation measures influence the course of the COVID-19 epidemic? *Lancet* **2020**, *395*, 931–934. [CrossRef]
34. Xiao, Y.; Torok, M.E. Taking the right measures to control COVID-19. *Lancet Infect. Dis.* **2020**. [CrossRef]
35. Chen, S.; Yang, J.; Yang, W.; Wang, C.; Bärnighausen, T. COVID-19 control in China during mass population movements at New Year. *Lancet* **2020**, *395*, 764–766. [CrossRef]
36. Bedford, J.; Enria, D.; Giesecke, J.; Heymann, D.L.; Ihekweazu, C.; Kobinger, G.; Lane, H.C.; Memish, Z.; Oh, M.; Sall, A.A.; et al. COVID-19: Towards controlling of a pandemic. *Lancet* **2020**, *395*, 1015–1018. [CrossRef]
37. Acuña-Villaorduña, C.; Jones-López, E.C.; Fregona, G.; Marques-Rodrigues, P.; Gaeddert, M.; Geadas, C.; Hadad, D.J.; White, L.F.; Molina, L.P.D.; Vinhas, S.; et al. Intensity of exposure to pulmonary tuberculosis determines risk of tuberculosis infection and disease. *Eur. Respir. J.* **2018**, *51*, 1701578. [CrossRef]
38. Cilloni, L.; Fu, H.; Vesga, J.F.; Dowdy, D.; Pretorius, C.; Ahmedov, S.; Nair, S.A.; Mosneaga, A.; Masini, E.O.; Suvanand, S.; et al. The potential impact of the COVID-19 pandemic on tuberculosis: A modelling analysis. *medRxiv* **2020**. [CrossRef]

39. Singh, M.; Mynak, M.; Kumar, L.; Mathew, J.; Jindal, S. Prevalence and risk factors for transmission of infection among children in household contact with adults having pulmonary tuberculosis. *Arch. Dis. Child.* **2005**, *90*, 624–628. [CrossRef]
40. Lalor, M.K.; Anderson, L.F.; Hamblion, E.L.; Burkitt, A.; Davidson, J.A.; Maguire, H.; Abubakar, I.; Thomas, H.L. Recent household transmission of tuberculosis in England, 2010–2012: Retrospective national cohort study combining epidemiological and molecular strain typing data. *BMC Med.* **2017**, *15*, 105. [CrossRef]
41. Saunders, M.J.; Wingfield, T.; Datta, S.; Montoya, R.; Ramos, E.; Baldwin, M.R.; Bio, E.R.; Baldwin, M.R.; Tovar, M.A.; Evans, B.E.W.; et al. A household-level score to predict the risk of tuberculosis among contacts of patients with tuberculosis: A derivation and external validation prospective cohort study. *Lancet Infect. Dis.* **2020**, *20*, 110–122. [CrossRef]
42. Ragonnet, R.; Trauer, J.M.; Geard, N.; Scott, N.; McBryde, E.S. Profiling Mycobacterium tuberculosis transmission and the resulting disease burden in the five highest tuberculosis burden countries. *BMC Med.* **2019**, *17*, 208. [CrossRef]
43. McCreesh, N.; White, R.G. An explanation for the low proportion of tuberculosis that results from transmission between household and known social contacts. *Sci. Rep.* **2018**, *8*, 5382. [CrossRef]
44. Karim, S.S.A.; Churchyard, G.J.; Karim, Q.A.; Lawn, S.D. HIV infection and tuberculosis in South Africa: An urgent need to escalate the public health response. *Lancet* **2009**, *374*, 921–933. [CrossRef]
45. Nunn, P.; Williams, B.; Floyd, K.; Dye, C.; Elzinga, G.; Raviglione, M. Tuberculosis control in the era of HIV. *Nat. Rev. Immunol.* **2005**, *5*, 819–826. [CrossRef] [PubMed]
46. UN. *Policy Brief: The Impact of COVID-19 on Children*; UN: New York, NY, USA, 2020.
47. WHO. *Who Operational Handbook on Tuberculosis: Module 1: Prevention: Tuberculosis Preventive Treatment*; World Health Organization: Geneva, Switzerland, 2020.
48. Qin, C.; Zhou, L.; Hu, Z.; Zhang, S.; Yang, S.; Tao, Y.; Xie, C.; Ma, K.; Shang, K.; Wang, W.; et al. Dysregulation of immune response in patients with COVID-19 in Wuhan, China. *Clin. Infect. Dis.* **2020**. [CrossRef]
49. Shi, Y.; Wang, Y.; Shao, C.; Huang, J.; Gan, J.; Huang, X.; Bucci, E.; Piacentini, M.; Ippolito, G.; Melino, G.; et al. COVID-19 infection: The perspectives on immune responses. *Nature* **2020**, *27*, 1451–1454. [CrossRef]
50. Singh, V.; Sharma, B.B.; Patel, V. Pulmonary sequelae in a patient recovered from swine flu. *Lung India Off. Organ Indian Chest Soc.* **2012**, *29*, 277. [CrossRef]
51. Noymer, A. The 1918–19 influenza pandemic affected tuberculosis in the United States: Reconsidering Bradshaw, Smith, and Blanchard. *Biodemogr. Soc. Biol.* **2008**, *54*, 125–133. [CrossRef]
52. Pawlowski, A.; Jansson, M.; Sköld, M.; Rottenberg, M.E.; Källenius, G. Tuberculosis and HIV co-infection. *PLoS Pathog.* **2012**, *8*, e1002464. [CrossRef]
53. Barnes, P.F.; Bloch, A.B.; Davidson, P.T.; Snider, D.E., Jr. Tuberculosis in patients with human immunodeficiency virus infection. *N. Engl. J. Med.* **1991**, *324*, 1644–1650. [CrossRef]
54. Sumner, A.; Hoy, C.; Ortiz-Juarez, E. *Estimates of the Impact of COVID-19 on Global Poverty*; United Nations University: Helsinki, Finland, 2020; Volume 43.
55. Lancet, T. *Tackling Poverty in Tuberculosis Control*; Elsevier: Amsterdam, The Netherlands, 2005.
56. Spence, D.P.; Hotchkiss, J.; Williams, C.S.; Davies, P.D. Tuberculosis and poverty. *BMJ* **1993**, *307*, 759–761. [CrossRef]
57. Oxlade, O.; Murray, M. Tuberculosis and poverty: Why are the poor at greater risk in India? *PLoS ONE* **2012**, *7*, e47533. [CrossRef]
58. WHO. *WHO Guidelines on Tuberculosis Infection Prevention and Control: 2019 Update: World Health Organization*; World Health Organization: Geneva, Switzerland, 2019.

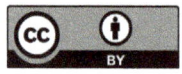

© 2020 by the authors. Licensee MDPI, Basel, Switzerland. This article is an open access article distributed under the terms and conditions of the Creative Commons Attribution (CC BY) license (http://creativecommons.org/licenses/by/4.0/).

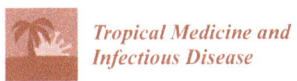

Article

Investing in Operational Research Capacity Building for Front-Line Health Workers Strengthens Countries' Resilience to Tackling the COVID-19 Pandemic

Rony Zachariah [1,*], Selma Dar Berger [2], Pruthu Thekkur [2,3], Mohammed Khogali [1], Karapet Davtyan [4], Ajay M. V. Kumar [2,3,5], Srinath Satyanarayana [3], Francis Moses [6], Garry Aslanyan [1], Abraham Aseffa [1], Anthony D. Harries [2,7] and John C. Reeder [1]

1. UNICEF, UNDP, World Bank, WHO Special Programme for Research and Training in Tropical Disease (TDR), 1211 Geneva, Switzerland; khogalim@who.int (M.K.); aslanyang@who.int (G.A.); armidiea@who.int (A.A.); reederj@who.int (J.C.R.)
2. Center for Operational Research, International Union against Tuberculosis and Lung Disease (The Union), 75006 Paris, France; sberger@theunion.org (S.D.B.); pruthu.tk@theunion.org (P.T.); akumar@theunion.org (A.M.V.K.); adharries@theunion.org (A.D.H.)
3. Center for Operational Research, The Union South-East Asia (USEA), New Delhi 110016, India; SSrinath@theunion.org
4. Country Health Policies and Systems, World Health Organization Regional Office for Europe, 2100 Copenhagen, Denmark; kdavtyan@who.int
5. Community Medicine, Yenepoya Medical College (Deemed to Be University), Yenepoya, Mangalore 575018, India
6. Reproductive Health and Family Planning Program, Ministry of Health and Sanitation, Freetown 23222, Sierra Leone; franqoline@gmail.com
7. London School of Hygiene and Tropical Medicine, Keppel Street, London WC1 7HT, UK
* Correspondence: zachariahr@who.int; Tel.: +41-79-72-88-488

Received: 27 June 2020; Accepted: 15 July 2020; Published: 16 July 2020

Abstract: (1) Introduction. The Structured Operational Research and Training IniTiative (SORT IT) supports countries to build operational research capacity for improving public health. We assessed whether health workers trained through SORT IT were (1) contributing to the COVID-19 pandemic response and if so, (2) map where and how they were applying their SORT IT skills. (2) Methods. An online questionnaire survey of SORT IT alumni trained between 2009 and 2019. (3) Results. Of 895 SORT IT alumni from 93 countries, 652 (73%) responded to the survey and 417 were contributing to the COVID-19 response in 72 countries. Of those contributing, 307 (74%) were applying their SORT IT skills to tackle the pandemic in 60 countries and six continents including Africa, Asia, Europe, South Pacific and North/South America. Skills were applied to all the pillars of the emergency response with the highest proportions of alumni applying their skills in data generation/analysis/reporting (56%), situation analysis (55%) and surveillance (41%). Skills were also being used to mitigate the health system effects of COVID-19 on other diseases (27%) and in conducting research (26%). (4) Conclusion. Investing in people and in research training ahead of public health emergencies generates downstream dividends by strengthening health system resilience for tackling pandemics. It also strengthens human resources for health and the integration of research within health systems.

Keywords: COVID-19; operational research; health systems; SORT IT; pandemics; training

1. Introduction

"The operational research training I received from TDR and its partners has been invaluable as it has enabled me to transfer the skills I acquired while conducting research on Ebola to my current work on COVID-19"—Dr James Squire, Ministry of Health, Sierra Leone.

These words coming from a front-line doctor who led the 2014/2015 Ebola outbreak response at its epicenter in Kailahun district in Sierra Leone merit reflection. Dr Squire is now leading the Ministry of Health's efforts to enhance surveillance systems that generate real-time, high-quality and disaggregated data for tackling Coronavirus disease 2019 (COVID-19). Encouragingly, he is applying the research skills he gained through the Structured Operational Research and Training InitiaTive (SORT IT) to his current work on COVID-19, but how exactly are these skills being applied? Such information would help inform the wider gains of investing in research training.

SORT IT is a global partnership-based initiative led by TDR, The Special Programme for Research and Training in Tropical Diseases, and implemented with various partners including ministries of health, non-governmental organizations (NGOs) and academic institutions [1]. It supports countries to build operational research capacity for strengthening health care delivery systems, improving programme performance and promoting public health [1,2]. The model is unique in that it targets front-line health workers and other programme staff, embraces "on the job" learning and simultaneously combines research training with research implementation [3].

In line with a WHO call that "all nations should be producers and consumers of research and research capacity be strengthened close to the supply of and demand for health services" [4], SORT IT has trained participants from 93 countries [5]. With 70% of research studies influencing policy and practice, SORT IT examines what works or does not work in real-world settings and introduces solutions to improve health care [6].

In the light of the COVID-19 pandemic, the link between this training programme and its role in strengthening health system resilience to respond to pandemics merits examination. We therefore assessed (1) whether SORT IT alumni are contributing to the COVID-19 pandemic response and if so, (2) map where and how they are applying their SORT IT skills.

2. Methods

We carried out a semi-structured questionnaire-based survey on all SORT IT alumni trained from the start of the SORT IT programme (in 2009) until December 2019. E-mails of alumni were sourced from a SORT IT web-based alumni network and a training database. Between March and April 2020, each alumnus received a SurveyMonkey link (surveymonkey.co.uk) to access the questionnaire.

The questionnaire was pre-tested and included information on demographics, whether the person was currently involved with the COVID-19 response and if so, whether he/she was applying the skills gained from the SORT IT training to the pandemic response. If the response to the latter was "yes", the person was asked to specify the area(s) where the skills were being applied and provide some illustrative information. Up to two reminders were sent if responses were not received within 7 days. Where e-mails were invalid, social media links (Facebook Messenger, Skype and Whats App) were used to update contact details and send reminders.

The SORT IT programme covered various aspects of the research cycle such as research prioritization, formulation of the research question, study protocol writing, efficient data capture and analysis, manuscript writing and knowledge management [1]. SORT IT also has an in-built system to gather information for improving the quality and performance of the training programme [1]. Survey responders were all adults, participation was voluntary, data were anonymized, there were no personal identifiers and no sensitive personal questions were included that could risk psychological or social harm. This was thus considered a minimal risk study and the Ethics Advisory Group of the International Union Against Tuberculosis and Lung Disease, Paris, France (which oversees ethics reviews for the SORT IT global partnership), determined that ethics clearance was not required for this study. The survey data was exported to Microsoft Excel and used for data analysis.

3. Results

The survey covered 84 SORT IT courses with 895 alumni from 93 countries. A total of 652 (73%) alumni (female = 45%) responded to the survey (Figure 1). Of those who responded, 417 from 72 countries were actively involved in the COVID-19 response and 307 (74%) from 60 countries were applying their skills acquired from SORT IT courses to tackle the pandemic (Figure 2). The top five Low-and Middle Income-Countries (LMIC) where alumni were applying their skills included India (70), Myanmar (32), Zimbabwe (26), Kenya (19), Pakistan (18) and China (6). SORT IT Alumni were also using their acquired skills in high-income countries (HIC) including Australia, Belgium, Canada, Italy, Japan, USA, and the United Kingdom (Figure 2).

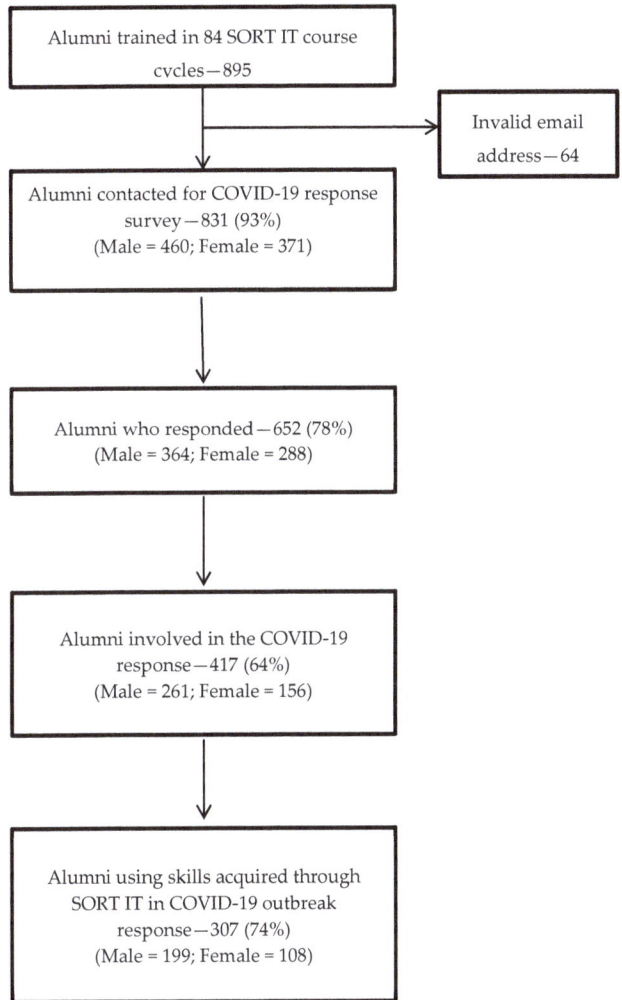

Figure 1. Flowchart showing response rate, involvement in COVID-19 and utilization of skills acquired through the Structured Operational Research and Training InitiaTive (SORT IT, 2009–2019).

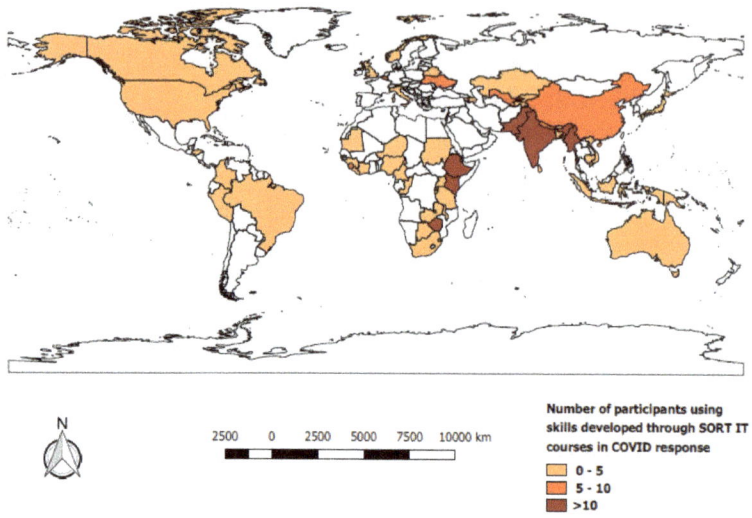

(SORT IT: Structured Operational Research and Training InitiaTive).

Africa (22 countries): Zimbabwe (26), Kenya (19), Ethiopia (13), Sierra Leone (8), Uganda (5), Guinea (4), Malawi (4), South Africa (3), Sudan (3), eSwatini (2), Nigeria (2), Rwanda (2), Botswana (1), Burundi (1), Republic of Cameroon (1), Côte d'Ivoire (1), Democratic Republic of the Congo (1), Liberia (1), Mauritania (1), Niger (1), United Republic of Tanzania (1), Zambia (1)

Asia (16 countries): India (70), Myanmar (32), Pakistan (18), Nepal (8), China (6), Uzbekistan (6), Bhutan (5), Kyrgyzstan (3), Bangladesh (2), Tajikistan (2), Cambodia (1), Indonesia (1), Japan (1), Kazakhstan (1), Sri Lanka (1), Vietnam (1)

Europe (8 countries): Belgium (6), Ukraine (6), Armenia (3), Italy (2), Azerbaijan (1), Belarus (1), Norway (1), United Kingdom (1)

South Pacific (7 countries): Federated States of Micronesia (4), Fiji (3), Papua New Guinea (3), Kiribati (2), Palau (2), Republic of the Marshall Islands (1), Guam (1)

South America (3 countries): Colombia (2), Brazil (1), Peru (1)

North America (3 countries): Canada (2), United States America (2) Honduras (1) Australia (2).

Figure 2. Geographic mapping of 307 SORT IT alumni applying their acquired SORT IT skills in 60 countries to tackle the COVID-19 pandemic.

Table 1 shows various areas of the COVID-19 emergency response where SORT IT alumni were applying their skills with some illustrative quotes. Skills were being applied in all the pillars of the outbreak response, namely: situation analysis, surveillance, emergency preparedness, case management and data generation and reporting. The three areas with the highest proportion of alumni applying their skills were data generation, analysis and reporting (56%), situation analysis (55%) and surveillance (41%). Alumni were also applying their skills in mitigating the health system effects of COVID-19 on diseases such as tuberculosis, HIV and non-communicable diseases (27%) and in conducting COVID-19 related research (26%).

In total, alumni from 85 countries responded, in 72 countries they were involved in the COVID-19 response and in 60 countries they were applying their skills gained through SORT IT.

Table 1. Categories of the COVID-19 pandemic response where trainees applied skills gained through the Structured Operational Research and Training Initiative (SORT IT, 2009–2019). Illustrative quotes are provided for each category (N=307).

Categories of the COVID-19 Response	Applying SORT IT Skills n (%)	Illustrative Quotes from Trainees around the Globe
Situation analysis	168 (55)	I was able to conduct a situation analysis on the Taftan border of Baluchistan and establish measures for screening, management and reporting of COVID-19—Pakistan I conducted a situational analysis in preparedness of health facilities to respond to COVID-19. I looked at availability of IPC equipment/supplies, staff capacity in case identification and management, and IPC practices to prevention spread—Uganda
Epidemic surveillance	126 (41)	I helped introduce a mobile health surveillance tool (TeCHO+) that is being used by community health workers to screen over 30 million people for COVID-19 in Gujarat—India I was able to adapt the District Health Information System (DHIS2) to set up a surveillance and tracking system in my country—Bhutan
Emergency preparedness and response	118 (38)	I am part of the rapid investigation team of MoH/WHO for outbreak investigation, emergency preparedness and response for Rohingya refugees in Cox's Bazar—Bangladesh The SORT IT knowledge helped me develop a mixed method study on health system preparedness to respond to the COVID-19 pandemic. It also helped my team to have an analysis plan to improve understanding of the findings by policy makers—Guinea
Infection, prevention and control (IPC) including health worker safety	145 (47)	The knowledge I acquired from the SORT IT training on Infection, Prevention and Control is being applied to the COVID-19 response—Zambia I was able to conduct a survey on the status of preparedness of health care workers for COVID-19—Kazakhstan
Clinical management (screening, diagnosis and clinical care)	82 (27)	I am leading a team in 3 districts Hospitals and 42 health centers on screening, protocol development and trainings—Rwanda I reviewed literature, analyzed data from quarantine centers and appraised the Ministry of Health and the Prime Minister's office on decisions regarding duration of quarantine and follow up thereafter—Bhutan
Data generation analysis and reporting	173 (56)	I was able to do data analysis of all surveillance reports received from the 35 facilities in a sub-county—Kenya I am developing a mobile reporting application for suspected COVID-19 patients. The code-books learnt from SORT IT are very useful for the software development—Myanmar

Table 1. Cont.

Categories of the COVID-19 Response	Applying SORT IT Skills n (%)	Illustrative Quotes from Trainees around the Globe
Operational or clinical research	79 (26)	My team are helping projects in different parts of the world to develop "simple" tools to efficiently capture relevant COVID-19 data to be used for operational research—Médecins Sans Frontières—BelgiumAs a research analyst for homeless shelters, the data analysis and writing skills I learnt, and the application of operational research principles are critical for my current work—Canada
Mitigating COVID-19 effect on other diseases (TB, HIV/AIDS, NCDs)	83 (27)	I was able to use routine programme data to highlight significant declines in uptake of routine antenatal services and specific measures are being taken to address this in the community and at health facilities—Sierra LeoneI was able to instruct health staff in the endocrine and diabetic clinics on Infection, Prevention and Control measures and re-arranged scheduling to reduce health worker exposure to COVID-19—Sri Lanka
Others	23 (8)	I am better at thinking more logically which is useful in all that I do—United KingdomI was able to organize courses, seminars and meetings with health authorities and to prepare flow charts for patient care—Honduras

TB: Tuberculosis; HIV/AIDS: Human Immune Deficiency Virus/Acquired Immune Deficiency Syndrome; NCDS: Non-Communicable Diseases. Many participants reported using several skills, and hence numbers and percentages are more than 488 and 100% respectively.

4. Discussion

This is one of the first studies showing that SORT IT provides skillsets and core competencies that can be used transversally in building health system resilience at the time of a pandemic. Encouragingly, about seven in every ten individuals involved with COVID-19 reported applying their SORT IT acquired skills in 60 countries, including both LMICs and HICs.

These findings show that SORT IT has equipped front-line health workers not only with research skills, but also with a skill-set needed to respond to the unprecedented COVID-19 pandemic [7]. This proves the down-stream benefits of investing in operational research capacity building. The wide geographic coverage with no dichotomy between LMICS and HICs shows that such skills are universally applicable and likely to enhance global solidarity in tackling future outbreaks and pandemics.

There might have been a perception by some donors that investing in research capacity building is a luxury that is divorced from public health action. Much funding for research training also lies with academic institutions and is not accessible to implementers from disease control programmes [3,8,9]. It is time for a *volte-face*.

The strengths of this study are that SORT IT alumni in 93 countries were contacted and specific efforts were made to validate invalid e-mails, thereby limiting non-responders. As the SORT IT programme has a robust built-in monitoring and evaluation system, we were able to make use of this existing system to gather both quantitative and qualitative information. Study limitations include a response rate of 73%, which under the circumstances is still acceptable to good, the self-reported nature of the response, the potential social desirability bias and, considering the continued expansion of the COVID-19 pandemic, possible underestimation in our figures.

There are a few other salient observations. First, skills are being applied beyond research to all the vital pillars of the outbreak response. While SORT IT teaches multiple and practical skills for activities such as generating and utilizing data, conducting operational research and using evidence to influence policy and/or practice, several transversal skills are acquired at the same time [1]. For example, skills are developed in fostering stakeholder engagement, performing situation analysis in programme settings, prioritizing health issues, ensuring quality-assured data capture and analysis, critically reviewing the scientific literature, scientific writing to the standards of a medical journal and managing knowledge. It is therefore not surprising that those who were trained through the SORT IT programme acquired a "tool-kit" of skills that can then be applied to several areas of the outbreak response.

Second, the three areas where acquired skills were particularly used were data generation, situation analysis and setting up surveillance systems. The generation of high quality, timely and disaggregated data is essential for ensuring that countries tackling COVID-19 become "data rich, information rich and action rich"—a fundamental goal of the SORT IT programme [2]. Conducting a sound situation analysis and setting up robust surveillance systems are crucial in any outbreak: these help to feel and monitor the pulse of an outbreak and prevent responders from thinking and acting blindly.

Third, with the lock-down and restricted movements imposed by COVID-19, individuals with chronic diseases such as tuberculosis, HIV/AIDS and non-communicable diseases will understandably face hurdles in accessing diagnostic and treatment facilities and adhering to follow-up schedules [10]. It is encouraging that SORT IT alumni were using their skills in offsetting these negative health system effects.

Finally, following the 2014/2015 Ebola outbreak, WHO spearheaded global efforts to avert epidemics by making Research and Development (R&D) "outbreak-ready" [7]. While this will accelerate R&D on vaccines, drugs, and diagnostics, finding out "how to deliver" these innovations in an equitable manner is imperative [8]. SORT IT could play an important role in such operational research.

In conclusion, the results of this study demonstrate the value of investing in people and in research training ahead of public health emergencies. Clearly, building upstream operational research capacity has generated downstream dividends in strengthening health system resilience for tackling pandemics. In addition, it strengthens human resources for health (HRH) and the integration of research within health systems. In summary, it allows the health system to have the right people in the right place at the right time.

Author Contributions: All authors were involved with the conception and design, R.Z., S.D.B., P.T., M.K. were involved with data collection, analysis and interpretation while K.D., A.M.V.K., S.S., F.M., G.A., A.A., A.D.H. and J.C.R. were involved with interpretation. R.Z. wrote the first draft of the manuscript, which was revised by all and all authors have read and agreed to the published version of the manuscript.

Funding: This research received no specific external funding.

Acknowledgments: TDR and partners can conduct their work thanks to the commitment and support from a variety of funders. These include our long-term core contributors from national governments and international institutions, as well as designated funding for specific projects within our current priorities. A full list of TDR donors is available on our website at: https://www.who.int/tdr/about/funding/en/. We are grateful to all these donors and particularly those who have supported research training activities, which allow health workers to save lives on the frontlines of the COVID-19 public health emergency. We are also grateful to all the SORT IT alumni who have responded to this survey despite their tight schedules and for their invaluable work in tackling COVID-19.

Conflicts of Interest: We have no conflict of interest to declare.

Data Availability Statement: De-identified study data are available on reasonable request from the corresponding author (zachariahr@who.int). A justification for its further use should be provided.

References

1. Ramsay, A.; Harries, A.D.; Zachariah, R.; Bissell, K.; Hinderaker, S.G.; Edginton, M.; Enarson, D.A.; Satyanarayana, S.; Kumar, A.M.V.; Hoa, N.B.; et al. The Structured Operational Research and Training Initiative for public health programmes. *Public Health Action* **2014**, *4*, 79–84. [CrossRef] [PubMed]
2. Harries, A.; Khogali, M.; Kumar, A.M.V.; Satyanarayana, S.; Takarinda, K.C.; Karpati, A.; Olliaro, P.; Zachariah, R. Building the capacity of public health programmes to become data rich, information rich and action rich. *Public Health Action* **2018**, *8*, 34–36. [CrossRef] [PubMed]
3. Rujumba, J. Byamugisha, R. Publishing operational research from 'real life' programme data: A better form of accountability. *Trop. Med. Int. Health* **2011**, *17*, 133–134. [CrossRef] [PubMed]
4. WHO. *The World Health Report 2013: Research for Universal Health Coverage*; World Health Organization: Geneva, Switzerland, 2013; Available online: http://apps.who.int/iris/bitstream/10665/85761/2/9789240690837_eng.pdf (accessed on 13 March 2014).
5. TDR. SORT IT Coverage and Outputs. Available online: https://www.who.int/tdr/capacity/strengthening/sort/en/ (accessed on 4 April 2020).
6. Kumar, A.M.; Shewade, H.D.; Tripathy, J.P.; Guillerm, N.; Tayler-Smith, K.; Berger, S.D.; Bissell, K.; Reid, A.J.; Zachariah, R.; Harries, A.D. Does research through Structured Operational Research and Training (SORT IT) courses impact policy and practice? *Public Health Action* **2016**, *6*, 44–49. [CrossRef] [PubMed]
7. Shamasunder, S.; Holmes, S.M.; Goronga, T.; Carrasco, H.; Katz, E.; Frankfurter, R.; Keshavjee, S. COVID-19 reveals weak health systems by design: Why we must re-make global health in this historic moment. *Glob. Public Health* **2020**, 1–7. [CrossRef]
8. Walley, J.; Khan, M.A.; Shah, S.K.; Witter, S.; Wei, X. How to get research into practice: First get practice into research. *Bull. World Health Organ.* **2007**, *85*, 424. [CrossRef] [PubMed]
9. Chalmers, I.; Glasziou, P. Avoidable waste in the production and reporting of research evidence. *Obstet. Gynecol.* **2009**, *114*, 1341–1345. [CrossRef]
10. Adepoju, P. Tuberculosis and HIV responses threatened by COVID-19. *Lancet HIV* **2020**, *7*, e319–e320. [CrossRef]

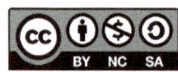

© 2020 by World Health Organization; Licensee MDPI, Basel, Switzerland. This is an open access article distributed under the terms of the Creative Commons Attribution IGO License (http://creativecommons.org/licenses/by/3.0/igo/legalcode), which permits unrestricted use, distribution, and reproduction in any medium, provided the original work is properly cited. In any reproduction of this article there should not be any suggestion that WHO or this article endorse any specific organisation or products. The use of the WHO logo is not permitted.

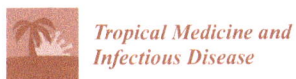 *Tropical Medicine and Infectious Disease*

Case Report

Treatment of Severe COVID-19 with Tocilizumab Mitigates Cytokine Storm and Averts Mechanical Ventilation during Acute Respiratory Distress: A Case Report and Literature Review

Faryal Farooqi [1,*], Naveen Dhawan [1], Richard Morgan [1], John Dinh [1], Kester Nedd [1] and George Yatzkan [2]

1. Department of Internal Medicine, Larkin Community Hospital, South Miami, FL 33143, USA; naveendhawan@hotmail.com (N.D.); morgan@larkinhospital.com (R.M.); Jdinh@larkinhospital.com (J.D.); knedd01@gmail.com (K.N.)
2. Department of Pulmonary Medicine, Larkin Community Hospital, South Miami, FL 33143, USA; georgeyatzkan@yahoo.com
* Correspondence: faryalifarooqi@gmail.com or ffarooqi@larkinhospital.com

Received: 21 May 2020; Accepted: 2 July 2020; Published: 3 July 2020

Abstract: COVID-19, caused by the novel severe acute respiratory coronavirus 2 (SARS-CoV-2), emerged in Wuhan, China, in 2019 and has resulted in the current pandemic. The disease continues to pose a major therapeutic challenge. Patient mortality is ultimately caused by acute respiratory distress syndrome (ARDS). Cytokine release syndrome (or "cytokine storm") is likely to be a contributing factor to ARDS in many patients. Because interleukin 6 (IL-6) is known to play a key role in inflammation, IL-6 receptor inhibitors such as tocilizumab may potentially treat COVID-19 by attenuating cytokine release. We present the case of a 48-year-old male with severe COVID-19, on the verge of meeting intubation requirements, who needed progressive oxygen support for respiratory distress. The patient was treated with a non-weight-based dosage of tocilizumab to prevent the onset of a cytokine storm. We chose to administer an IL-6 inhibitor because of the gradually increasing levels of acute phase reactants identified on serial blood draws, as well as his declining respiratory status. The treatment was well-tolerated in conjunction with standard drug therapies for COVID-19 (hydroxychloroquine, azithromycin, and zinc). The patient subsequently experienced marked improvements in his respiratory symptoms and overall clinical status over the following days. We believe that tocilizumab played a substantial role in his ability to avert clinical decline, particularly the need for mechanical ventilation. Ultimately, the patient was downgraded from the ICU and discharged within days. We highlight the potential of IL-6 inhibitors to prevent the progression of respiratory disease to a point requiring ventilator support. This case underscores the potential importance of early serial measurements of IL-6 and cytokine storm-associated acute phase reactants, such as ferritin, D-dimer, and C-reactive protein, in guiding clinical decision-making in the management of patients with suspected COVID-19. **Conclusion:** The early, proactive identification of serum acute phase reactants should be implemented in the treatment of COVID-19 in order to screen for a primary contributor to mortality—the cytokine storm. This screening, when followed by aggressive early treatment for cytokine storm, may have optimal therapeutic benefits and obviate the need for mechanical ventilation, thereby decreasing mortality. Additionally, we review current evidence regarding cytokine release syndrome in COVID-19 and the use of IL-6 receptor inhibition as a therapeutic strategy, and examine other reported cases in the literature describing IL-6 antagonist treatment for patients with COVID-19.

Keywords: COVID-19; SARS-CoV-2; IL-6 inhibitors; tocilizumab; cytokine release syndrome; cytokine storm

1. Introduction

The novel coronavirus disease 2019 (COVID-19) outbreak started in December 2019 in Wuhan, China, and has emerged as a major pandemic [1,2]. Severe acute respiratory syndrome coronavirus (SARS-CoV-2), an enveloped positive-stranded RNA virus, was later identified as the causative agent [3,4]. As of April 28, 2020, there were more than 3,000,000 reported cases and 200,00 deaths from COVID-19 worldwide [5]. The case-fatality rate of COVID-19 has been estimated to be 2–3%, although estimates vary [6]. Patients with severe cases develop pneumonia that can lead to acute respiratory distress syndrome (ARDS) [3]. Respiratory failure secondary to ARDS in patients with COVID-19 is the most common cause of death [7].

Currently, no specific effective drug treatment or vaccine is available for COVID-19 [8,9]. Therapeutic management is supportive, but some repurposed off-label anti-HIV and anti-viral medications are currently in use, including hydroxychloroquine, remdesevir, lopinavir/ritonavir, and interleukin 6 (IL-6) receptor inhibitors, in addition to convalescent plasma therapy [9–12]. Although several trials are underway, the use of these drugs remains to be substantiated by large, randomized clinical studies; to date, they have only shown promise in anecdotal experiences and circumstantial evidence mostly derived from studies conducted in vitro or in patients in single-arm studies with limited sample sizes and nonrandomized subject populations, which have yielded mixed results [10,13–18].

A major clinical feature of COVID-19 is lung-centric pathology resulting in respiratory deterioration, and the most common cause of death is acute respiratory failure due to ARDS [3,19]. According to current data, only 5% of all COVID-19 infections result in ARDS requiring mechanical ventilation, because most infected individuals experience complete recovery [20]. However, 25% of all patients with COVID-19 are believed to clinically progress and acquire critical complications, including ARDS, in which patients may quickly deteriorate and succumb to respiratory failure [21]. In particular, the survival rate among patients who require ventilator support remains poor. In a recent study on ICU patients with COVID-19 in Wuhan, China, only 21% of patients requiring non-invasive mechanical ventilation and 14% of patients requiring invasive mechanical ventilation survived [22]. Therefore, the early management of respiratory symptoms to prevent progression to ARDS and avert the need for mechanical ventilation is critical for preventing mortality.

Cytokine storm, a hyperinflammatory state mediated by the release of cytokines, is known to be a key cause of ARDS [21]. In this regard, disrupting cytokine storm is an important potential therapeutic approach [21]. Interleukin 6 (IL-6), a multifunctional mediator of inflammation, is widely believed to play a pivotal role in the development of cytokine storm and to eventually cause the ARDS and interstitial pneumonia seen in severe COVID-19 [7,20,23,24]. The attenuation of IL-6 through receptor blockade has been hypothesized to blunt the cytokine storm responsible for respiratory disease progression [20].

Promising results of a recent single-arm trial of 21 patients with severe COVID-19 in China in February 2020 showed clinical improvements after therapy with the IL-6 receptor antagonist tocilizumab. Consequently, the Chinese National Health Commission included tocilizumab in the 7th edition of its guide for COVID-19 diagnosis and treatment [20,21,25]. Italian guidelines followed suit and began to suggest the use of tocilizumab in cases of rapid radiologic and clinical deterioration [26,27]. Other trials are currently underway worldwide to better understand the potential therapeutic effects of IL-6 receptor inhibitors for COVID-19 treatment [28,29]. Currently, 23 trials are investigating the use of tocilizumab worldwide [28]. Additionally, ten trials are underway to investigate the role of the IL-6 receptor inhibitor sarilumab for treating COVID-19 [29].

Here, we present the case of a patient with severe COVID-19 who was administered tocilizumab, combined with generally accepted therapy at the time (hydroxychloroquine, azithromycin, and zinc), in an ICU setting. From a clinical standpoint, cytokine storm development was observed, as the patient required incremental increases in oxygen therapy (L/min) just prior to tocilizumab administration. He was on the verge of requiring intubation and mechanical ventilation, on the basis of his apparent respiratory distress and arterial blood gas measurements. Interestingly, the patient showed immediate improvement and did not require ventilatory support after he received the IL-6 inhibitor. He eventually recovered and was sufficiently stable for hospital discharge shortly thereafter. The present case highlights the importance of addressing a mounting cytokine storm in its early stages. Our findings imply that inhibition of the IL-6 receptor has profound benefits under certain circumstances of severe COVID-19.

2. Case Presentation

A 48-year-old male cruise ship worker with no significant past medical history presented to our hospital with shortness of breath and the production of sputum. He had reportedly tested positive for COVID-19 before arrival at our hospital. He described having felt sick for seven days while on a cruise ship, with an initial acute onset of symptoms that developed over the course of a day and rapid progression to dyspnea on exertion. He also reported a productive cough with yellow sputum, fever, occasional hemoptysis, nasal congestion, a sore throat, and concomitant nausea and vomiting during the few days before admission. The patient denied experiencing any similar previous episodes.

On hospital admission, the patient was hypoxic in the emergency department and was placed on a non-rebreather mask. Arterial blood gas analysis after admission revealed a pH of 7.44, PCO_2 of 34, PO_2 of 113, and SaO_2 of 98.2% (with a 15% non-rebreather mask). When the non-rebreather mask was momentarily removed, desaturation occurred, and the SaO_2 decreased to 88%.

A chest X-ray revealed infiltrates visible as bilateral hazy opacities (in the right lung more than the left lung), thus suggesting possible multifocal pneumonia or pulmonary edema due to ARDS, along with cardiomegaly. Laboratory results revealed elevated acute phase reactants (erythrocyte sedimentation rate (ESR) 50, C-reactive protein (CRP) > 16, ferritin 672, and lactate dehydrogenase (LDH) 460) and lymphopenia (lymphocyte count 1.2). Additionally, the blood laboratory results showed transaminitis, with elevated aspartate aminotransferase (AST) at 58 and normal alanine aminotransferase (ALT) at 34.

The increased levels of acute phase reactants, an inflammatory biomarker profile elevated from baseline, and lymphopenia supported our suspicion of cytokine storm as a feature of COVID-19 [30]. The broader differential included acute hypoxic respiratory failure and early onset multifocal viral pneumonia with impending ARDS. Importantly, some of the primary acute phase reactants believed to be associated with cytokine storm include ferritin, D-dimer, CRP, troponin, and LDH [31–33]. The clinical values of ferritin, D-dimer, and CRP, in addition to the ESR, which is a general marker of inflammation, were closely monitored on a regular basis. Lymphocyte counts were regularly assessed as lymphopenia, which is also believed to be associated with cytokine storm in COVID-19 [31–33]. Oxygen saturation was also carefully monitored each day. To confirm SARS-CoV-2 infection, we conducted a nasopharyngeal swab test. The real-time reverse-transcriptase polymerase chain reaction (RT-PCR) assay results later revealed a positive result on day 5.

The treatment included high-flow oxygen, hydroxychloroquine, azithromycin, zinc, guaifenesin, acetaminophen, meropenem, vitamin c, cefepime, albuterol, atrovent, mucomyst, dexamethasone, and methylprednisolone. Additionally, the patient received two doses of tocilizumab (*Actemra*) at 500 mg administered 12 h apart. One dose was administered during the night of day 1, and a subsequent dose was administered the following morning. Overnight, the patient remained on the non-rebreather mask with 98% saturation.

On day 2, the patient began to feel fatigued and experienced greater difficulty breathing. Because the patient had not improved on the non-rebreather mask, he was switched to BiPAP with 100% oxygen. The IL-6 levels were elevated (66 pg/mL). The acute phase reactants remained elevated: D-dimer 2027, ferritin 588.1, ESR 100 (representing an increase), and CRP > 16. AST remained elevated (55), whereas ALT was normal (40). The lymphocyte count was 1.1.

On day 3, the laboratory results revealed leukocytosis (WBC 13.1). Both AST (48) and ALT (50) remained elevated. The acute phase reactants remained high (CRP trended downward but remained elevated (14.4), ESR 102, D-dimer 2660, and ferritin 824.8 (representing an increase)). The lymphocyte counts remained low (1.12). Troponin was measured on that day and was found to be low (<0.05). The patient's oxygen saturation remained low (88–89%), and then rose to 93% and later to 96%. The patient remained on BiPAP overnight and was then shifted to a non-rebreather mask and finally a nasal canula.

On day 4, the patient became more stable. He reported mild shortness of breath with no acute complaints. He was taken off the BiPAP and put on the 100% non-rebreather mask. The O_2 saturation was 99% peripherally. The acute phase reactants, although still elevated, had improved markedly from the previous day (CRP 4.7, ESR 89, D-dimer 1388, and ferritin 584.2). AST remained normal (27), and ALT was elevated (45). The lymphocyte counts were within normal limits (1.4). Leukocytosis persisted (WBC 16.7).

On day 5, the patient was stable and experienced only mild shortness of breath and no other complaints. He was still on a non-rebreather at 50%. The O_2 saturation was 96%. The acute phase reactant levels remained elevated, but most values showed improvement (D-dimer 1093, ESR 40, and CRP 3.6 (representing a decrease), and ferritin 682 (representing an increase from the previous day)). The lymphocyte count was 1.3. ALT was elevated (54), and AST was normal (29). The WBC level was 14.2. A chest X-ray revealed diminished infiltrates as patchy opacities compared with imaging on day 2 (Figure 1).

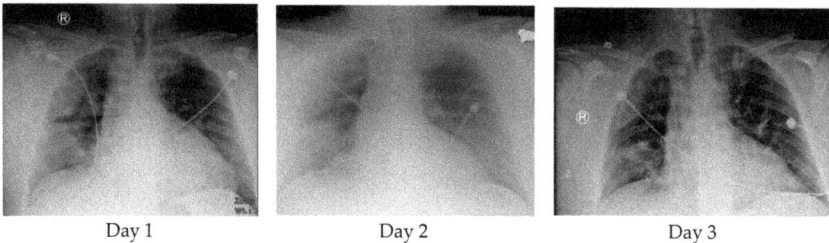

Figure 1. Chest X-rays on day 1, day 2, and day 5. Tocilizumab was administered as two doses of 500 mg Q12 (during the night of day 1 and the morning of day 2).

On day 6, the patient remained stable with even respiration and unlabored breathing. He continued on the non-rebreather mask at 98–99% levels. All acute phase reactant levels had decreased (CRP 1.5, ESR 25, D-dimer 724, and ferritin 564.1). ALT (37) and AST (25) were both normal. Lymphocyte (3.0) and WBC (9.03) counts were in normal ranges.

On day 7, the patient's condition further improved. The acute phase reactants had mostly further improved; CRP (1.1), D-dimer (811), and ferritin (538.3) remained at elevated levels, and ESR was in a normal range at 10. The lymphocyte count was 1.15. ALT remained elevated (43), and AST was normal (25). The patient continued on a non-rebreather mask and was transferred out of the ICU unit. The remainder of his hospital stay was unremarkable. He eventually fully recovered and was discharged from our hospital on day 17. The patient's clinical progression, as shown by acute phase reactants (ferritin, D-dimer, and CRP), the lymphocyte count, ESR, and O_2 saturation, are depicted in Figure 2.

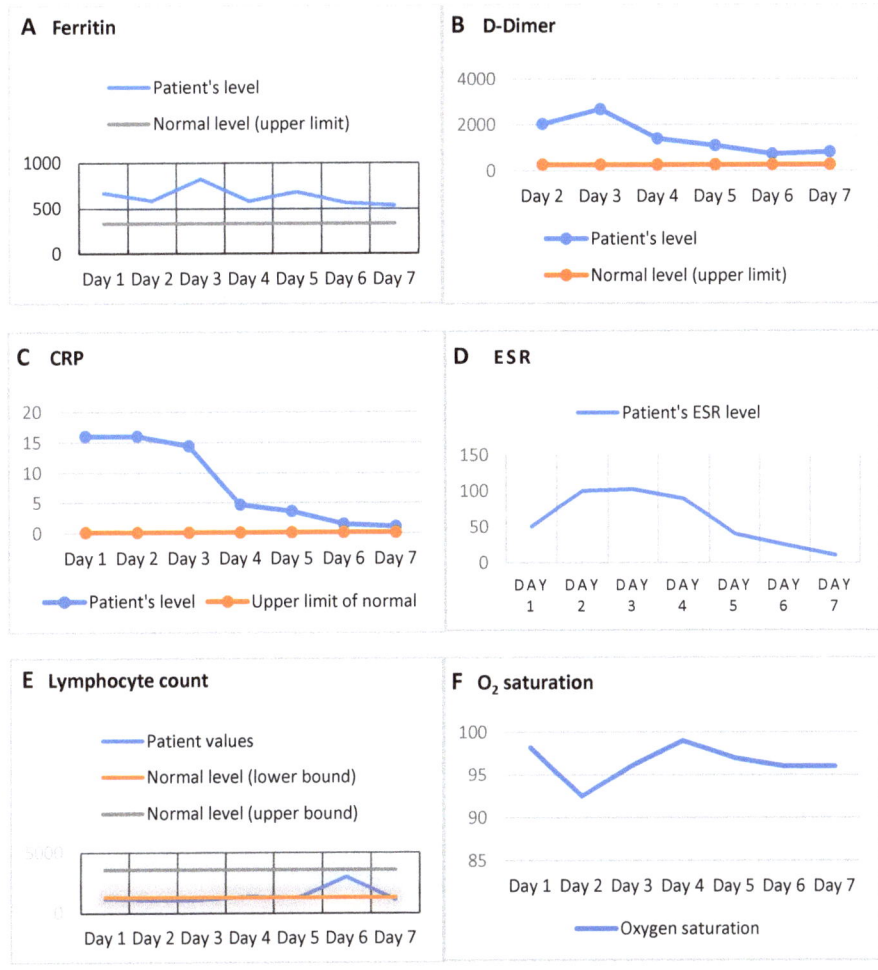

Figure 2. Line charts of trends in acute phase reactant biomarkers of cytokine storm—ferritin, D-dimer, and C-reactive protein (CRP) levels—along with the lymphocyte count and O_2 saturation during the hospital stay (day 1 refers to the first day of the hospital stay). The acute phase reactants displayed an overall decline from peak levels. (**A**) Ferritin levels. (**B**) D-Dimer trends (levels first measured on day 2 of the hospital stay). (**C**) CRP levels, which were >16 for days 1 and 2 of the hospital stay. (**D**) Erythrocyte sedimentation rate (ESR) levels (reference interval 0–15). (**E**) Lymphocyte count. (**F**) Oxygen saturation (SO_2, pulse oximetry) levels during the hospital stay. The patient was initially started on a non-rebreather mask and then switched to BiPAP on day 3.

3. Discussion

3.1. COVID-19 Pathophysiology and Cytokine Storm

Cytokine storm is seen in a variety of syndromes, including macrophage activation syndrome (MAS), hemophagocytic lymphohistiocytosis (HLH), and chimeric antigen receptor (CAR) T-cell therapy (used to treat lymphomas and leukemias) associated with hyperinflammation (known as cytokine release syndrome) [3,34–38]. MAS is a rare and potentially life-threatening condition entailing a cytokine storm in which macrophage and lymphocyte interactions are dysregulated, thus leading to cytokine release [39]. HLH is a critical condition marked by hyperinflammation, hemophagocytosis, and histiocyte proliferation, and is classified as either familial HLH or secondary HLH [40]. One potential mechanism for the cytokine storm in HLH disorders may be an increase in cytokines, including TNFα, IL-1, interferon gamma (IFN-γ), IL-6, sTNFRs, and soluble IL-2R (sIL-2R), as a consequence of dysregulated interactions between lymphocytes and macrophages [39]. Patients with COVID-19 exhibit clinical attributes similar to secondary HLH: hyperferritinemia, cytopenia, and ARDS [12].

The inflammatory cytokine storm observed in COVID-19 shares features with MAS and HLH, but has some distinguishing characteristics [3]. In COVID-19, compared with MAS, the increases in ferritin are not as high, and organ damage is primarily restricted to the lungs [38]. The clinical attributes of patients with COVID-19 also mirror those in cytokine release syndrome, which arise as a consequence of CAR-T cell therapies for certain lymphomas [20]. Importantly, not all patients with COVID-19 undergo cytokine storm; this phenomenon only occurs in a certain subset of severe cases [12]. The classic clinical picture of a patient with cytokine storm involves rapid respiratory deterioration [41,42]. Our patient began to decline and demonstrated symptoms of respiratory distress (labored breathing) on the first day of admission, and had reportedly been experiencing symptoms for 7 days prior.

Cytokine storm instigates a robust immune-driven attack on the body, leading to ARDS (and multi-organ failure) and ultimately causing morbidity in severe COVID-19 [43,44]. The pathophysiology of cytokine storm is not fully understood, but is currently thought to be based on the mechanisms of inflammatory disorders, including MAS and cytokine release syndrome. Initially, SARS-CoV-2 binds angiotensin converting enzyme 2 (ACE-2) receptors and then invades the respiratory epithelium [37,45]. Dendritic cells and alveolar macrophages are activated because of the presence of SARS-CoV-2 and subsequently release IL-6, which is also secreted by the respiratory epithelium [37,45]. A cascade of the cytokines IL-1B, IL-12, and TNF-α results, and their secretion induces WBCs to release cytokines, thus effectively perpetuating an inflammatory cycle [12,45]. These cytokines also enter the circulation and cause systemic multi-system pathology [46].

The robust hyperinflammatory cytokine response induces the apoptosis of endothelial and epithelial cells in the lungs, resulting in tissue injury, leakage and edema, and ARDS [46,47]. As immune cells destroy alveolar tissue, permeability increases, thus resulting in fluid entry into the alveoli; less oxygen enters the blood, because alveolar type I cells are diminished, and a loss of surfactant leads to alveolar collapse. These responses together impair normal gas exchange [3,48]. Additionally, cytokines cause vasodilation, thereby contributing to a build-up of fluid in the alveoli, diluting surfactant, and causing alveolar collapse; as alveolar type I and alveolar type II cells are destroyed, the alveoli collapse, and ARDS ensues [48].

An increased synthesis of collagen and TGF-α and deposition of fibrin are also observed in the development of ARDS [3]. Features of ARDS additionally include alveolar exudate, edema, and cellular infiltration, thus resulting in damaged alveoli and limited gas exchange [21]. Xu et al. [44] have described post-mortem biopsies of COVID-19 patients with ARDS in China that showed classic ARDS-related features, such as pneumocyte desquamation, the formation of hyaline membranes, and pulmonary edema. Additionally, the presence of lymphocyte-dominated mononuclear inflammatory infiltrate in the interstitium was observed bilaterally [44]. Because of the high numbers of mononuclear lymphocytes, these T-cells have been thought to potentially enter the pulmonary circulation and trigger an inflammatory storm [21].

ARDS and severe illness in patients with COVID-19 usually develop 1–2 weeks after the onset of symptoms [49]. Our understanding of ARDS in COVID-19 is still evolving. It has been suggested that COVID-19 may be characterized by a unique form of ARDS, marked by a feature not seen in classic ARDS: the seemingly preserved compliance and respiratory mechanics relative to the high degree of hypoxemia [50]. Figure 3 depicts the alveolar changes that occur in severe COVID-19.

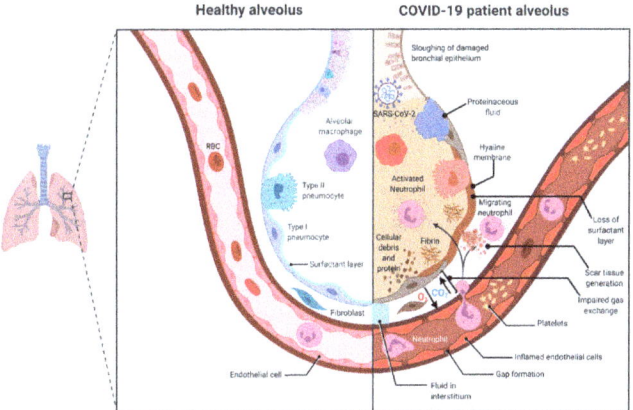

Figure 3. Alveolar changes due to cytokine syndrome-induced acute respiratory distress syndrome (ARDS) in severe coronavirus disease 2019 (COVID-19), according to current understanding [3,48,50,51]. This model is based in part on hypotheses (because our understanding of ARDS remains incomplete), along with reported pathological findings in COVID-19-related ARDS from post-mortem biopsies. Many of the features are hallmark characteristics of conventional ARDS. Nonetheless, COVID-19 is increasingly believed to display an atypical form of ARDS [50].

3.2. Diagnostic and Prognostic Roles of Serum Markers for Severe COVID-19 and Cytokine Storm

The onset of the hyperinflammation in cytokine storm may be evidenced by coagulopathy, cytopenia, tissue damage, the inflammation of liver tissue, and the activation of macrophages and hepatocytes [38]. Therefore, laboratory findings potentially suggesting the onset of cytokine storm in patients with COVID-19 may include increased levels of acute phase markers (such as D-dimer, CRP, LDH, ferritin, and troponin), low platelets, decreased fibrinogen, lymphopenia, thrombocytopenia, increased LDH, and transaminitis (elevated AST and ALT) [31–33,38]. Lymphopenia is a commonly reported feature of COVID-19 cytokine storm, and given that the cytokine storm must be orchestrated by other leukocytes (not T cells), an elevated WBC count is also common, suggesting that lymphopenia with leukocytosis may be a key feature in the differential diagnosis of COVID-19 [51]. In our patient, lymphopenia was observed on day 1, and on day 3 the patient developed leukocytosis. Elevated CRP and ferritin levels are key in the diagnosis of MAS and HLH. Recent studies have suggested a similar marker profile in severe COVID-19. Interestingly, cytokine storm in COVID-19 differs from that associated with other viruses as the increase in ferritin in COVID-19 is relatively modest [38]. Ferritin has been suggested as a prognostic indicator for cytokine storm in COVID-19 [38,52].

Serum inflammatory biomarkers may have a role in assessing disease progression, since a poor prognosis in COVID-19 appears to be correlated with abnormal serum markers and clinical attributes of cytokine storm [38]. A recent retrospective observational study of 21 patients in China comparing the attributes of moderate versus severe COVID-19 found that severe cases are more often typified by hypoalbuminemia and lymphopenia, with relatively high levels of ALT, LDH, and CRP, and particularly high levels of TNF-α, IL-2R, IL-6, and IL-10 [53]. One recent meta-analysis of 21 COVID-19-related studies on 3377 patients has shown that the levels of interleukin 10 (IL-10), IL-6, and ferritin strongly correlate with disease severity [30]. The study also showed that patients who experienced severe disease and even mortality had thrombocytopenia, lymphocytopenia, and higher WBC counts compared with those with moderate disease and disease resolution [30]. Mehta et al. [12] have suggested that inflammatory biomarkers, including ESR, decreased platelets, and increased ferritin, should be used by clinicians to risk-stratify patients who might benefit from immunomodulating treatments (such as IL-6 inhibitors). One recent study of 343 hospitalized patients with COVID-19 in Wuhan showed that D-dimer levels above 2.0 μg/mL on admission were predictive of mortality, thereby suggesting a potential prognostic role of D-dimer [54].

Therefore, an early assessment of these biomarkers may be critical, since rapidly identifying an emerging cytokine storm and targeting immune dysregulation in patients with COVID-19 before the rapid progression to ARDS has the potential to avoid the need for mechanical ventilation, given the low rates of survival among patients with COVID-19 who are placed on ventilators [22,38]. Experience in MAS and cytokine release syndrome has shown that intervening at an early stage of disease may be important for avoiding irreversible damage to tissue [38].

3.3. The Role of IL-6 in Cytokine Storm and COVID-19

IL-6 is a pleiotropic cytokine in the glycoprotein-130 (gp130) family of cytokines [55,56]. It has a myriad of physiological functions, including the production of acute phase reactants, stimulation of immunoglobulin production by activated B cells, regulation of bone homeostasis, lipid oxidation, glucose metabolism, and regulation of energy expenditure and appetite [56–59]. The mechanistic and multifunctional complexity of IL-6 is underscored by its anti-inflammatory effects (production of acute phase reactants from liver and epithelial cell regeneration), in addition to its pro-inflammatory properties (inflammatory cell recruitment, disrupted differentiation of regulatory T-cells, and inhibition of inflammatory cell apoptosis) [37,60]. Therefore, the role of IL-6 in COVID-19 is complex and not fully elucidated [3]. For instance, theoretically, the high IL-6 levels in COVID-19 pneumonia have been suggested to have beneficial or deleterious effects, since IL-6 in other infections can enhance viral replication or suppression in experimental models [3,61]. However, emphasis has been placed on its mainly pro-inflammatory nature in COVID-19, as confirmed by clinical reports on patients with COVID-19.

IL-6 plays a major role in various inflammatory and autoimmune disorders [62]. Importantly, an excessive generation of IL-6 during infections and tissue injury is believed to be responsible for cytokine release syndrome [59]. IL-6 dysregulation leads to the activation of complement and coagulation, inducing vascular leakage [24,63–65]. The activation of IL-6 is thought to be the key feature of the progression of COVID-19 pneumonia to ARDS and hyperinflammation [45].

IL-6 peak levels have been associated with pulmonary disease progression in COVID-19 [66]. Importantly, on day 2, our patient showed elevated IL-6 levels. In a recent retrospective cohort study of 201 patients in Wuhan, China, Wu et al. [67] reported a statistically significant correlation between IL-6 and mortality.

Interestingly, a role of IL-6 as a prognostic marker for COVID-19 has also been suggested. One recent meta-analysis of studies involving a total of 264 patients with COVID-19 in China reported that patients with severe COVID-19 have higher IL-6/IFN-γ ratios than those with more moderate conditions, thus suggesting that the IL-6 and IFN-γ levels may serve as a possible prognostic tool in managing patients with COVID-19 [68].

Figure 4 illustrates the proposed inflammatory sequence of the cytokine storm observed in COVID-19 and the key role played by IL-6.

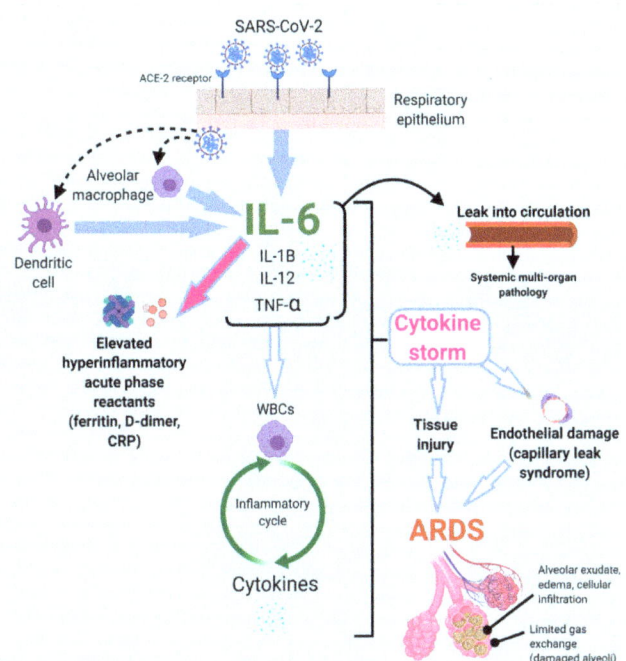

Figure 4. Proposed model of the cytokine storm in severe COVID-19, revealing the mechanistic complexity of the cytokine cascade and subsequent pathology [3,21,37,45,46,69]. The model is primarily based on current knowledge of cytokine storm, as seen in macrophage activation syndrome (MAS), hemophagocytic lymphohistiocytosis (HLH), and chimeric antigen receptor (CAR) T-cell therapy. Notably, cytokine storm in both MAS and HLH displays increased levels of cytokines interleukin (IL)-1, IL-2, IL-18, macrophage colony stimulating factor (M-CSF), interferon-γ, and tumor necrosis factor (TNF) α, in addition to IL-6, although definitive causality due to all these cytokines has not been determined [23].

3.4. IL-6 Signal Transduction Pathway

IL-6 signaling occurs through a complex sequence of induction. There are two forms of the IL-6 receptor: a membrane-bound IL-6 receptor (IL-6R) and a soluble IL-6 receptor (sIL-6R) [70] IL-6 signaling primarily occurs through two modes: the classic signaling pathway mediated by membrane-bound IL-6R and the trans-signaling pathway mediated by sIL-6R [56,59]. Membrane-bound IL-6R is mainly found on hepatocytes, certain epithelial cells, megakaryocytes, and some groups of leukocytes; thus, the classic signaling pathway only occurs in these locations [55,71]. In contrast, the trans-signaling pathway can occur in all cells of the body, because it primarily requires the presence of the gp130 receptor protein, which is expressed in all cells [60].

In the classic signaling pathway, IL-6 binds membrane-bound IL-6R on the membrane of target cells and then interacts with the gp130 receptor to form a complex [55,70]. The activation of gp130 leads to the downstream activation of the Janus activated kinase-signal transducer and activator of transcription (JAK/STAT) pathway by influencing JAK (which is constitutively bound to the gp130 cytoplasmic domain), thereby inducing STAT3 phosphorylation (activation of STAT3) [56,70]. Therefore, IL-6's interaction with its receptor ultimately leads to the activation of STAT3. The JAK/STAT3 complex translocates to the nucleus, where it activates transcription and consequently leads to the expression of acute phase proteins, which are a main feature of inflammation; their induction may have homeostatic effects [56,60].

This JAK/STAT pathway is regulated through negative feedback by suppressors of cytokine synthesis (SOCS-1 and SOCS-3) [56,59]. SOCS-1 binds activated JAK and SOCS-3 binds phosphorylated gp130, thus halting JAK activation [56]. Notably, IL-6R signaling also activates the JAK-SHP2 mitogen activated protein kinase (MAP-kinase) pathway, in addition to the JAK-STAT signaling pathway, thereby resulting in the activation of several transcription factors [56,59]. In the trans-signaling pathway, the binding of IL-6 to sIL-6R in cells that lack surface expression of the IL-6 receptor results in coupling with gp130, which in turn leads to signal transduction [56,70]. This pathway is hypothesized to be pro-inflammatory [60].

3.5. Potential Therapeutic Role of IL-6 Receptor Inhibition in COVID-19

IL-6 receptor inhibition has promise as a therapeutic strategy because it results in a blockade of signal transduction and gene expression [70]. IL-6 and its interactions with the IL-6 receptor stimulate the release of various acute phase proteins (including fibrinogen, CRP, hepcidin, and serum amyloid A) and promote inflammation. Therefore, the blockade of this interaction can be used to attenuate systemic inflammation in immune disorders such as Castleman disease and rheumatoid arthritis [59,72].

For example, two IL-6 receptor inhibitors used to treat rheumatoid arthritis are tocilizumab and sarilumab [33]. Tocilizumab is a humanized monoclonal antibody (IgG1k subclass) that acts against both IL-6R and sIL-6R receptors and is traditionally used to treat rheumatoid arthritis, systemic juvenile idiopathic arthritis, Castleman disease, and other autoimmune disorders [37,73–75]. The U.S. FDA cleared tocilizumab in 2017 for the treatment of cytokine release syndrome resulting from CAR-T cell therapy [37]. Figure 5 depicts the IL-6 signaling pathway and the role of tocilizumab in IL-6 receptor antagonism.

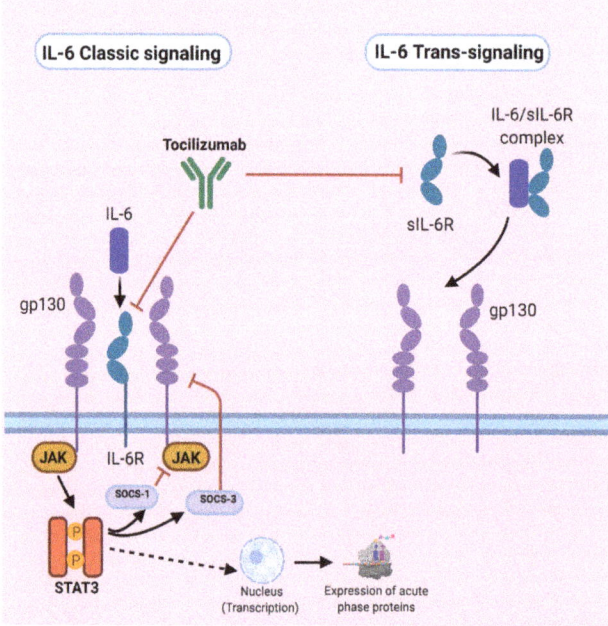

Figure 5. IL-6 classic and trans-signaling pathways, with a model of tocilizumab-mediated therapeutic receptor antagonism [21,55,56,60,70,76]. The diagram displays the normal sequences of the classic and trans-signaling pathways. Tocilizumab acts on both pathways (on the IL-6 receptor in the classic pathway and the soluble IL-6 receptor in the trans-signaling pathway). Note: IL-6 also uses trans presentation (in which IL-6 and membrane-bound IL-6R on dendritic cells are presented to gp130-expressing T-cells in proximity) as the third mode of signal transduction, but this pathway is not shown here [56,75].

In the U.S., tocilizumab is sold under the trade name Actemra, whereas in Europe, its trade name is RoActemra [73]. Tocilizumab has an additional use in treating the cytokine release syndrome that specifically results from CAR T-cell therapy used in B-cell malignancies [33,34]. Therefore, tocilizumab and sarilumab have been suggested to have therapeutic potential in patients with COVID-19 when there is suspicion of a cytokine storm according to elevated acute phase reactant markers (e.g., ferritin, D-dimer, CRP, and LDH), as was the case in our patient [31–33].

Accordingly, on day 1 of admission, we initiated an intravenous (IV) administration of tocilizumab. For the treatment for CAR-T therapy-initiated cytokine release syndrome, a conventional IV infusion of tocilizumab (alone or with corticosteroids) is indicated with a weight-based dose at 8 mg/kg for patients weighing at least 30 kg, which corresponded to a dose of 1005 mg in our patient [77]. We administered two smaller doses (500 mg each) with a 12 hour interval not based on weight, given the experimental nature of its use in COVID-19 and to mitigate any adverse effects. The National Health Commission of China's official guidelines in the "Chinese Clinical Guidance for COVID-19 Pneumonia Diagnosis and Treatment" suggest using tocilizumab in patients who display widespread lung lesions and disease in severe stages with elevated IL-6 levels; its use is contraindicated in patients with ongoing infections, particularly tuberculosis [25]. The first dose has been suggested to be introduced at 4–8 mg/kg (but the suggested dose is 400 mg diluted to 100 mL in addition to 0.9% normal saline with more than 1 hour of infusion time) [25]. These guidelines also recommend that if patients have a suboptimal response after the first dose, a second administration with the same dose can be performed after 12 hours, with a maximum of two administrations [25]. Additionally, it has been recommend that a single dose does not exceed 800 mg [25]. Therefore, the dosing regimen for our patient was similar to this recommended dosing protocol, but with a slightly higher dose per administration.

Importantly, IL-6 inhibitors attenuate the immune response, increasing the risk of opportunistic infections, leukopenia, and liver injury [73,78]. Some known adverse effects of tocilizumab include liver disease, allergic reactions, anaphylaxis, stomach and abdominal pain, skin and soft tissue infections, neutropenia, and hypercholesterolemia [73,79]. Reactivation of tuberculosis can occur, although this has been reported to be less common than that after treatment with tumor necrosis factor inhibitors [73]. Additionally, a possible association between tocilizumab and osteonecrosis of the jaw has been reported [80]. However, our patient did not exhibit any noticeable symptoms due to tocilizumab. Notably, IL-6 inhibitors may be cost-prohibitive [81]. Clinicians should weigh the benefits and limitations of tocilizumab therapy compared with other currently used drugs for the management of COVID-19 (Table 1).

Table 1. Comparison of tocilizumab with other drugs currently in use or under investigation for the treatment of patients with COVID-19.

Drug	General Use	Efficacy in COVID-19	Adverse Effects	Special Attributes
Tocilizumab [21,73,74,79,80]	Rheumatoid arthritis, systemic juvenile idiopathic arthritis, and polyarticular juvenile idiopathic arthritis	Anecdotal experiences suggesting a therapeutic benefit Several trials underway Large, randomized controlled studies needed	Liver disease, allergic reactions, anaphylaxis, rash, stomach and abdominal pain, skin and soft tissue infections, neutropenia, hypercholesterolemia, and possibly jaw osteonecrosis	Recombinant monoclonal antibody used for blockade of the proinflammatory cytokine IL-6 receptor Potential reactivation of tuberculosis and increased risk of infections Not usable for all patients Use potentially limited to severe COVID-19 (e.g., ICU cases) Expensive and possibly cost-prohibitive
Hydroxychloroquine [18,82,83]	Malaria prophylaxis and treatment, and systemic lupus erythematosus	Potential antiviral properties Demonstrated drug efficacy against SARS in vitro Efficacy for COVID-19 yet to be demonstrated In vivo and in vitro studies on COVID-19 currently underway	Ocular complications (corneal deposits, retinopathy), cardiotoxicity (cardiomyopathy and conduction abnormalities), cutaneous and neurologic effects, GI complications, abnormal liver function, and hepatic failure	Long half-life Increased potential for adverse effects when combined with azithromycin (which can also cause heart conduction abnormalities)
Lopinavir-Ritonavir [14,84,85]	HIV (lopinavir)	No benefit shown in a major recent randomized controlled trial of 199 severe COVID-19 hospitalized patients Demonstrated activity of lopinavir against coronavirus in vitro Decreased risk of ARDS or death due to SARS after treatment with lopinavir+ritonavir combined with ribavirin	GI effects (diarrhea, nausea, and vomiting), dizziness, drowsiness, headaches, hypertriglyceridemia, changes in body fat, and severe allergic reactions	Protease inhibition (lopinavir)
Remdesivir [15,16,86–88]	Ebola (still under investigation)	Efficacy to be determined for COVID-19 Decreased viral titers in mice infected with Middle East respiratory syndrome Phase III trial completed for use in Ebola, but no benefit shown in 2019 trial during Ebola outbreak in the Democratic Republic of Congo	Increased liver enzymes (potential liver damage), nausea, and vomiting	Disruption of viral replication by inhibiting RNA polymerase Currently in "compassionate use" for patients with COVID-19 in the U.S. and Europe
Convalescent plasma [10,17,89]	Previously used in SARS1 (2003) and MERS; also used as post-exposure prophylaxis in various infectious disease outbreaks	Limited anecdotal reports suggesting possible benefit in patients with COVID-19 Larger trials currently underway	Allergic and anaphylactic reactions, transfusion-related acute lung injury, circulatory overload (transfusion associated), infection transmission, and hemolytic transfusion reactions	Passive antibody administration

3.6. Evidence and Reports of Tocilizumab Use for COVID-19

Our experience at a small-sized urban community hospital mirrors the positive results reported in other cases in the literature. The first report that sparked considerable attention in China described 21 patients with severe COVID-19 at two different Chinese hospitals who received one administration of tocilizumab in conjunction with standard therapy; all patients reported dramatic clinical improvements [90]. The patients received a single 400 mg tocilizumab dose and standard recommended therapy with lopinavir, methylprednisolone, oxygen treatment, and symptom relief medications. The fever declined in several days, and marked improvement was observed in all patients. Lymphocyte and CRP levels decreased after tocilizumab therapy. Fifteen patients showed a decreased oxygen intake, and one patient no longer needed oxygen therapy. Twenty patients were discharged (average of 13.5 days after tocilizumab therapy), and one was removed from the ICU [21]. No adverse effects were reported. As a result, the National Health Commission of China officially added tocilizumab to its guidelines in the "Chinese Clinical Guidance for COVID-19 Pneumonia Diagnosis and Treatment" [21,25].

Luo et al. [13] conducted a retrospective study of 15 patients with COVID-19 in Wuhan, China. The study assessed 15 patients with COVID-19 (12 males and three females with a median age of 73 years) treated with tocilizumab (eight patients were given a combination with methylprednisolone). Ten patients were administered a single dose and two were given double doses of tocilizumab. Serum acute phase reactants CRP and IL-6 were measured before and after therapy. Two patients were "moderately ill," and the rest were in a serious or critical condition. Ten patients had at least one co-morbidity. The CRP levels decreased in all patients. The IL-6 levels decreased in most (11) patients. Mortality was seen in three patients and disease exacerbation occurred in two patients. The remaining ten patients showed stabilization. A total of four critically ill patients were given a single dose; three patients died and one experienced disease aggravation. The authors concluded that tocilizumab may have benefits. The study further suggested that a single dose of tocilizumab (even when used with glucocorticoids) may not be sufficient for improvement in critical patients, whereas repeated doses may result in improvement. The limitations of the study were its retrospective and observational nature, small sample size, and non-randomized sample, with a substantial number of patients with comorbidities. Doses of tocilizumab varied among patients, some of whom received a double dose and approximately half of whom received methylprednisolone in addition to tocilizumab.

Other reports have described patients treated with tocilizumab with hydroxychloroquine without other major drugs, similar to our patient. De Luna et al. [91] have reported the case of a 45-year-old patient with COVID-19 in France who had sickle cell anemia with acute chest syndrome and pneumonia, and who was administered tocilizumab (in addition to hydroxychloroquine) and showed subsequent improvement. He presented on day 1 with an oxygen saturation of 91%, and then deteriorated to 80% oxygen saturation on day 2, at which time he was administered IV tocilizumab (8 mg/kg dose), in addition to the ongoing hydroxychloroquine (200 mg every 8 hours) and supplemental oxygen. On day 3, he showed improvement. In our patient, tocilizumab was administered in conjunction with ongoing hydroxychloroquine and other standard medications on day 1, followed by a second dose 12 hours later on the morning of day 2. Our patient also showed major improvement after tocilizumab administration, although we administered two doses rather than one.

Fontana et al. [92] have also described the successful use of tocilizumab in conjunction with hydroxychloroquine (with other immunosuppressive drugs) in a 61-year-old man with a previous kidney transplant for ESRD from chronic interstitial nephritis and an extensive past medical history (nodal marginal zone lymphoma, pulmonary embolism, Parkinson's disease, and neurogenic bladder). The patient was admitted for a continual fever and shivering, and over the course of the hospital stay, was diagnosed with COVID-19. His arterial pO_2 declined to 57 mmHg, and low-flowing oxygen via a nasal canula was started. Hydroxychloroquine (200 mg, twice per day) was administered, and the ongoing cyclosporine dose was decreased by half. Two days later, because of the lack of improvement, cyclosporine was withdrawn, and the methylprednisolone dose was increased to 16 mg daily. After 324 mg subcutaneous administration of tocilizumab, the patient's fever resolved, the arterial pO$_2$ improved progressively, and oxygen therapy was discontinued. The IL-6 levels increased 6 days after tocilizumab administration (to 619.11 pg/mL), probably because of receptor inhibition as opposed to a lack of drug efficacy. The patient was discharged on day 22 without a fever and with 95% peripheral oxygen saturation on ambient air.

Importantly, this is the only case in the literature showing possible adverse effects of tocilizumab administration: leukopenia, neutropenia, and pseudomonas infection. However, these were treated and adequately managed. IV immunoglobulins (IVIG) were administered to alleviate ensuing leukopenia with neutropenia, which was thought to have arisen from tocilizumab administration. The patient's leukocyte count increased. Meropenem was re-introduced after a urine culture showing multi-drug resistant *Pseudomonas aeruginosa*, which might have resulted from tocilizumab treatment, given that secondary bacterial infections are a known adverse effect. Furthermore, the patient had several comorbidities and, as a transplant patient, was already being treated with cyclosporine. Therefore, the role of tocilizumab in his outcome is difficult to determine. Additionally, because he had also been treated with hydroxychloroquine, IVIG, methylprednisolone, and azithromycin, the role of any individual drug cannot be established.

In other case reports, patients were also treated with several drugs in conjunction with tocilizumab, and they often had distinct comorbidities. Zhang et al. [93] have described the case of a 60-year-old male COVID-19 patient in Wuhan, China, with multiple myeloma who received tocilizumab and showed clinical improvement. He initially received moxifloxacin, umifenovir, and chemotherapy. He was later given methylprednisolone after experiencing chest tightness and shortness of breath. On day 9, he was intravenously administered one dose of tocilizumab. On day 12, he no longer felt chest tightness. The IL-6 levels decreased overall, with a slight momentary rebound elevation. On day 19, his CT scan showed a diminished classic ground-glass appearance. He was successfully discharged.

Other studies have reported patients who were also administered two or more doses of tocilizumab and improved. Michot et al. [94] have described the case of a 42-year-old male with metastatic sarcamatoid clear cell renal carcinoma who developed COVID-19 and showed improvement after two doses of tocilizumab. During the hospital stay, he received lopinavir-ritonavir on day 7 for 5 days. On day 8, he experienced sudden dyspnea and a decrease in oxygen saturation. The tocilizumab was administered in two doses of 8 mg/kg with an 8-hour interval in between. The patient showed clinical improvement, his fever regressed, and he had decreased oxygen requirements. His CRP levels dramatically decreased. Importantly, these positive results must be viewed by considering that the patient already had an immunosuppressed status due to cancer, and that because he received lopinavir-ritonavir, any benefit from this drug alone or the combination remains unclear.

Cellina et al. [95] have characterized the case of 64-year-old man with no comorbidities who developed COVID-19 and experienced dyspnea and decreased oxygen saturation at 90% on day 6 of his hospital stay. On day 7, he was started on assisted ventilation, and tocilizumab was administered in two doses of 8 mg/kg, with 12 hours between doses (days 7 and 8). On day 9, the CRP and WBC count declined, and his condition improved. He was weaned off ventilatory support. On day 14, his CT revealed improvements.

Similarly, Di Giambenedetto et al. [26] have reported the successful resolution of clinical symptoms in three male hospitalized patients with COVID-19 (71, 45, and 53 years of age) after treatment with tocilizumab. Clinical improvement was seen in all three patients. In one patient (71-year-old male) who was given two doses of tocilizumab, there was a resolution of fever, the oxygen saturation improved, and the CRP returned to a normal range. In the second patient (45-year-old male) treated with two doses of tocilizumab in addition to antiviral treatment, there was clinical improvement, fever resolution, and a decrease in CRP levels after tocilizumab infusion. In the third patient (53-year-old) treated with three doses of tocilizumab, dyspnea resolved, the oxygen saturation improved, and the CRP levels decreased.

In one investigation by Jacobs et al. [96], over the course of 24 days, 32 patients with COVID-19 were placed on extracorporeal membrane oxygen (ECMO), followed by the administration of adjunctive drugs. Five survived, and two of the five survivors were treated with tocilizumab or sarilumab. However, the clinical details of these patients and the specifics of drug administration have not been described. This study had a small sample size and was observational and retrospective. Additionally, other factors might have contributed to the outcomes (e.g., the use of ECMO).

In another observational study, Giamarellos-Bourboulis et al. [97] administered tocilizumab to six patients who were part of a group of 54 patients with COVID-19 under study for immune dysregulation and immune responses. The plasma of these patients was also studied. The absolute lymphocyte levels in the six patients decreased after tocilizumab therapy. The introduction of tocilizumab in plasma-enriched cell medium partially restored HLA-DR expression on cells. Importantly, IL-6 is believed to be the cause of decreased HLA-DR on CD14 monocytes [97]. Severe respiratory failure is associated with a significant decrease in HLA-DR expression on CD14 monocytes [97]. Therefore, the investigators suggested that tocilizumab partially relieves the immune dysregulation seen in COVID-19.

However, one patient described in the literature by Ferrey et al. [98] remained in a critical condition after tocilizumab therapy. He was a 56-year-old male with end-stage renal disease dependent on hemodialysis and with hypertension, who developed severe COVID-19. He developed ARDS and was intubated. He was given hydroxychloroquine in conjunction with standard drugs for ARDS and septic shock. On day 6, he received tocilizumab. The authors report that he remained in a critical condition at the time of the case report (his care was ongoing). Importantly, the patient had other notable comorbidities, which may have influenced his outcome.

Interestingly, the experience reported for one patient with COVID-19 by Minhai et al. [99] may even suggest a potential prophylactic role of tocilizumab in preventing severe COVID-19. The authors report the case of a 57-year-old female patient in Switzerland who experienced systemic sclerosis, insulin-dependent type 2 diabetes mellitus, and obesity, and who was already being administered tocilizumab (8 mg/kg every 4 weeks IV) before presenting to the hospital 4 weeks after the last tocilizumab dose with symptoms of COVID-19. She was quarantined at home and monitored, and she received no drug administration (her scheduled tocilizumab infusion for systemic sclerosis was postponed). Ultimately, she only developed a mild form of COVID-19 and subsequently recovered. The authors postulate that the pre-COVID-19 administration of tocilizumab might have led to a mild form of the disease and might possibly have prevented severe COVID-19, particularly given the patient's several comorbidities, which placed her at high risk of developing severe COVID-19. Therefore, in contrast to other patients, this patient had received tocilizumab before SARS-CoV-2 infection. Nonetheless, a definitive role of tocilizumab in preventing severe COVID-19 in this patient cannot be established. Notably, she was already immunosuppressed because of her comorbidities.

The relative sudden recovery in nearly all of these reported cases after tocilizumab administration during respiratory deterioration suggests that tocilizumab may have a therapeutic benefit. Only a certain subset of patients might strongly benefit from tocilizumab. Interestingly, only one case showed any adverse effect of tocilizumab, thus suggesting the relative safety of this treatment, although potential adverse effects might still occur. Moreover, tocilizumab might have an optimal therapeutic effect when used concomitantly with other drugs. Future studies should explore which patients are most likely to benefit from tocilizumab, determine whether its sole use or combined therapy yields the most optimal effect, and identify the most effective dosing regimens.

In addition, only one case involved a patient placed on mechanical ventilation and subsequently administered tocilizumab for successful recovery; all other patients were administered the drug at a time when their respiratory function was declining, but they had not yet been placed on mechanical ventilation, thus suggesting that tocilizumab might work most effectively at the time of emergence of a cytokine storm. Precise identification of the optimal time period in which to administer tocilizumab is critical, and further investigations may shed light on the most suitable time to use the drug. The case described by Minhai et al. [99] suggests the need for studies examining the potential role of tocilizumab in preventing severe COVID-19. A summary of existing cases in the literature that describe tocilizumab use in patients with COVID-19 is shown in Table 1.

Our case report has some notable limitations. The patient was concomitantly treated with several drugs (including hydroxychloroquine and azithromycin) that might have influenced his clinical course. Therefore, we cannot definitely ascertain whether any one drug agent or the combination played a role in his recovery. Additionally, because most patients with SARS-CoV-2 infection recover (the case-fatality rate is low, at an estimated 2–3%), determining whether the introduction of tocilizumab might be solely responsible for lung recovery is challenging.[6] However, given that the patient was declining with deteriorating respiratory symptoms, and that sharp recovery and relief was observed after tocilizumab administration, tocilizumab may have had a role in the patient's clinical improvement.

4. Conclusions

We present the case of a patient with COVID-19 whose condition improved after the use of tocilizumab, obviating the need for mechanical ventilation. He tolerated tocilizumab well and did not experience any known adverse effects. Our experience appears to mirror other cases in the literature that suggest a potential efficacious role of IL-6 receptor inhibition in attenuating cytokine release syndrome in patients with severe COVID-19.

Avoiding the need for mechanical ventilation is a key therapeutic strategy in COVID-19 management. Current evidence suggests that approximately 79–86% of patients who require ventilator support experience mortality [22]. Therefore, the period of time before respiratory decline to the point at which ventilator support is needed may be especially important during the COVID-19 disease course. Therefore, although all reports to date are anecdotal and evidence is circumstantial, there may be a role for early aggressive immunosuppressive management to avert the need for ventilator support; this time period may be crucial for recovery and for preventing progression to ARDS, which can cause irreversible lung damage.

Our case highlights the importance of the early recognition of the cytokine storm and of prompt immunosuppressive measures to halt disease progression. The early identification of clinical deterioration (as assessed by levels of cytokine storm-associated acute phase reactants) and subsequent aggressive management of patients with severe COVID-19 during the onset of respiratory decline may be key for preventing mortality. As suggested by both our experience and anecdotal cases described in the literature, acute phase reactant proteins may play an important role in the diagnosis and prognosis in severe COVID-19. Future studies are needed to determine their potential in risk stratification. According to the results of recent studies, clinicians should consider initiating measurements of IL-6 levels, the WBC count, lymphocytes, platelets, ferritin, D-dimer, CRP, and LDH for the risk stratification of cytokine storm [30–33].

The efficacy of combination therapy of IL-6 inhibitors with other drugs, such as hydroxychloroquine (in conjunction with azithromycin) and zinc, or other currently used COVID-19 treatments requires further investigation. Several therapies when used in concert might potentially attenuate disease pathology. We administered a smaller dose of tocilizumab than is typically used in patients with cytokine release syndrome, but slightly higher than the amounts used in previous studies. Therefore, our experience may shed light on the need for optimal therapeutic doses, which must still be established. Further investigations should explore the potential of dosages not based on weight to determine whether this approach would yield different therapeutic results. According to the literature describing cases in which variable dosing led to recovery, determining whether a single or multiple dose is most effective in COVID-19 is also needed. The optimal timing of use remains to be determined. Additionally, not all patients may be candidates for IL-6 inhibitor treatment. Decisions to administer the drug should consider co-morbidities, such as inactive tuberculosis, in conjunction with the patient's current immune status.

Therapeutic horizons in the treatment for COVID-19 may entail various methods for preventing or disrupting disease progression in ARDS. Further investigations are warranted to shed light on alternative potential therapeutic targets for cytokine storm disruption, particularly in the IL-6 signaling pathway. For example, inhibitors of the JAK/STAT signaling pathway, which could help decrease the levels of cytokines (including IL-6 and IFN-γ) observed in severe COVID-19, have been suggested as a potential therapy [49,100]. However, to date, IL-6 receptor inhibition has garnered substantial attention in the scientific community worldwide, and the upcoming results of current trials of tocilizumab may provide a clearer picture of its efficacy. Until large randomized-controlled studies reveal conclusive evidence of the large-scale efficacy of IL-6 receptor inhibition as a viable therapeutic option in patients with severe COVID-19, clinicians should consider the anecdotal cases of the successful aversion of both cytokine storm and disease progression through the use of these drugs. Such decisions, however, must be made with caution and a consideration of the potential adverse immunomodulatory effects of IL-6 receptor inhibitor therapy. Despite the potential adverse effects of IL-6, the use of tocilizumab in conjunction with other immune-mediating medications may be a promising treatment for severe COVID-19.

Informed consent was obtained from the patient to describe and publish his case.

Author Contributions: Attending physician, G.Y.; conceptualization, F.F.; writing—original draft preparation, F.F., N.D.; writing—review and editing, F.F., N.D., G.Y., J.D., K.N., and R.M.; supervision/staff doctor/patient diagnosis, F.F., G.Y., J.D., R.M., and K.N. All authors have read and agreed to the published version of the manuscript.

Funding: The research received no external funding.

Acknowledgments: The authors are grateful to the hospital staff for their assistance. We thank Marcos Sanchez for his guidance.

Conflicts of Interest: The authors declare no conflict of interest.

References

1. WHO Novel Coronavirus-China. Available online: https://www.who.int/csr/don/12-january-2020-novel-coronavirus-china/en/ (accessed on 20 April 2020).
2. Zhou, P.; Yang, X.L.; Wang, X.G.; Hu, B.; Zhang, L.; Zhang, W.; Si, H.R.; Zhu, Y.; Li, B.; Huang, C.L.; et al. A pneumonia outbreak associated with a new coronavirus of probable bat origin. *Nature* **2020**, *579*, 270–273. [CrossRef] [PubMed]
3. McGonagle, D.; Sharif, K.; O'Regan, A.; Bridgewood, C. The Role of Cytokines including Interleukin-6 in COVID-19 induced Pneumonia and Macrophage Activation Syndrome-Like Disease. *Autoimmun. Rev.* **2020**, *19*, 102537. [CrossRef]
4. Rabaan, A.A.; Al-Ahmed, S.H.; Haque, S.; Sah, R.; Tiwari, R.; Malik, Y.S.; Dhama, K.; Yatoo, M.I.; Bonilla-Aldana, D.K.; Rodriguez-Morales, A.J. SARS-CoV-2, SARS-CoV, and MERS-COV: A comparative overview. *Infez. Med.* **2020**, *28*, 174–184. [PubMed]
5. COVID-19 Coronavirus Pandemic. Available online: https://www.worldometers.info/coronavirus/ (accessed on 28 April 2020).
6. Cascella, M.; Rajnik, M.; Cuomo, A.; Dulebohn, S.C.; Di Napoli, R. *Features, Evaluation and Treatment Coronavirus (COVID-19)*; StatPearls Publishing: Treasure Island, FL, USA, 2020.
7. Bizzarri, M.; Lagana, A.S.; Aragona, D.; Unfer, V. Inositol and pulmonary function. Could myo-inositol treatment downregulate inflammation and cytokine release syndrome in SARS-CoV-2? *Eur. Rev. Med. Pharmacol. Sci.* **2020**, *24*, 3426–3432.
8. Sun, P.; Lu, X.; Xu, C.; Sun, W.; Pan, B. Understanding of COVID-19 based on current evidence. *J. Med. Virol.* **2020**. [CrossRef] [PubMed]
9. Scavone, C.; Brusco, S.; Bertini, M.; Sportiello, L.; Rafaniello, C.; Zoccoli, A.; Berrino, L.; Racagni, G.; Rossi, F.; Capuano, A. Current pharmacological treatments for COVID-19: What's next? *Br. J. Pharmacol.* **2020**. [CrossRef]
10. Ye, M.; Fu, D.; Ren, Y.; Wang, F.; Wang, D.; Zhang, F.; Xia, X.; Lv, T. Treatment with convalescent plasma for COVID-19 patients in Wuhan, China. *J. Med. Virol.* **2020**. [CrossRef]
11. Kalil, A.C. Treating COVID-19-Off-Label Drug Use, Compassionate Use, and Randomized Clinical Trials During Pandemics. *JAMA* **2020**. [CrossRef]

12. Mehta, P.; McAuley, D.F.; Brown, M.; Sanchez, E.; Tattersall, R.S.; Manson, J.J.; Hlh Across Speciality Collaboration. COVID-19: Consider cytokine storm syndromes and immunosuppression. *Lancet* **2020**, *395*, 1033–1034. [CrossRef]
13. Luo, P.; Liu, Y.; Qiu, L.; Liu, X.; Liu, D.; Li, J. Tocilizumab treatment in COVID-19: A single center experience. *J. Med. Virol.* **2020**. [CrossRef] [PubMed]
14. Chu, C.M.; Cheng, V.C.; Hung, I.F.; Wong, M.M.; Chan, K.H.; Chan, K.S.; Kao, R.Y.; Poon, L.L.; Wong, C.L.; Guan, Y.; et al. Role of lopinavir/ritonavir in the treatment of SARS: Initial virological and clinical findings. *Thorax* **2004**, *59*, 252–256. [CrossRef] [PubMed]
15. Lu, H. Drug treatment options for the 2019-new coronavirus (2019-nCoV). *Biosci. Trends* **2020**, *14*, 69–71. [CrossRef] [PubMed]
16. Agostini, M.L.; Andres, E.L.; Sims, A.C.; Graham, R.L.; Sheahan, T.P.; Lu, X.; Smith, E.C.; Case, J.B.; Feng, J.Y.; Jordan, R.; et al. Coronavirus Susceptibility to the Antiviral Remdesivir (GS-5734) Is Mediated by the Viral Polymerase and the Proofreading Exoribonuclease. *mBio* **2018**, *9*. [CrossRef] [PubMed]
17. Pandey, S.; Vyas, G.N. Adverse effects of plasma transfusion. *Transfusion* **2012**, *52*, 65S–79S. [CrossRef]
18. Sinha, N.; Balayla, G. Hydroxychloroquine and COVID-19. *Postgrad. Med. J.* **2020**, 1–6. [CrossRef]
19. Ruan, Q.; Yang, K.; Wang, W.; Jiang, L.; Song, J. Clinical predictors of mortality due to COVID-19 based on an analysis of data of 150 patients from Wuhan, China. *Intensive Care Med.* **2020**. [CrossRef] [PubMed]
20. Buonaguro, F.M.; Puzanov, I.; Ascierto, P.A. Anti-IL6R role in treatment of COVID-19-related ARDS. *J. Transl. Med.* **2020**, *18*, 165. [CrossRef]
21. Fu, B.; Xu, X.; Wei, H. Why tocilizumab could be an effective treatment for severe COVID-19? *J. Transl. Med.* **2020**, *18*, 164. [CrossRef]
22. Yang, X.; Yu, Y.; Xu, J.; Shu, H.; Xia, J.; Liu, H.; Wu, Y.; Zhang, L.; Yu, Z.; Fang, M.; et al. Clinical course and outcomes of critically ill patients with SARS-CoV-2 pneumonia in Wuhan, China: A single-centered, retrospective, observational study. *Lancet Respir. Med.* **2020**. [CrossRef]
23. Schulert, G.S.; Grom, A.A. Pathogenesis of macrophage activation syndrome and potential for cytokine-directed therapies. *Annu. Rev. Med.* **2015**, *66*, 145–159. [CrossRef]
24. Garcia Roche, A.; Diaz Lagares, C.; Elez, E.; Ferrer Roca, R. Cytokine release syndrome. Reviewing a new entity in the intensive care unit. *Med. Intensiva* **2019**, *43*, 480–488. [CrossRef] [PubMed]
25. Chinese Clinical Guidance for COVID-19 Pneumonia Diagnosis and Treatment (7th Edition). Available online: https://www.elotus.org/promo-files/COVID-19_resources/Guidance%20for%20Corona%20Virus%20Disease%202019%20(English%207th%20Edition%20Draft).pdf (accessed on 26 April 2020).
26. Di Giambenedetto, S.; Ciccullo, A.; Borghetti, A.; Gambassi, G.; Landi, F.; Visconti, E.; Zileri Dal Verme, L.; Bernabei, R.; Tamburrini, E.; Cauda, R.; et al. Off-label Use of Tocilizumab in Patients with SARS-CoV-2 Infection. *J. Med. Virol.* **2020**. [CrossRef] [PubMed]
27. Vidant Health Tocilizumab and COVID-19. Available online: https://www.vidanthealth.com/getattachment/COVID-19-Updates/For-Physicians/Tocilizumab-and-COVID-19-v3-April-10-2020.pdf?lang=en-US (accessed on 28 April 2020).
28. NIH. Available online: https://clinicaltrials.gov/ct2/results?cond=Covid-19&term=Tocilizumab&cntry=&state=&city=&dist=&Search=Search (accessed on 23 April 2020).
29. NIH. Available online: https://clinicaltrials.gov/ct2/results?term=sarilumab%2C+sars-cov-2&cond=COVID-19 (accessed on 23 April 2020).
30. Henry, B.M.; de Oliveira, M.H.S.; Benoit, S.; Plebani, M.; Lippi, G. Hematologic, biochemical and immune biomarker abnormalities associated with severe illness and mortality in coronavirus disease 2019 (COVID-19): A meta-analysis. *Clin. Chem. Lab. Med.* **2020**. [CrossRef]
31. Chau, V.Q.; Oliveros, E.; Mahmood, K.; Singhvi, A.; Lala, A.; Moss, N.; Gidwani, U.; Mancini, D.M.; Pinney, S.P.; Parikh, A. The Imperfect Cytokine Storm: Severe COVID-19 with ARDS in Patient on Durable LVAD Support. *JACC Case Rep.* **2020**, in press. [CrossRef] [PubMed]
32. Tisoncik, J.R.; Korth, M.J.; Simmons, C.P.; Farrar, J.; Martin, T.R.; Katze, M.G. Into the eye of the cytokine storm. *Microbiol. Mol. Biol. Rev.* **2012**, *76*, 16–32. [CrossRef]
33. Clerkin, K.J.; Fried, J.A.; Raikhelkar, J.; Sayer, G.; Griffin, J.M.; Masoumi, A.; Jain, S.S.; Burkhoff, D.; Kumaraiah, D.; Rabbani, L.; et al. Coronavirus Disease 2019 (COVID-19) and Cardiovascular Disease. *Circulation* **2020**, *141*, 1648–1655. [CrossRef]

34. Kotch, C.; Barrett, D.; Teachey, D.T. Tocilizumab for the treatment of chimeric antigen receptor T cell-induced cytokine release syndrome. *Expert Rev. Clin. Immunol.* **2019**, *15*, 813–822. [CrossRef]
35. Crayne, C.B.; Albeituni, S.; Nichols, K.E.; Cron, R.Q. The Immunology of Macrophage Activation Syndrome. *Front. Immunol.* **2019**, *10*, 119. [CrossRef]
36. Giavridis, T.; van der Stegen, S.J.C.; Eyquem, J.; Hamieh, M.; Piersigilli, A.; Sadelain, M. CAR T cell-induced cytokine release syndrome is mediated by macrophages and abated by IL-1 blockade. *Nat. Med.* **2018**, *24*, 731–738. [CrossRef]
37. Zhang, C.; Wu, Z.; Li, J.W.; Zhao, H.; Wang, G.Q. The cytokine release syndrome (CRS) of severe COVID-19 and Interleukin-6 receptor (IL-6R) antagonist Tocilizumab may be the key to reduce the mortality. *Int. J. Antimicrob. Agents* **2020**, *55*, 105954. [CrossRef]
38. Henderson, L.A.; Canna, S.W.; Schulert, G.S.; Volpi, S.; Lee, P.Y.; Kernan, K.F.; Caricchio, R.; Mahmud, S.; Hazen, M.M.; Halyabar, O.; et al. On the alert for cytokine storm: Immunopathology in COVID-19. *Arthritis Rheumatol.* **2020**, *72*, 1059–1063. [CrossRef]
39. Osugi, Y.; Hara, J.; Tagawa, S.; Takai, K.; Hosoi, G.; Matsuda, Y.; Ohta, H.; Fujisaki, H.; Kobayashi, M.; Sakata, N.; et al. Cytokine production regulating Th1 and Th2 cytokines in hemophagocytic lymphohistiocytosis. *Blood* **1997**, *89*, 4100–4103. [CrossRef] [PubMed]
40. Atteritano, M.; David, A.; Bagnato, G.; Beninati, C.; Frisina, A.; Iaria, C.; Bagnato, G.; Cascio, A. Haemophagocytic syndrome in rheumatic patients. A systematic review. *Eur. Rev. Med. Pharm. Sci.* **2012**, *16*, 1414–1424.
41. Brumfiel, G. Why Some COVID-19 Patients Crash: The Body's Immune System Might Be to Blame. Available online: https://www.npr.org/sections/health-shots/2020/04/07/828091467/why-some-covid-19-patients-crash-the-bodys-immune-system-might-be-to-blame (accessed on 27 April 2020).
42. Hamblin, J. Why Some People Get Sicker than Others. Available online: https://www.theatlantic.com/health/archive/2020/04/coronavirus-immune-response/610228/ (accessed on 27 April 2020).
43. Li, X.; Geng, M.; Peng, Y.; Meng, L.; Lu, S. Molecular immune pathogenesis and diagnosis of COVID-19. *J. Pharm. Anal.* **2020**. [CrossRef] [PubMed]
44. Xu, Z.; Shi, L.; Wang, Y.; Zhang, J.; Huang, L.; Zhang, C.; Liu, S.; Zhao, P.; Liu, H.; Zhu, L.; et al. Pathological findings of COVID-19 associated with acute respiratory distress syndrome. *Lancet Respir. Med.* **2020**, *8*, 420–422. [CrossRef]
45. Lipworth, B.; Chan, R.; Lipworth, S.; RuiWen Kuo, C. Weathering the Cytokine Storm in Susceptible Patients with Severe SARS-CoV-2 Infection. *J. Allergy Clin. Immunol. Pract.* **2020**. [CrossRef]
46. Cytokine Storm. Available online: https://www.sinobiological.com/resource/cytokines/cytokine-storm (accessed on 27 April 2020).
47. Ye, Q.; Wang, B.; Mao, J. Cytokine Storm in COVID-19 and Treatment. *J. Infect.* **2020**. [CrossRef]
48. Routley, N. Visualizing What COVID-19 Does to Your Body. Available online: https://www.visualcapitalist.com/visualizing-what-covid-19-does-to-your-body/ (accessed on 26 April 2020).
49. Huang, C.; Wang, Y.; Li, X.; Ren, L.; Zhao, J.; Hu, Y.; Zhang, L.; Fan, G.; Xu, J.; Gu, X.; et al. Clinical features of patients infected with 2019 novel coronavirus in Wuhan, China. *Lancet* **2020**, *395*, 497–506. [CrossRef]
50. Gattinoni, L.; Coppola, S.; Cressoni, M.; Busana, M.; Rossi, S.; Chiumello, D. Covid-19 Does Not Lead to a "Typical" Acute Respiratory Distress Syndrome. *Am. J. Respir. Crit. Care Med.* **2020**. [CrossRef]
51. Shi, Y.; Wang, Y.; Shao, C.; Huang, J.; Gan, J.; Huang, X.; Bucci, E.; Piacentini, M.; Ippolito, G.; Melino, G. COVID-19 infection: The perspectives on immune responses. *Cell Death Differ.* **2020**, *27*, 1451–1454. [CrossRef]
52. Terpos, E.; Ntanasis-Stathopoulos, I.; Elalamy, I.; Kastritis, E.; Sergentanis, T.N.; Politou, M.; Psaltopoulou, T.; Gerotziafas, G.; Dimopoulos, M.A. Hematological findings and complications of COVID-19. *Am. J. Hematol.* **2020**. [CrossRef] [PubMed]
53. Chen, G.; Wu, D.; Guo, W.; Cao, Y.; Huang, D.; Wang, H.; Wang, T.; Zhang, X.; Chen, H.; Yu, H.; et al. Clinical and immunological features of severe and moderate coronavirus disease 2019. *J. Clin. Investig.* **2020**, *130*, 2620–2629. [CrossRef] [PubMed]
54. Zhang, L.; Yan, X.; Fan, Q.; Liu, H.; Liu, X.; Liu, Z.; Zhang, Z. D-dimer levels on admission to predict in-hospital mortality in patients with Covid-19. *J. Thromb. Haemost.* **2020**, *18*, 1324–1329. [CrossRef] [PubMed]
55. Liu, X.; Teichtahl, A.J.; Wicks, I.P. Interleukin-6 in rheumatoid arthritis from the laboratory to the bedside. *Curr. Pharm. Des.* **2015**, *21*, 2187–2197. [CrossRef]

56. Kang, S.; Tanaka, T.; Narazaki, M.; Kishimoto, T. Targeting Interleukin-6 Signaling in Clinic. *Immunity* **2019**, *50*, 1007–1023. [CrossRef]
57. Pedersen, B.K.; Febbraio, M.A. Muscle as an endocrine organ: Focus on muscle-derived interleukin-6. *Physiol. Rev.* **2008**, *88*, 1379–1406. [CrossRef]
58. Kishimoto, T.; Hibi, M.; Murakami, M.; Narazaki, M.; Saito, M.; Taga, T. The molecular biology of interleukin 6 and its receptor. *Ciba Found. Symp.* **1992**, *167*, 5–16.
59. Jordan, S.C.; Choi, J.; Kim, I.; Wu, G.; Toyoda, M.; Shin, B.; Vo, A. Interleukin-6, A Cytokine Critical to Mediation of Inflammation, Autoimmunity and Allograft Rejection: Therapeutic Implications of IL-6 Receptor Blockade. *Transplantation* **2017**, *101*, 32–44. [CrossRef]
60. Rose-John, S. IL-6 trans-signaling via the soluble IL-6 receptor: Importance for the pro-inflammatory activities of IL-6. *Int. J. Biol. Sci.* **2012**, *8*, 1237–1247. [CrossRef]
61. Velazquez-Salinas, L.; Verdugo-Rodriguez, A.; Rodriguez, L.L.; Borca, M.V. The Role of Interleukin 6 During Viral Infections. *Front. Microbiol.* **2019**, *10*, 1057. [CrossRef]
62. Gottschalk, T.A.; Tsantikos, E.; Hibbs, M.L. Pathogenic Inflammation and Its Therapeutic Targeting in Systemic Lupus Erythematosus. *Front. Immunol.* **2015**, *6*, 550. [CrossRef] [PubMed]
63. Lee, D.W.; Gardner, R.; Porter, D.L.; Louis, C.U.; Ahmed, N.; Jensen, M.; Grupp, S.A.; Mackall, C.L. Current concepts in the diagnosis and management of cytokine release syndrome. *Blood* **2014**, *124*, 188–195. [CrossRef] [PubMed]
64. Godel, P.; Shimabukuro-Vornhagen, A.; von Bergwelt-Baildon, M. Understanding cytokine release syndrome. *Intensive Care Med.* **2018**, *44*, 371–373. [CrossRef]
65. Tanaka, T.; Narazaki, M.; Kishimoto, T. Immunotherapeutic implications of IL-6 blockade for cytokine storm. *Immunotherapy* **2016**, *8*, 959–970. [CrossRef] [PubMed]
66. Russell, B.; Moss, C.; George, G.; Santaolalla, A.; Cope, A.; Papa, S.; Van Hemelrijck, M. Associations between immune-suppressive and stimulating drugs and novel COVID-19-a systematic review of current evidence. *Ecancermedicalscience* **2020**, *14*, 1022. [CrossRef] [PubMed]
67. Wu, C.; Chen, X.; Cai, Y.; Xia, J.; Zhou, X.; Xu, S.; Huang, H.; Zhang, L.; Zhou, X.; Du, C.; et al. Risk Factors Associated With Acute Respiratory Distress Syndrome and Death in Patients With Coronavirus Disease 2019 Pneumonia in Wuhan, China. *JAMA Intern. Med.* **2020**. [CrossRef] [PubMed]
68. Lagunas-Rangel, F.A.; Chavez-Valencia, V. High IL-6/IFN-gamma ratio could be associated with severe disease in COVID-19 patients. *J. Med. Virol.* **2020**. [CrossRef] [PubMed]
69. Walker, J.; Hopkins, J.S. Haywire Immune Response Eyed in Coronavirus Deaths, Treatment. *Wall Street J.* **2020**. Available online: https://www.wsj.com/articles/haywire-immune-response-eyed-in-coronavirus-deaths-treatment-11586430001?mod=searchresults&page=1&pos=1 (accessed on 2 July 2020).
70. Kishimoto, T. Interleukin-6: Discovery of a pleiotropic cytokine. *Arthritis Res. Ther.* **2006**, *8*, S2. [CrossRef]
71. Kishimoto, T. IL-6: From its discovery to clinical applications. *Int. Immunol.* **2010**, *22*, 347–352. [CrossRef]
72. Garbers, C.; Heink, S.; Korn, T.; Rose-John, S. Interleukin-6: Designing specific therapeutics for a complex cytokine. *Nat. Rev. Drug Discov.* **2018**, *17*, 395–412. [CrossRef] [PubMed]
73. Sheppard, M.; Laskou, F.; Stapleton, P.P.; Hadavi, S.; Dasgupta, B. Tocilizumab (Actemra). *Hum. Vaccines Immunother.* **2017**, *13*, 1972–1988. [CrossRef]
74. European Medicine Agency. *Assessment Report For RoActemra*, 1st ed.; European Medicines Agency: London, UK, 2009. Available online: http://www.ema.europa.eu/docs/en_GB/document_library/EPAR_-_Public_assessment_report/human/000955/WC500054888.pdf (accessed on 17 April 2020).
75. Narazaki, M.; Kishimoto, T. The Two-Faced Cytokine IL-6 in Host Defense and Diseases. *Int. J. Mol. Sci.* **2018**, *19*, 3528. [CrossRef] [PubMed]
76. Garbers, C.; Aparicio-Siegmund, S.; Rose-John, S. The IL-6/gp130/STAT3 signaling axis: Recent advances towards specific inhibition. *Curr. Opin. Immunol.* **2015**, *34*, 75–82. [CrossRef] [PubMed]
77. Genentech Actemra, Highlights of Prescribing Information. Available online: https://www.gene.com/download/pdf/actemra_prescribing.pdf (accessed on 19 April 2020).
78. Rose-John, S.; Winthrop, K.; Calabrese, L. The role of IL-6 in host defence against infections: Immunobiology and clinical implications. *Nat. Rev. Rheumatol.* **2017**, *13*, 399–409. [CrossRef]
79. Tocilizumab Solution. Available online: https://www.webmd.com/drugs/2/drug-153516/tocilizumab-intravenous/details (accessed on 17 April 2020).

80. Bennardo, F.; Buffone, C.; Giudice, A. New therapeutic opportunities for COVID-19 patients with Tocilizumab: Possible correlation of interleukin-6 receptor inhibitors with osteonecrosis of the jaws. *Oral Oncol.* **2020**, 104659. [CrossRef]
81. Tocilizumab (Actemra): Adult Patients with Moderately to Severly Active Rheumatoid Arthritis [Internet] Table 1, Cost-Comparison Table or Biologic Disease-Modifying Drugs for Rheumatoid Arthritis. Available online: https://www.ncbi.nlm.nih.gov/books/NBK349513/table/T43/ (accessed on 28 April 2020).
82. Ponticelli, C.; Moroni, G. Hydroxychloroquine in systemic lupus erythematosus (SLE). *Expert Opin. Drug Saf.* **2017**, *16*, 411–419. [CrossRef]
83. Costedoat-Chalumeau, N.; Dunogue, B.; Morel, N.; Le Guern, V.; Guettrot-Imbert, G. Hydroxychloroquine: A multifaceted treatment in lupus. *Presse Med.* **2014**, *43*, e167–e180. [CrossRef]
84. Cao, B.; Wang, Y.; Wen, D.; Liu, W.; Wang, J.; Fan, G.; Ruan, L.; Song, B.; Cai, Y.; Wei, M.; et al. A Trial of Lopinavir-Ritonavir in Adults Hospitalized with Severe Covid-19. *N. Engl. J. Med.* **2020**. [CrossRef]
85. Lopinavir-Ritonavir. Available online: https://www.webmd.com/drugs/2/drug-19938-3294/lopinavir-ritonavir-oral/lopinavir-ritonavir-solution-oral/details (accessed on 17 April 2020).
86. Sheahan, T.P.; Sims, A.C.; Leist, S.R.; Schafer, A.; Won, J.; Brown, A.J.; Montgomery, S.A.; Hogg, A.; Babusis, D.; Clarke, M.O.; et al. Comparative therapeutic efficacy of remdesivir and combination lopinavir, ritonavir, and interferon beta against MERS-CoV. *Nat. Commun.* **2020**, *11*, 222. [CrossRef]
87. Kupferschmidt, K.; Cohen, J. Race to find COVID-19 treatments accelerates. *Science* **2020**, *367*, 1412–1413. [CrossRef] [PubMed]
88. Cunha, J.P. Remdesivir (RDV). Available online: https://www.rxlist.com/consumer_remdesivir_rdv/drugs-condition.htm (accessed on 17 April 2020).
89. Bloch, E.M.; Shoham, S.; Casadevall, A.; Sachais, B.S.; Shaz, B.; Winters, J.L.; van Buskirk, C.; Grossman, B.J.; Joyner, M.; Henderson, J.P.; et al. Deployment of convalescent plasma for the prevention and treatment of COVID-19. *J. Clin. Investig.* **2020**, *130*, 2757–2765. [CrossRef] [PubMed]
90. Xu, X.; Han, M.; Li, T.; Sun, W.; Wang, D.; Fu, B.; Zhou, Y.; Zheng, X.; Yang, Y.; Li, X.; et al. Effective Treatment of Severe COVID-19 Patients with Tocilizumab. Available online: file:///C:/Users/Naveen%20Dhawan/Downloads/202003.00026v1%20(1).pdf (accessed on 26 April 2020).
91. De Luna, G.; Habibi, A.; Deux, J.F.; Colard, M.; d'Alexandry d'Orengiani, A.; Schlemmer, F.; Joher, N.; Kassasseya, C.; Pawlotsky, J.M.; Ourghanlian, C.; et al. Rapid and Severe Covid-19 Pneumonia with Severe Acute Chest Syndrome in a Sickle Cell Patient Successfully Treated with Tocilizumab. *Am. J. Hematol.* **2020**, *95*, 876–878. [CrossRef] [PubMed]
92. Fontana, F.; Alfano, G.; Mori, G.; Amurri, A.; Lorenzo, T.; Ballestri, M.; Leonelli, M.; Facchini, F.; Damiano, F.; Magistroni, R.; et al. COVID-19 pneumonia in a kidney transplant recipient successfully treated with Tocilizumab and Hydroxychloroquine. *Am. J. Transpl.* **2020**, *20*, 1902–1906. [CrossRef] [PubMed]
93. Zhang, X.; Song, K.; Tong, F.; Fei, M.; Guo, H.; Lu, Z.; Wang, J.; Zheng, C. First case of COVID-19 in a patient with multiple myeloma successfully treated with tocilizumab. *Blood Adv.* **2020**, *4*, 1307–1310. [CrossRef] [PubMed]
94. Michot, J.M.; Albiges, L.; Chaput, N.; Saada, V.; Pommeret, F.; Griscelli, F.; Balleyguier, C.; Besse, B.; Marabelle, A.; Netzer, F.; et al. Tocilizumab, an anti-IL6 receptor antibody, to treat Covid-19-related respiratory failure: A case report. *Ann. Oncol.* **2020**, *31*, 961–964. [CrossRef] [PubMed]
95. Cellina, M.; Orsi, M.; Bombaci, F.; Sala, M.; Marino, P.; Oliva, G. Favorable changes of CT findings in a patient with COVID-19 pneumonia after treatment with tocilizumab. *Diagn. Interv. Imaging* **2020**, *101*, 323–324. [CrossRef]
96. Jacobs, J.P.; Stammers, A.H.; St Louis, J.; Hayanga, J.W.A.; Firstenberg, M.S.; Mongero, L.B.; Tesdahl, E.A.; Rajagopal, K.; Cheema, F.H.; Coley, T.; et al. Extracorporeal Membrane Oxygenation in the Treatment of Severe Pulmonary and Cardiac Compromise in COVID-19: Experience with 32 patients. *ASAIO J.* **2020**, *66*, 722–730. [CrossRef]
97. Giamarellos-Bourboulis, E.J.; Netea, M.G.; Rovina, N.; Akinosoglou, K.; Antoniadou, A.; Antonakos, N.; Damoraki, G.; Gkavogianni, T.; Adami, M.E.; Katsaounou, P.; et al. Complex Immune Dysregulation in COVID-19 Patients with Severe Respiratory Failure. *Cell Host Microbe* **2020**, *27*, 992–1000. [CrossRef]
98. Ferrey, A.J.; Choi, G.; Hanna, R.M.; Chang, Y.; Tantisattamo, E.; Ivaturi, K.; Park, E.; Nguyen, L.; Wang, B.; Tonthat, S.; et al. A Case of Novel Coronavirus Disease 19 in a Chronic Hemodialysis Patient Presenting with Gastroenteritis and Developing Severe Pulmonary Disease. *Am. J. Nephrol.* **2020**, *51*, 337–342. [CrossRef]

99. Mihai, C.; Dobrota, R.; Schroder, M.; Garaiman, A.; Jordan, S.; Becker, M.O.; Maurer, B.; Distler, O. COVID-19 in a patient with systemic sclerosis treated with tocilizumab for SSc-ILD. *Ann. Rheum. Dis.* **2020**, *79*, 668–669. [CrossRef] [PubMed]
100. Stebbing, J.; Phelan, A.; Griffin, I.; Tucker, C.; Oechsle, O.; Smith, D.; Richardson, P. COVID-19: Combining antiviral and anti-inflammatory treatments. *Lancet Infect. Dis.* **2020**, *20*, 400–402. [CrossRef]

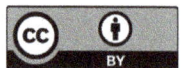 © 2020 by the authors. Licensee MDPI, Basel, Switzerland. This article is an open access article distributed under the terms and conditions of the Creative Commons Attribution (CC BY) license (http://creativecommons.org/licenses/by/4.0/).

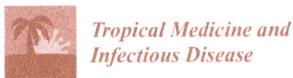 *Tropical Medicine and Infectious Disease*

Commentary

Challenges in Tuberculosis Clinical Trials in the Face of the COVID-19 Pandemic: A Sponsor's Perspective

I.D. Rusen

Senior Vice President, Research Division, Vital Strategies, New York, NY 10005, USA; IRusen@vitalstrategies.org

Received: 24 April 2020; Accepted: 14 May 2020; Published: 27 May 2020

Abstract: The COVID-19 pandemic has caused unforeseen and extreme changes in societal and health system functioning not previously experienced in most countries in a lifetime. The impact of the pandemic on clinical trials can be especially profound given their complexities and operational requirements. The STREAM Clinical Trial is the largest trial for MDR-TB ever conducted. Currently operating in seven countries, the trial had 126 participants on treatment and 312 additional participants in active follow up as of March 31, 2020. Areas of particular concern during this global emergency include treatment continuity, supply chain management and participant safety monitoring. This commentary highlights some of the challenges faced due to the pandemic and the steps taken to protect the safety of trial participants and the integrity of the trial.

Keywords: MDR-TB; clinical trials; COVID-19

The COVID-19 pandemic has caused unforeseen and extreme changes in societal and health system functioning not previously experienced in most countries in a lifetime [1]. The disruptions have been dynamic-varying by time and geography-which adds to their unpredictable effect. The negative impact of COVID-19 on tuberculosis (TB) programs has recently been reported with models predicting 126,100 excess TB deaths over the next five years for every one month of COVID-related lockdown [2]. Clinical trial implementation is especially challenging in this pandemic environment, requiring sponsors to adhere to trial protocols and regulatory requirements as closely as possible while ensuring the safety of trial participants and staff.

Tuberculosis clinical trials carry inherent challenges at the best of times. Locations with the highest tuberculosis burden often have less resilient regulatory infrastructure, complex operational environments and more limited clinical trial experience [3]. During an unexpected and large-scale disruption like COVID-19, the impact of these weaknesses becomes more magnified.

STREAM is the largest multi-country trial for multidrug-resistant tuberculosis (MDR-TB) ever conducted. Conceived by the Union and global partners with initial funding from USAID, the trial has recruited over 1000 patients to two distinct stages. Results from STREAM Stage 1 were published in 2019 and 2020 [4,5], and recruitment was recently completed for the second stage in January, 2020. As of March 31, 2020, 126 participants remain on MDR-TB treatment with 21 of those in the intensive phase of treatment and 312 participants remain in active follow-up.

Stage 2 of STREAM is a registration trial [6], which adds complexity to implementation. It incorporates central safety and microbiology testing, requiring regular export of biological samples. In addition, a contract research organization (CRO) is employed to conduct onsite monitoring and source data verification to ensure data quality.

The COVID-19 pandemic has had an important impact on the implementation of STREAM. Key challenges faced by STREAM (and similar trials) together with the responses of the trial team to date, are outlined in this commentary.

Early in the COVID-19 outbreak, working with our main implementing partner, Medical Research Council Clinical Trials Unit at University College London, a STREAM-COVID-19 Task Force was formed to identify and address the risks and challenges arising due to the pandemic. A continuity plan was developed, and the task force met (and continues to meet) weekly to respond to the rapidly changing circumstances.

Enhanced communication with trial sites was initiated to provide timely guidance to the sites, and also ensure that the Task Force was aware of any pandemic-related issues faced by sites. Sites were provided educational material on TB and COVID-19 and were requested to inform the central trial team of any unforeseen challenges. Additional site resources were considered upon request, such as office space away from health care facilities. Importantly, there were no reported shortages of personal protective equipment (PPE). Sites have also been directed to maintain regular communication with all trial participants. Participants are to be informed of potential changes to their follow-up schedules, as well as other site-specific changes. Importantly all participants were reassured about their care during the trial and instructed to raise any concerns with the trial team.

Areas requiring particular attention of the Task Force included:

1. Care and Treatment Continuity

While treatment continuity is a priority in most clinical trials, the urgency is heightened in tuberculosis trials due to the nature of the disease. Treatment interruption is associated with poor outcomes and development of further drug resistance [7]. The long treatment regimens required for tuberculosis complicate efforts to prevent interruptions under normal conditions, let alone during a pandemic. For the small number of participants still receiving an injectable agent, the potential challenges are even greater in terms of travel required to receive their treatment.

Most STREAM trial sites are now under various levels of 'stay at home' orders which discourage or prevent movement of participants to trial sites for follow-up visits, including collection of medicine (Table 1). Even where country policies allow travel for medical reasons, this may require a government-issued permit for internal movement and lack of available public transportation may still prevent participants from attending clinics. Furthermore, limiting participant exposure to the health system and potential coronavirus exposure is an important consideration.

Table 1. STREAM Stage 2 countries and current status of participants and restrictions on travel and import/export.

Country	Participants on Treatment	Participants in Follow Up	Movement Restrictions Preventing Clinic Visits	Restrictions on Import/Export
Ethiopia	Yes	Yes	No	Yes
Georgia	No	Yes	No	No
India	Yes	Yes	Yes	Yes
Moldova	Yes	Yes	No	No
Mongolia	Yes	Yes	No	Yes
South Africa	No	Yes	Yes	Yes
Uganda	Yes	Yes	Yes	Yes

as of 15 April 2020.

These factors require clinical trial sponsors to balance the need for routine treatment management against the possible negative impacts of participant travel to clinics. In the STREAM trial, arrangements have been made for delivery of medicines to the homes of participants who consent and, where necessary, nearby health centers have also been mobilized for administration of injectable agents. To prevent risks to treatment continuity should circumstances further restrict clinic visits or delivery of supplies, the amount of drug provided has been increased. To date, adequate supplies of medicines have been assured for all participants. Video communication has been introduced at most trial sites and has proven feasible for most participants. This enhanced communication supports both treatment adherence, as well as safety monitoring (as described below).

2. Supply Chain

Supply chain disruptions also pose a potentially significant challenge during a pandemic. As borders close to travel, including, at times, cargo deliveries, replenishment of medicine stocks can be disrupted. Even domestic travel disruption can threaten continuity of trial supplies where a central depot is utilized in larger countries. The situation can be aggravated if expiration dates of medicines are relatively short and/or by cumbersome importation requirements because frequent replenishments are all the more challenging when timelines for importation are extended. Depending on the duration of restrictions that prevent/extend timelines for importation of medicines, alternative options for medicine procurement, including (where possible) local procurement and borrowing from other local sources (e.g., the National Tuberculosis Program) must be explored.

Supply chain interruptions of laboratory and other supplies (e.g., materials for medicine re-packaging and kits for central laboratory testing) may also occur but pose less serious risks to the trial.

3. Participant Safety Monitoring (Including Export of Safety and Microbiology Samples)

Participant safety is always paramount. However, under current conditions, safety monitoring may be interrupted. This is because the risk of exposure to coronavirus in transit to or at health centers may outweigh the monitoring benefits of in-person clinic visits or because local restrictions on movement may prevent participants from attending scheduled clinic visits, or both. Furthermore, restrictions on the export of blood samples can make it necessary to conduct safety testing locally, rather than at central laboratories, and some local laboratories may not have the capacity to conduct all protocol safety assessments. Comprehensive review of local laboratory capacity has been limited by the rapid timeline of transition from central to local laboratories. In most instances, sites have transitioned to their own institution laboratories that routinely serve the tuberculosis programs. Accreditation has been ensured for external private laboratories when utilized for trial samples. Export restrictions may also interrupt transport of microbiology samples for central testing, but these do not carry immediate risk, since microbiology for immediate participant management is already performed locally.

In the STREAM trial, sites are conducting frequent, remote monitoring by phone, including video monitoring wherever possible. Where more intensive monitoring is required for participants identified at greater risk, e.g., ECG monitoring for participants with a previously identified QT prolongation, arrangements have been made to transport participants to the site for necessary assessments and interventions to ensure safety, including local blood analysis. Sputum collection continues wherever possible either during in-person clinic visits or through home collection during the treatment and the immediate follow-up period, as these results may impact on optimal treatment management for participants. Sputum collection in the later follow-up period is generally being rescheduled (provided participants are well) to reduce COVID risks for participants and staff.

The trial continues to store blood and microbiology specimens for future export, provided storage and stability requirements can be met.

Accurate diagnosis of TB patients with respiratory symptoms against the backdrop of other respiratory illnesses, such as COVID-19, can present a clinical challenge. Fortunately, most participants in STREAM have completed, or are approaching the end of, the intensive phase of treatment and TB-related respiratory symptoms should be limited to the small number of participants experiencing treatment failure. Participants presenting with respiratory symptoms will be assessed for both TB for COVID-19 in accordance with local guidelines and testing capacity. Any suspected or confirmed COVID-19 cases will be managed according to local guidelines and documented in a manner similar to other concurrent illnesses in the trial. Early reports of greater severity of COVID-19 illness amongst TB patients [8] heighten the need to prevent exposure of trial participants to the greatest extent possible.

Additional challenges related to trial implementation include: ensuring sufficient human resources at sites when local staff reassignment to COVID-related tasks is occurring and/or staff are personally impacted by COVID-19, continuing to conduct source data verification (SDV) when on-site monitoring by external partners cannot take place, and disruption of community engagement (CE) activities when in-person meetings are not possible.

The experience of the STREAM trial against the backdrop of the pandemic highlights the importance of contingency planning and risk mitigation both before and during unanticipated crises. While some of the challenges highlighted are specific to clinical trial implementation, many issues and potential solutions presented apply equally to operational research of MDR-TB regimens. Guidance from regulatory agencies has been especially useful to clarify acceptable responses to the very real challenges arising out of the pandemic [9,10]. Careful documentation of protocol deviations related to the pandemic is essential and these deviations will be reported to local and global ethics committees, as well as ultimately to regulatory authorities. The trial team will continue to closely monitor the status of the pandemic across trial sites and adapt accordingly to ensure the integrity of the trial, as well as the safety of all participants and site staff.

Ethics Statement: Ethics approval not required.

Funding: STREAM Stage 1 was funded by The United States Agency for International Development (USAID), with additional support from the United Kingdom Medical Research Council (MRC) and the United Kingdom Department for International Development (DFID). STREAM Stage 2 is being funded by USAID and Janssen Pharmaceuticals, the maker of bedaquiline, with additional support from MRC and DFID.

Acknowledgments: The Sponsor acknowledges the extraordinary efforts of all trial partners and especially the site staff and trial participants during this challenging period.

Conflicts of Interest: The authors declare no conflict of interest.

References

1. Gates, B. Responding to COVID-19—A Once-in-a-Century Pandemic? *N. Engl. J. Med.* **2020**. [CrossRef] [PubMed]
2. Stop TB Partnership (2020) The potential impact of the COVID-19 response on tuberculosis in high-burden countries: A modelling analysis. Available online: http://www.stoptb.org/assets/documents/news/Modeling%20Report_1%20May%202020_FINAL.pdf (accessed on 19 April 2020).
3. Alemayehu, C.; Mitchell, G.; Nikles, J. Barriers for conducting clinical trials in developing countries—A systematic review. *Int. J. Equity Health* **2018**, *17*, 37. [CrossRef]
4. Nunn, A.J.; Phillips, P.P.J.; Meredith, S.K.; Chiang, C.J.; STREAM Study Collaborators. A Trial of a Shorter Regimen for Rifampin-Resistant Tuberculosis. *N. Engl. J. Med.* **2019**, *380*, 1201–1213. [CrossRef] [PubMed]
5. Madan, J.J.; Rosu, L.; Tefera, M.G.; van Rensburg, C.; Evans, D.; Langley, I.; Tomeny, E.M.; Nunn, A.; Phillips, P.P.J.; Rusen, I.D.; et al. Economic evaluation of short treatment for multidrug-resistant tuberculosis, Ethiopia and South Africa: The STREAM trial. *Bull. World Health Organ.* **2020**, *98*, 306–314. [CrossRef]
6. ClinicalTrials. *The Evaluation of a Standard Treatment Regimen of Anti-tuberculosis Drugs for Patients with MDR-TB (STREAM)*; Identifier NCT02409290; National Library of Medicine: Bethesda, MD, USA, 2020. Available online: https://clinicaltrials.gov/ct2/show/record/NCT02409290 (accessed on 19 April 2020).
7. Alipanah, N.; Jarlsberg, L.; Miller, C.; Linh, N.N.; Falzon, D.; Jaramillo, E.; Nahid, P. Adherence interventions and outcomes of tuberculosis treatment: A systematic review and meta-analysis of trials and observational studies. *PLoS Med.* **2018**, *15*, e1002595. [CrossRef] [PubMed]
8. Liu, Y.; Bi, L.; Chen, Y.; Wang, Y.; Fleming, J.; Yu, Y.; Gu, Y.; Liu, C.; Fan, L.; Wanx, X.; et al. Active or latent tuberculosis increases susceptibility to COVID-19 and disease severity. *Medrxiv* **2020**. preprint. [CrossRef]

9. US Food and Drug Administration. FDA Guidance on Conduct of Clinical Trials of Medical Products during COVID-19 Public Health Emergency. 2020. Available online: https://www.fda.gov/regulatory-information/search-fda-guidance-documents/fda-guidance-conduct-clinical-trials-medical-products-during-covid-19-public-health-emergency (accessed on 25 March 2020).
10. South Africa Health Products Regulatory Authority (SAHPRA). SAHPRA Policy on Conduct of Clinical Trials of Health Products during the Current COVID-19 Pandemic. Available online: http://www.sahpra.org.za/wp-content/uploads/2020/03/SAHPRA-Communication_COVID_19-Final-25032020.pdf (accessed on 25 March 2020).

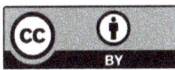

© 2020 by the author. Licensee MDPI, Basel, Switzerland. This article is an open access article distributed under the terms and conditions of the Creative Commons Attribution (CC BY) license (http://creativecommons.org/licenses/by/4.0/).

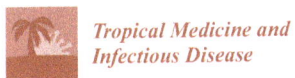

Review

Prognosis of COVID-19 in Patients with Liver and Kidney Diseases: An Early Systematic Review and Meta-Analysis

Tope Oyelade [1,*], Jaber Alqahtani [2] and Gabriele Canciani [1,3]

1 Institute for Liver and Digestive Health, Division of Medicine, University College London, London NW3 2PF, UK; gabriele.canciani20@gmail.com
2 School of Respiratory Medicine, University College London, London NW3 2PF, UK; jaber.alqahtani.18@ucl.ac.uk
3 School of Medicine, La Sapienza University, Rome 00185, Italy
* Correspondence: t.oyelade@ucl.ac.uk

Received: 26 April 2020; Accepted: 12 May 2020; Published: 15 May 2020

Abstract: The mortality and severity in COVID-19 is increased in patients with comorbidities. The aim of this study was to evaluate the severity and mortality in COVID-19 patients with underlying kidney and liver diseases. We retrieved data on the clinical features and primary composite end point of COVID-19 patients from Medline and Embase which had been released from inception by the April 16, 2020. The data on two comorbidities, liver diseases and chronic kidney disease, were pooled and statistically analysed to explain the associated severity and mortality rate. One hundred and forty-two abstracts were screened, and 41 full articles were then read. In total, 22 studies including 5595 COVID-19 patients were included in this study with case fatality rate of 16%. The prevalence of liver diseases and chronic kidney disease (CKD) were 3% (95% CI; 2–3%) and 1% (95% CI; 1–2%), respectively. In patients with COVID-19 and underlying liver diseases, 57.33% (43/75) of cases were severe, with 17.65% mortality, while in CKD patients, 83.93% (47/56) of cases were severe and 53.33% (8/15) mortality was reported. This study found an increased risk of severity and mortality in COVID-19 patients with liver diseases or CKD. This will lead to better clinical management and inform the process of implementing more stringent preventative measures for this group of patients.

Keywords: COVID-19; SARS-CoV-2; hepatitis B and C; cirrhosis; chronic kidney disease; alcohol-related liver disease; nonalcoholic steatohepatitis; necrosis

1. Introduction

The 2010 Global Burden of Disease reported that liver diseases were responsible for about 2 million deaths annually, with 50% of these associated with complications due to liver cirrhosis and the other half linked to hepatocellular carcinoma and viral hepatitis [1]. Cirrhosis is an end stage of chronic liver disease often preceded by hepatocellular necrosis and progressive fibrosis triggered by various agents including viral infections and chronic alcohol use [2]. Alcohol-related liver disease, nonalcoholic steatohepatitis and hepatitis B and C have been reported to be the main aetiologies of liver cirrhosis, with an up to 80% mortality rate recorded 1-year after decompensation [3,4]. Aside from mortality, the economic impact of liver-associated morbidity is also high, with associated disease-adjusted life years loss at over 41 million years globally. According to the World Health Organization (WHO) global health estimate of 2015, chronic liver disease ranks as the 16th highest cause of morbidity globally [5,6]. Despite the availability of vaccines for hepatitis B and the advances in clinical understanding and the management of chronic liver diseases, the global health burden of the disease increased between 1990 and 2017. This rise in health burden was attributed to ageing and an overall increase in the global population [4].

According to Kidney Disease Improving Global Outcome (KDIGO), chronic kidney disease (CKD) is a dysfunction of the kidney characterised by established histological damage or a suboptimal (<60 mL/min/1.73 m^2) glomerular filtration rate (GFR) persisting for at least 3 months [7]. Although the majority of CKD cases are linked to diabetes and hypertension [8], other risk factors, including genetics [9], recreational drugs and alcohol consumption [10], obesity [11], gender [12,13], age [12], lower birth weight [14], smoking status [15,16], ethnicity [17], family history of CKD [18] and acute kidney injury, have been studied [19,20]. In 2017, the number of deaths associated with CKD or CDK-related complications was estimated to be 1.2 million, accounting for 4.6% of global deaths [21]. Between 1990 and 2017, CKD rose as a cause of global mortality from the 17th to the 12th leading cause of death, with a 46% increase in the total number of deaths caused directly or indirectly by cardiovascular disease linked to kidney dysfunction [22]. While the relationship between COVID-19-induced acute kidney injury has been investigated previously [23], to the best of our knowledge, no studies have looked at the risk of COVID-19 in patients with all-form renal disease.

The severe acute respiratory syndrome coronavirus 2 (SARS-CoV-2) is a viral pathogen which is responsible for the coronavirus disease 2019 (COVID-19) [24]. Symptoms of COVID-19 include fever, fatigue, dry cough, dyspnoea and sore throat, with patients presenting with abnormal chest CT (Computed Tomography) scans in the form of pulmonary ground glass opacity changes [25,26]. COVID-19 was first reported in December 2019, with its possible origin linked to the Wuhan seafood market in China [27]. Since first being reported, SARS-CoV-2 has infected, as of 2nd of April, 2020, 896,450 people and caused 45,525 deaths worldwide, with these numbers rising daily [28]. So far, the risk factors associated with poor clinical outcomes (death or admission to an intensive care unit (ICU)) have been reported to be old age and several comorbidities associated with compromised immune system to help the patient fight the infection. The most common of these comorbidities are hypertension, diabetes, cardiovascular diseases and malignancies. These comorbidities, individually or in combination with age, were reported to be linked with poor prognoses [29]. Several studies have looked at the risk posed to patients with various chronic diseases by COVID-19. For instance, Alqahtani et al. 2020 looked at the risk of smoking status and chronic obstructive pulmonary disease (COPD) in COVID-19 patients, establishing an increased risk of death or admission to ICU for patients with COPD or smoking history infected with SARS-CoV-2 [30].

While COVID-19-induced liver and kidney injuries have been documented, to the best of our knowledge, there has been no report on the risk posed by COVID-19 infection in patients with a history of liver or renal disease. Understanding the risk to this subpopulation of patients will facilitate effective prevention decisions and clinical management. We aim here to understand the risks by looking at reported cases since the outbreak of COVID-19.

2. Methods

Preferred Reporting in Systematic Reviews and Meta-Analyses (PRISMA) guidelines were followed during the drafting of this review. We searched Medline and Embase from November 2019 to 10 April 2020 and later, on the 14 April 2020, an updated search was performed. The search strategy was designed to include all papers on COVID-19 published from 21 November 2019, when the first case of the disease was reported, up to right before this review was submitted (Table A1 in Appendix A).

2.1. Inclusion and Exclusion Criteria

Studies considered were those reporting the clinical characteristics of diagnosed COVID-19 patients with underlying kidney and/or liver diseases. To be eligible, studies had to also report clinical outcome in the form of disease severity (defined as admission to ICU or need for a respirator or intubation) as well as death. Excluded studies were those including COVID-19 patient clinical features but not liver or kidney diseases comorbidity, SARS (Severe Acute Respiratory Syndrome), MERS (Middle East Respiratory Syndrome) and other coronavirus infections, non-English manuscripts, reviews, qualitative studies, editorials and letters of correspondence.

2.2. Data Collection

Potential studies were initially screened by two of the authors (T.O. and J.A.), who scrutinised the title and abstract and came to a final decision on whether each study should be included. Included studies were then fully read by the authors to identify which of the included studies satisfied the inclusion criteria stated above. The references of the finally selected studies were then screened for other eligible studies. A third author was consulted throughout the selection period to resolve conflicts between the two authors. Selected reports were uploaded to Endnote, and duplicates were removed. The duplicate-free studies were uploaded to the Rayyan review software for screening based on title, abstract and then full text by two independent reviewers.

2.3. Quality Assessment

The quality of the included studies was independently assessed by two authors using a modified version of the Newcastle-Ottawa Scale (NOS) [31]. Accordingly, the modified NOS included three domains and six questions scored with a star if satisfied and no star if otherwise. The domains covered assessments of the quality of "Selection", "Ascertainment" and "Outcome". The "Selection" domain describes the adequacy of the sample sizes and representativeness of the study population. A sample size of ≥29 patients was considered adequate, as it represents the lower range of the included studies where clinical characteristics and outcomes were adequately presented. Studies including multiple centres were given an extra point. The "Ascertainment" domain evaluated the adequacy of the confirmatory test and mode of recording comorbidity. The use of polymerase chain reaction (PCR) tests for diagnosis, as recommended by the WHO [32], was scored, as well as the use of electronic medical records (EMRs) to confirm comorbidities. Verbal confirmation of comorbidities was considered inadequate. The "Outcome" domain scored the adequacy of how outcomes were reported and the follow-up period. Outcomes reported by qualified clinical staff and a follow-up of at least two weeks, as recommended by the European Centre for Disease Prevention and Control (ECDC), were scored (Table A1).

2.4. Data Extraction and Analysis

All analyses were performed using the Stata/SE15 software. The pooled prevalence of patients with CKD and liver diseases was analysed using the Metaprop procedure in Stata. Fixed and random effect models were used depending on the level of heterogeneity observed between the included studies. Forest plots were generated presenting the effect sizes (95% CI), percentage weights and the between-studies heterogeneity (I^2 Statistic, p-value, Figures 1 and 2). The prevalence and clinical outcomes of COVID-19 patients with CKD and liver diseases were synthesised from all included studies. Primary composite end points were disease severity and mortality. Disease severity was defined as extended hospital stay, admission to ICU or need for mechanical ventilation.

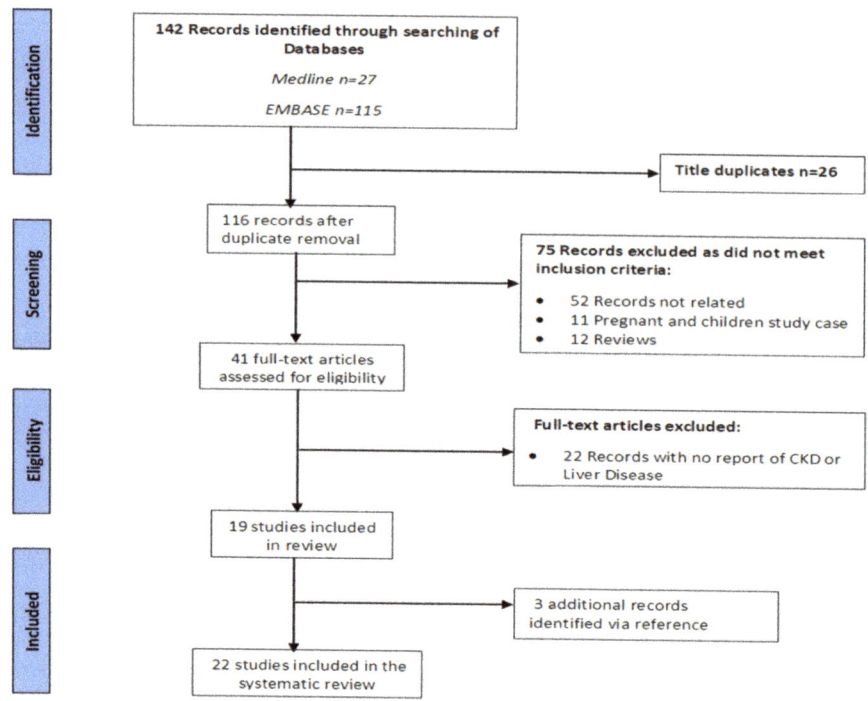

Figure 1. Risk of COVID-19 in patients with chronic liver and kidney diseases: a systematic review according to the Preferred Reporting Items for Systematic Reviews and Metanalyses diagram.

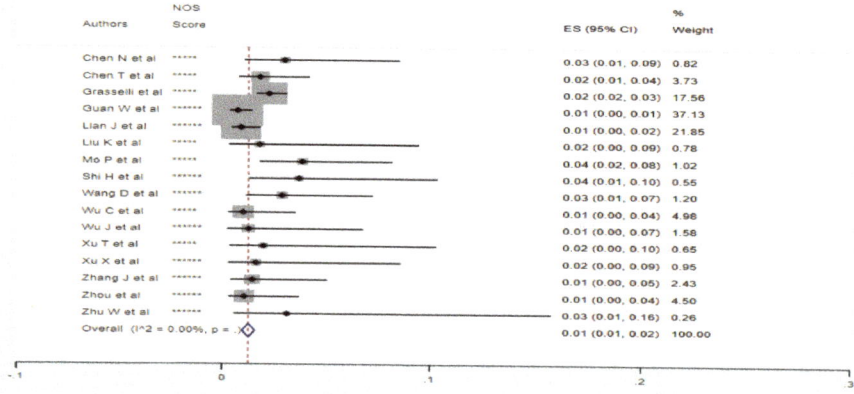

Figure 2. Pooled prevalence of patients with chronic renal diseases diagnosed with COVID-19. The red dotted line represents the overall effect size of the studies (0.01). The lateral edges of the blue diamond represent the limits of the 95% confidence intervals (0.01, 0.02). ES = Effect Size, NOS = Newcastle-Ottawa Score.

3. Results

The initial database search generated 142 papers, from which 26 duplicates were removed. After the title and abstract were screened, 75 papers were excluded and 41 included based on the inclusion criteria. After the full-text reviews, another 22 studies were excluded, resulting in 19 studies with the desired criteria. All the references of the 19 included studies were then screened for studies relevant to the review; three more studies were included from the references, making a total of 22 studies (Figure 1). The modified NOS assessment performed showed a low risk of bias in the included studies (Table A1).

3.1. Description of Included Studies

The total number of confirmed COVID-19 cases included in this study was 5595, of which 2045 (36.55%) were female. Where reported, 147/5305 (2.77%) and 83/5038 (1.65%) had comorbidities of liver diseases and CKD respectively. The mean ±SD (range) of the sample sizes of all included studies was 254.32 ± 385.76 (29–1591). One of the studies was conducted in Italy and the rest in China. Fifteen of the 22 studies, comprising 4367 patients, reported mortality. Where reported, the mortality was 710/4367 (16.26%) in this review. The mean (±SD) follow-up time was 30.55 ± 13.24 days. The clinical characteristics of the liver diseases and CKD, including the stages and aetiology, were not provided in all the studies (Table 1).

3.2. Prevalence of Renal Diseases in Confirmed COVID-19 Cases

The prevalence of CKDs in patients diagnosed with COVID-19 was 1% (95% CI; 1–2%). A random effect model was initially used to pool the studies. However, this was changed to the fixed effect model because of the observed low level of between-studies heterogeneity ($I^2 = 27.60\%$, $p = 0.15$; Data not shown).

3.3. Disease Outcome for Renal Diseases Patients with COVID-19

In all, 5 studies including 3123 COVID-19 patients, 56 of which had CKD, reported severity. Where reported, the severity of COVID-19 was 83.93% (47/56) in patients with underlying CKD. Only 3 studies, including 15 COVID-19 patients with CKD, reported mortality. The mortality in patients with CKD diagnosed with COVID-19 was 53.33% (8/15) (Table 1).

3.4. Prevalence of Liver Diseases in Confirmed COVID-19 Cases

The prevalence of liver diseases in patients diagnosed with COVID-19 is 3% (95% CI; 2–3%). A random effect model was used for pooling the studies because of the observed low level of between-studies heterogeneity ($I^2 = 46.62\%$, $p = 0.01$) (Figure 3).

Table 1. Characteristics of the studies included. Severity is defined as extended hospital stay, need for ICU or mechanical ventilation. Mortality is defined as death associated with COVID-19.

Authors	Country	Study Type	Sample Size	Female (%)	Mortality (%)	Follow-up Time (Days)	Liver Patients (%)	Liver Severity (%)	Liver Deaths (%)	Renal Patients (%)	Renal Severity (%)	Renal Death (%)
Chen J et al. [33]	China-Shanghai	Retrospective Analysis	249	123/249 (49.40)	2/249 (0.80)	16	2/249 (0.80)	-	-	-	-	-
Chen L et al. [34]	China-Wuhan	Retrospective Analysis	29	8/29 (27.59)	26/29 (89.66)	15	2/29 (6.90)	-	-	-	-	-
Chen N et al. [35]	China-Wuhan	Descriptive Analysis	99	32/99 (32.32)	11/99 (11.11)	20	-	-	-	3/99 (3.03)	-	-
Chen T et al. [36]	China-Wuhan	Retrospective Analysis	274	103/274 (37.59)	113/274 (41.24)	30	11/274 (4.02)	-	5/11 (45.46)	5/274 (1.83)	-	4/5 (80.00)
Grasselli et al. [37]	Italy-Multicentre	Retrospective Analysis	1591	287/1591 (18.04)	405/1591 (25.46)	34	28/1591 (1.76)	28/28 (100.00)	-	36/1591 (2.26)	36/36 (100.00)	-
Guan W et al. [38]	China-Multicentre	Retrospective Analysis	1099	459/1099 (41.77)	15/1099 (1.37)	49	23/1099 (2.09)	1/23 (4.35)	1/23 (4.35)	8/1099 (0.73)	3/8 (37.50)	2/8 (25.00)
Huang C et al. [25]	China-Wuhan	Prospective Analysis	41	11/41 (26.83)	-	32	1/41 (2.44)	-	-	-	-	-
Huang Y et al. [39]	China-Wuhan	Retrospective Analysis	34	20/34 (58.82)	-	39	1/34 (2.94)	-	-	-	-	-
Lian J et al. [40]	China-Zhejiang	Retrospective Analysis	788	381/788 (48.35)	-	26	31/788 (3.93)	-	-	7/788 (0.89)	-	-
Liu K et al. [41]	China-Hainan	Retrospective Analysis	56	25/56 (44.64)	3/56 (5.36)	46	1/56 (1.79)	-	-	1/56 (1.79)	-	-
Mo P et al. [42]	China-Wuhan	Retrospective Analysis	155	69/155 (44.52)	22/155 (14.19)	36	7/155 (4.52)	5/7 (71.43)	-	6/155 (3.87)	4/6 (66.67)	-
Shi H et al. [43]	China-Wuhan	Descriptive Analysis	81	39/81 (48.15)	3/81 (3.70)	47	7/81 (8.64)	-	-	3/81 (3.70)	-	-
Wan S et al. [44]	China-Chongqing	Retrospective Analysis	135	63/135 (46.67)	1/135 (0.74)	16	2/135 (1.48)	1/2 (50.00)	-	-	-	-
Wang D et al. [45]	China-Wuhan	Retrospective Analysis	138	63/138 (45.65)	6/138 (4.35)	34	4/138 (2.90)	-	-	4/138 (2.90)	2/4 (50.00)	-
Wang Z et al. [46]	China-Wuhan	Retrospective Analysis	69	37/69 (53.62)	5/69 (7.25)	19	1/69 (1.45)	-	-	-	-	-
Wu C et al. [47]	China-Wuhan	Retrospective Analysis	201	73/201 (36.32)	44/201 (21.89)	63	7/201 (3.48)	-	-	2/201 (1.00)	-	-
Wu J et al. [48]	China-Jiangsu	Retrospective Analysis	80	41/80 (51.25)	-	23	1/80 (1.25)	-	-	1/80 (1.25)	-	-
Xu T et al. [49]	China-Changzhou	Retrospective Analysis	51	26/51 (50.98)	-	35	1/51 (1.96)	-	-	1/51 (1.96)	-	-

Table 1. Cont.

Authors	Country	Study Type	Sample Size	Female (%)	Mortality (%)	Follow-up Time (Days)	Liver Patients (%)	Liver Severity (%)	Liver Deaths (%)	Renal Patients (%)	Renal Severity (%)	Renal Death (%)
Xu X et al. [50]	China-Zhejiang	Retrospective Analysis	62	27/62 (43.55)	-	16	7/62 (11.29)	4/7 (57.14)	-	1/62 (1.61)	-	-
Zhang J et al. [51]	China-Wuhan	Retrospective Analysis	140	69/140 (49.29)	-	34	8/140 (5.71)	4/8 (50.00)	-	2/140 (1.43)	2/2 (100.00)	-
Zhou et al. [52]	China-Wuhan	Retrospective Analysis	191	72/191 (37.70)	54/191 (28.27)	15	-	-	-	2/191 (1.05)	-	2/2 (100.00)
Zhu W et al. [53]	China-Anhui	Retrospective Analysis	32	17/32 (53.13)	-	27	2/32 (6.3)	-	-	1/32 (3.13)	-	-
Total			5595	2045/5595 (36.55)	710/4367 (16.26)	672	147/5305 (2.77)	43/75 (57.33)	6/34 (17.65)	83/5038 (1.65)	47/56 (83.93)	8/15 (53.33)

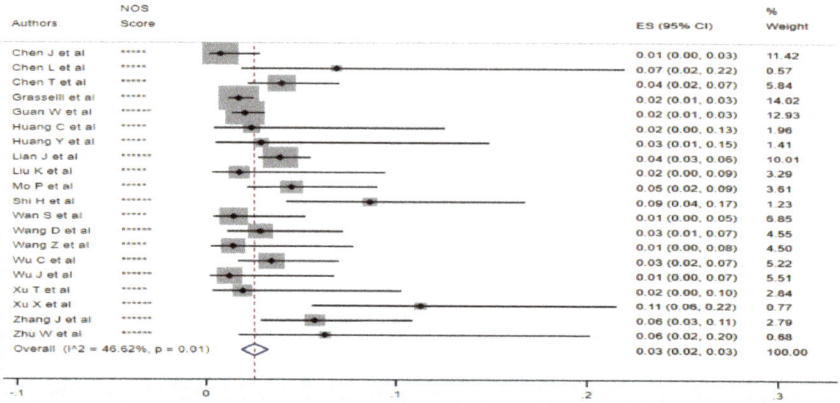

Figure 3. Pooled prevalence of patients with liver diseases (Chronic Liver Diseases, Hepatitis B/C infections) diagnosed with COVID-19. The red dotted line represents the overall effect size of the studies (0.03). The edges of the blue diamond represent 95% confidence intervals (0.02, 0.03). ES = Effect Size, NOS = Newcastle-Ottawa Score.

4. Discussion

We report here, for the first time, the prevalence, severity and mortality of patients diagnosed with COVID-19 with underlying chronic kidney disease and liver diseases. Our outcomes show that the overall prevalence of CKD and Liver Diseases in COVID-19 are 1% and 3% respectively. We also report a COVID-19 severity of 83.93% (47/56) in patients with CKD and 57.33% (43/75) in patients with liver diseases. The rate of mortality in COVID-19 patients with CKD and Liver diseases was found to be 53.33% (8/15) and 17.65% (6/34) respectively.

The presence of comorbidities is associated with poor prognoses in patients with COVID-19, with higher mortality rates and severity. The most common comorbidities reported so far in severe cases have been hypertension, diabetes, cardiovascular diseases, cerebrovascular diseases and COPD [29]. However, how these diseases contribute to the COVID-19 outcome remains unclear.

Biomarkers of liver injuries have been reported to increase in patients with COVID-19 [25,35,45], although, no virus was found in the liver tissue of patients who died from the disease [54]. This is to be expected, as angiotensin II-converting enzyme (ACE2) receptor, a key player in the "docking" and replication of the SARS-CoV-2 virus, is not expressed in hepatocytes. However, ACE2 expression has been reported in cholangiocytes [55], leading to the suggestion that the binding of SARS-CoV-2 to the epithelial cells of the biliary tree may cause biliary dysfunction [56]. Zhang et al. also suggested that the transient liver injuries observed in COVID-19 patients may be associated with drug toxicity, cytokine storm or hypoxia [56]. While many studies have reported liver dysfunction in COVID-19 [25,35,45], the mechanistic link between the two remains to be established.

Furthermore, CKD have been associated with inflammation and dysregulation of the immune system [57]. This dysregulation of immune function, which may exist in patients with underlying CKD, may explain the increased severity and mortality due to COVID-19. The levels of ACE2 receptor in the kidney have been previously reported to be altered in patients with human kidney diseases [58]. In a recent study by Fan et al., it was reported that ACE2 receptor is overexpressed in the tubular cells of patients with CKD. Alteration in kidney functions, characterised by increased serum creatinine and urea nitrogen, was also reported in patients with COVID-19 [59]. Taken together, the alterations in ACE2 receptor expression may explain the observed kidney dysfunction in COVID-19 and provide the answer to why patients with CKD are vulnerable to the SARS-CoV-2 virus.

This study is limited by several factors. Firstly, some included studies did not report comorbidities. Where comorbidities were specified, the criteria for defining severity were not uniform. Some studies included only patients with primary composite outcomes, while some did not report mortality. Lastly, the aetiology and pathophysiological characteristics of the comorbidities were not documented.

Indeed, this review involved an in-depth literature search followed by a systematic analysis of data involving a total of 5595 patients with confirmed COVID-19. For the first time, we have established the potential risk of COVID-19 in liver disease and CKD patients, which indicates an increased vulnerability of this subpopulation.

The most important clinical implication of this study is that Liver disease and CKD patients are potentially highly vulnerable to COVID-19 and should be considered for remote consultation and the most stringent social isolation to prevent infection. Future studies should investigate how liver diseases and CKD contribute to poor prognoses in COVID-19.

5. Conclusions

We report a potential increased risk of severity and mortality in COVID-19 patients with liver diseases and CKD. This study will facilitate better clinical management and inform the process of implementing more stringent preventative measures for this group of patients.

Author Contributions: Conceptualization, T.O. and J.A.; methodology, T.O.; software, T.O.; validation, T.O., J.A., G.C.; formal analysis, T.O.; investigation, T.O.; resources, T.O.; data curation, T.O., G.C.; writing—original draft preparation, T.O.; writing—review and editing, T.O., J.A., G.C.; visualization, G.C.; supervision, T.O.; project administration, T.O. All authors have read and agreed to the published version of the manuscript.

Funding: This research received no external funding.

Conflicts of Interest: The authors declare no conflict of interest.

Appendix A

```
Database: Ovid MEDLINE(R) and Epub Ahead of Print, In-Process & Other Non-Indexed
Citations, Daily and Versions(R) <1946 to April 10, 2020>
Search Strategy:
--------------------------------------------------------------------
1    COVID-19.mp. (3190)
2    2019 novel coronavirus.mp. (363)
3    2019 coronavirus.mp. (46)
4    2019-nCoV.mp. (460)
5    SARS-CoV-2.mp. (1009)
6    Wuhan Coronavirus.mp. (14)
7    1 or 2 or 3 or 4 or 5 or 6 (3655)
8    clinical characteristic*.mp. [mp=title, abstract, original title, name of substance word,
subject heading word, floating sub-heading word, keyword heading word, organism
supplementary concept word, protocol supplementary concept word, rare disease
supplementary concept word, unique identifier, synonyms] (67298)
9    clinical Characteristics.mp. (66591)
10   clinical features.mp. (100583)
11   clinical feature*.mp. [mp=title, abstract, original title, name of substance word, subject
heading word, floating sub-heading word, keyword heading word, organism supplementary
concept word, protocol supplementary concept word, rare disease supplementary concept
word, unique identifier, synonyms] (104280)
12   8 or 9 or 10 or 11 (166495)
13   7 and 12 (181)
14   limit 13 to english language (159)
15   limit 14 to humans (27)

*****************************
```

Figure A1. Medline Search Strategy.

Table A1. Quality Assessment.

First Author	SELECTION		ASCERTAINMENT		OUTCOME		OVERALL
	Sample Size Adequate	Population Representative (Multicentre)	Test Adequate	Comorbidity Confirmation Adequate (EMR)	Outcome Reported Adequately (Clinical Staff)	Follow-up Long Enough (≥2 Weeks)	OVERALL (≥4 Stars = Lower Risk of Bias)
Chen J et al.	*		*	*	*	*	*****
Chen L et al.	*		*	*	*	*	*****
Chen N et al.	*		*	*	*	*	****
Chen T et al.	*		*	*	*	*	*****
Grasselli et al.	*	*	*		*	*	*****
Guan W et al.	*	*	*	*	*	*	******
Huang C et al.	*		*	*	*	*	*****
Huang Y et al.	*		*	*	*	*	*****
Lian J et al.	*	*	*	*	*	*	******
Liu K et al.	*		*	*	*	*	*****
Mo P et al.	*		*	*	*	*	*****
Shi H et al.	*	*	*	*	*	*	******
Wan S et al.	*		*	*	*	*	*****
Wang D et al.	*	*	*	*	*	*	******
Wang Z et al.	*		*	*	*	*	*****
Wu C et al.	*		*	*	*	*	*****
Wu J et al.	*	*	*	*	*	*	******
Xu T et al.	*		*	*	*	*	*****
Xu X et al.	*	*	*	*	*	*	******
Zhang J et al.	*		*	*	*	*	*****
Zhou et al.	*	*	*	*	*	*	******
Zhu W et al.	*	*	*	*	*	*	******

```
Database: Embase <1980 to 2020 Week 15>
Search Strategy:
--------------------------------------------------------------------------------
1     COVID-19.mp. (1687)
2     2019 novel coronavirus.mp. (450)
3     2019 coronavirus.mp. (34)
4     2019-nCoV.mp. (374)
5     SARS-CoV-2.mp. (561)
6     Wuhan Coronavirus.mp. (12)
7     1 or 2 or 3 or 4 or 5 or 6 (2218)
8     clinical characteristic*.mp. [mp=title, abstract, heading word, drug trade name, original
title, device manufacturer, drug manufacturer, device trade name, keyword, floating
subheading word, candidate term word] (111691)
9     clinical Characteristics.mp. or exp clinical feature/ (742652)
10    clinical feature*.mp. [mp=title, abstract, heading word, drug trade name, original title,
device manufacturer, drug manufacturer, device trade name, keyword, floating subheading
word, candidate term word] (721829)
11    8 or 9 or 10 (798804)
12    7 and 11 (139)
13    limit 12 to english language (127)
14    limit 13 to human (115)

*****************************
```

Figure A2. Embase Search Strategy.

References

1. Mokdad, A.A.; Lopez, A.D.; Shahraz, S.; Lozano, R.; Mokdad, A.H.; Stanaway, J.; Murray, C.J.; Naghavi, M. Liver cirrhosis mortality in 187 countries between 1980 and 2010: A systematic analysis. *BMC Med.* **2014**, *12*, 145. [CrossRef] [PubMed]
2. Anthony, P.P.; Ishak, K.G.; Nayak, N.C.; Poulsen, H.E.; Scheuer, P.J.; Sobin, L.H. The morphology of cirrhosis. Recommendations on definition, nomenclature, and classification by a working group sponsored by the World Health Organization. *J. Clin. Pathol.* **1978**, *31*, 395–414. [CrossRef] [PubMed]
3. Fleming, K.M.; Aithal, G.P.; Card, T.R.; West, J. All-cause mortality in people with cirrhosis compared with the general population: A population-based cohort study. *Liver Int.* **2012**, *32*, 79–84. [CrossRef] [PubMed]
4. Sepanlou, S.G.; Safiri, S.; Bisignano, C.; Ikuta, K.S.; Merat, S.; Saberifiroozi, M.; Poustchi, H.; Tsoi, D.; Colombara, D.V.; Abdoli, A.; et al. The global, regional, and national burden of cirrhosis by cause in 195 countries and territories, 1990-2017: A systematic analysis for the Global Burden of Disease Study 2017. *Lancet Gastroenterol. Hepatol.* **2020**, *5*, 245–266. [CrossRef]
5. WHO. *Global Health Estimates 2015: Deaths by Cause, Age, Sex, by Country and by Region, 2000–2015*; World Health Organization: Geneva, Switzerland, 2016.
6. Asrani, S.K.; Devarbhavi, H.; Eaton, J.; Kamath, P.S. Burden of liver diseases in the world. *J. Hepatol.* **2019**, *70*, 151–171. [CrossRef]
7. Levin, A.S.P.; Bilous, R.W.; Coresh, J. Chapter 1: Definition and classification of CKD. *Kidney Int. Suppl.* **2013**, *3*, 19–62. [CrossRef]
8. McClellan, W.M.; Flanders, W.D. Risk factors for progressive chronic kidney disease. *J. Am. Soc. Nephrol.* **2003**, *14*, S65–S70. [CrossRef]
9. Kottgen, A.; Glazer, N.L.; Dehghan, A.; Hwang, S.J.; Katz, R.; Li, M.; Yang, Q.; Gudnason, V.; Launer, L.J.; Harris, T.B.; et al. Multiple loci associated with indices of renal function and chronic kidney disease. *Nat. Genet.* **2009**, *41*, 712–717. [CrossRef]
10. Perneger, T.V.; Whelton, P.K.; Klag, M.J. Risk of kidney failure associated with the use of acetaminophen, aspirin, and nonsteroidal antiinflammatory drugs. *N. Engl. J. Med.* **1994**, *331*, 1675–1679. [CrossRef]
11. Chang, A.; Kramer, H. CKD progression: A risky business. *Nephrol. Dial. Transplant.* **2012**, *27*, 2607–2609. [CrossRef]
12. Iseki, K. Factors influencing the development of end-stage renal disease. *Clin. Exp. Nephrol.* **2005**, *9*, 5–14. [CrossRef] [PubMed]
13. Suleymanlar, G.; Utas, C.; Arinsoy, T.; Ates, K.; Altun, B.; Altiparmak, M.R.; Ecder, T.; Yilmaz, M.E.; Camsari, T.; Basci, A.; et al. A population-based survey of Chronic REnal Disease In Turke—The CREDIT study. *Nephrol. Dial. Transplant.* **2011**, *26*, 1862–1871. [CrossRef] [PubMed]

14. Lackland, D.T.; Egan, B.M.; Fan, Z.J.; Syddall, H.E. Low birth weight contributes to the excess prevalence of end-stage renal disease in African Americans. *J. Clin. Hypertens. (Greenwich)* **2001**, *3*, 29–31. [CrossRef] [PubMed]
15. Bleyer, A.J.; Shemanski, L.R.; Burke, G.L.; Hansen, K.J.; Appel, R.G. Tobacco, hypertension, and vascular disease: Risk factors for renal functional decline in an older population. *Kidney Int.* **2000**, *57*, 2072–2079. [CrossRef]
16. Orth, S.R.; Schroeder, T.; Ritz, E.; Ferrari, P. Effects of smoking on renal function in patients with type 1 and type 2 diabetes mellitus. *Nephrol. Dial. Transplant.* **2005**, *20*, 2414–2419. [CrossRef]
17. Nzerue, C.M.; Demissochew, H.; Tucker, J.K. Race and kidney disease: Role of social and environmental factors. *J. Natl. Med. Assoc.* **2002**, *94*, 28s–38s.
18. Song, E.Y.; McClellan, W.M.; McClellan, A.; Gadi, R.; Hadley, A.C.; Krisher, J.; Clay, M.; Freedman, B.I. Effect of community characteristics on familial clustering of end-stage renal disease. *Am. J. Nephrol.* **2009**, *30*, 499–504. [CrossRef]
19. Gonzalez-Quiroz, M.; Pearce, N.; Caplin, B.; Nitsch, D. What do epidemiological studies tell us about chronic kidney disease of undetermined cause in Meso-America? A systematic review and meta-analysis. *Clin. Kidney J.* **2018**, *11*, 496–506. [CrossRef]
20. Goldstein, S.L.; Devarajan, P. Acute kidney injury in childhood: Should we be worried about progression to CKD? *Pediatric Nephrol.* **2011**, *26*, 509–522. [CrossRef]
21. Bikbov, B.; Purcell, C.A.; Levey, A.S.; Smith, M.; Abdoli, A.; Abebe, M.; Adebayo, O.M.; Afarideh, M.; Agarwal, S.K.; Agudelo-Botero, M.; et al. Global, regional, and national burden of chronic kidney disease, 1990-2017: A systematic analysis for the Global Burden of Disease Study 2017. *Lancet* **2020**, *395*, 709–733. [CrossRef]
22. Cockwell, P.; Fisher, L.-A. The global burden of chronic kidney disease. *Lancet* **2020**, *395*. [CrossRef]
23. Wang, L.; Li, X.; Chen, H.; Yan, S.; Li, D.; Li, Y.; Gong, Z. Coronavirus Disease 19 Infection Does Not Result in Acute Kidney Injury: An Analysis of 116 Hospitalized Patients from Wuhan, China. *Am. J. Nephrol.* **2020**, *51*, 343–348. [CrossRef]
24. WHO. *Coronavirus Disease (COVID-2019) Situation Reports*; World Health Organization: Geneva, Switzerland, 2020.
25. Huang, C.; Wang, Y.; Li, X.; Ren, L.; Zhao, J.; Hu, Y.; Zhang, L.; Fan, G.; Xu, J.; Gu, X.; et al. Clinical features of patients infected with 2019 novel coronavirus in Wuhan, China. *Lancet* **2020**, *395*, 497–506. [CrossRef]
26. Chan, J.F.; Yuan, S.; Kok, K.H.; To, K.K.; Chu, H.; Yang, J.; Xing, F.; Liu, J.; Yip, C.C.; Poon, R.W.; et al. A familial cluster of pneumonia associated with the 2019 novel coronavirus indicating person-to-person transmission: A study of a family cluster. *Lancet* **2020**, *395*, 514–523. [CrossRef]
27. Wu, F.; Zhao, S.; Yu, B.; Chen, Y.M.; Wang, W.; Song, Z.G.; Hu, Y.; Tao, Z.W.; Tian, J.H.; Pei, Y.Y.; et al. A new coronavirus associated with human respiratory disease in China. *Nature* **2020**, *579*, 265–269. [CrossRef]
28. WHO. *Coronavirus Disease 2019 (COVID-19), Situation Report—73*; World Health Organization: Geneva, Switzerland, 2020.
29. Guan, W.J.; Liang, W.H.; Zhao, Y.; Liang, H.R.; Chen, Z.S.; Li, Y.M.; Liu, X.Q.; Chen, R.C.; Tang, C.L.; Wang, T.; et al. Comorbidity and its impact on 1590 patients with Covid-19 in China: A Nationwide Analysis. *Eur. Respir. J.* **2020**. [CrossRef]
30. Alqahtani, J.S.; Oyelade, T.; Aldhahir, A.M.; Alghamdi, S.M.; Almehmadi, M.; Alqahtani, A.S.; Quaderi, S.; Mandal, S.; Hurst, J.R. Prevalence, Severity and Mortality associated with COPD and Smoking in patients with COVID-19: A Rapid Systematic Review and Meta-Analysis. *PLoS ONE* **2020**, *15*, e0233147. [CrossRef]
31. Murad, M.H.; Sultan, S.; Haffar, S.; Bazerbachi, F. Methodological quality and synthesis of case series and case reports. *BMJ Evid. Based Med.* **2018**, *23*, 60–63. [CrossRef]
32. World Health Organization. *Laboratory Testing for Coronavirus Disease (COVID-19) in Suspected Human Cases: Interim Guidance, 19 March 2020*; World Health Organization: Geneva, Switzerland, 2020.
33. Chen, J.; Qi, T.; Liu, L.; Ling, Y.; Qian, Z.; Li, T.; Li, F.; Xu, Q.; Zhang, Y.; Xu, S.; et al. Clinical progression of patients with COVID-19 in Shanghai, China. *J. Infect.* **2020**. [CrossRef]
34. Chen, L.; Liu, H.G.; Liu, W.; Liu, J.; Liu, K.; Shang, J.; Deng, Y.; Wei, S. Analysis of clinical features of 29 patients with 2019 novel coronavirus pneumonia. *Zhonghua Jie He He Hu Xi Za Zhi* **2020**, *43*, E005. [CrossRef]
35. Chen, N.; Zhou, M.; Dong, X.; Qu, J.; Gong, F.; Han, Y.; Qiu, Y.; Wang, J.; Liu, Y.; Wei, Y.; et al. Epidemiological and clinical characteristics of 99 cases of 2019 novel coronavirus pneumonia in Wuhan, China: A descriptive study. *Lancet* **2020**, *395*, 507–513. [CrossRef]

36. Chen, T.; Wu, D.; Chen, H.; Yan, W.; Yang, D.; Chen, G.; Ma, K.; Xu, D.; Yu, H.; Wang, H.; et al. Clinical characteristics of 113 deceased patients with coronavirus disease 2019: Retrospective study. *BMJ* **2020**, *368*, m1091. [CrossRef]
37. Grasselli, G.; Zangrillo, A.; Zanella, A.; Antonelli, M.; Cabrini, L.; Castelli, A.; Cereda, D.; Coluccello, A.; Foti, G.; Fumagalli, R.; et al. Baseline Characteristics and Outcomes of 1591 Patients Infected With SARS-CoV-2 Admitted to ICUs of the Lombardy Region, Italy. *JAMA* **2020**. [CrossRef]
38. Guan, W.J.; Ni, Z.Y.; Hu, Y.; Liang, W.H.; Ou, C.Q.; He, J.X.; Liu, L.; Shan, H.; Lei, C.L.; Hui, D.S.C.; et al. Clinical Characteristics of Coronavirus Disease 2019 in China. *N. Engl. J. Med.* **2020**. [CrossRef]
39. Huang, Y.; Tu, M.; Wang, S.; Chen, S.; Zhou, W.; Chen, D.; Zhou, L.; Wang, M.; Zhao, Y.; Zeng, W.; et al. Clinical characteristics of laboratory confirmed positive cases of SARS-CoV-2 infection in Wuhan, China: A retrospective single center analysis. *Travel Med. Infect. Dis.* **2020**. [CrossRef]
40. Lian, J.; Jin, X.; Hao, S.; Cai, H.; Zhang, S.; Zheng, L.; Jia, H.; Hu, J.; Gao, J.; Zhang, Y.; et al. Analysis of Epidemiological and Clinical features in older patients with Corona Virus Disease 2019 (COVID-19) out of Wuhan. *Clin. Infect. Dis.* **2020**. [CrossRef]
41. Liu, K.; Chen, Y.; Lin, R.; Han, K. Clinical features of COVID-19 in elderly patients: A comparison with young and middle-aged patients. *J. Infect.* **2020**. [CrossRef]
42. Mo, P.; Xing, Y.; Xiao, Y.; Deng, L.; Zhao, Q.; Wang, H.; Xiong, Y.; Cheng, Z.; Gao, S.; Liang, K.; et al. Clinical characteristics of refractory COVID-19 pneumonia in Wuhan, China. *Clin. Infect. Dis.* **2020**. [CrossRef]
43. Shi, H.; Han, X.; Jiang, N.; Cao, Y.; Alwalid, O.; Gu, J.; Fan, Y.; Zheng, C. Radiological findings from 81 patients with COVID-19 pneumonia in Wuhan, China: A descriptive study. *Lancet Infect. Dis.* **2020**, *20*, 425–434. [CrossRef]
44. Wan, S.; Xiang, Y.; Fang, W.; Zheng, Y.; Li, B.; Hu, Y.; Lang, C.; Huang, D.; Sun, Q.; Xiong, Y.; et al. Clinical features and treatment of COVID-19 patients in northeast Chongqing. *J. Med. Virol.* **2020**. [CrossRef]
45. Wang, D.; Hu, B.; Hu, C.; Zhu, F.; Liu, X.; Zhang, J.; Wang, B.; Xiang, H.; Cheng, Z.; Xiong, Y.; et al. Clinical Characteristics of 138 Hospitalized Patients with 2019 Novel Coronavirus-Infected Pneumonia in Wuhan, China. *JAMA* **2020**. [CrossRef]
46. Wang, Z.; Yang, B.; Li, Q.; Wen, L.; Zhang, R. Clinical Features of 69 Cases with Coronavirus Disease 2019 in Wuhan, China. *Clin. Infect. Dis.* **2020**. [CrossRef]
47. Wu, C.; Chen, X.; Cai, Y.; Xia, J.; Zhou, X.; Xu, S.; Huang, H.; Zhang, L.; Zhou, X.; Du, C.; et al. Risk Factors Associated with Acute Respiratory Distress Syndrome and Death in Patients with Coronavirus Disease 2019 Pneumonia in Wuhan, China. *JAMA Intern. Med.* **2020**. [CrossRef]
48. Wu, J.; Liu, J.; Zhao, X.; Liu, C.; Wang, W.; Wang, D.; Xu, W.; Zhang, C.; Yu, J.; Jiang, B.; et al. Clinical Characteristics of Imported Cases of COVID-19 in Jiangsu Province: A Multicenter Descriptive Study. *Clin. Infect. Dis.* **2020**. [CrossRef]
49. Xu, T.; Chen, C.; Zhu, Z.; Cui, M.; Chen, C.; Dai, H.; Xue, Y. Clinical features and dynamics of viral load in imported and non-imported patients with COVID-19. *Int. J. Infect. Dis.* **2020**. [CrossRef]
50. Xu, X.W.; Wu, X.X.; Jiang, X.G.; Xu, K.J.; Ying, L.J.; Ma, C.L.; Li, S.B.; Wang, H.Y.; Zhang, S.; Gao, H.N.; et al. Clinical findings in a group of patients infected with the 2019 novel coronavirus (SARS-Cov-2) outside of Wuhan, China: Retrospective case series. *BMJ* **2020**, *368*, m792. [CrossRef]
51. Zhang, J.J.; Dong, X.; Cao, Y.Y.; Yuan, Y.D.; Yang, Y.B.; Yan, Y.Q.; Akdis, C.A.; Gao, Y.D. Clinical characteristics of 140 patients infected with SARS-CoV-2 in Wuhan, China. *Allergy* **2020**. [CrossRef]
52. Zhou, F.; Yu, T.; Du, R.; Fan, G.; Liu, Y.; Liu, Z.; Xiang, J.; Wang, Y.; Song, B.; Gu, X.; et al. Clinical course and risk factors for mortality of adult inpatients with COVID-19 in Wuhan, China: A retrospective cohort study. *Lancet* **2020**, *395*, 1054–1062. [CrossRef]
53. Zhu, W.; Xie, K.; Lu, H.; Xu, L.; Zhou, S.; Fang, S. Initial clinical features of suspected coronavirus disease 2019 in two emergency departments outside of Hubei, China. *J. Med. Virol.* **2020**. [CrossRef]
54. Xu, Z.; Shi, L.; Wang, Y.; Zhang, J.; Huang, L.; Zhang, C.; Liu, S.; Zhao, P.; Liu, H.; Zhu, L.; et al. Pathological findings of COVID-19 associated with acute respiratory distress syndrome. *Lancet Respir. Med.* **2020**, *8*, 420–422. [CrossRef]
55. Chai, X.; Hu, L.; Zhang, Y.; Han, W.; Lu, Z.; Ke, A.; Zhou, J.; Shi, G.; Fang, N.; Fan, J.; et al. Specific ACE2 Expression in Cholangiocytes May Cause Liver Damage After 2019-nCoV Infection. *BioRxiv* **2020**. [CrossRef]
56. Zhang, C.; Shi, L.; Wang, F.S. Liver injury in COVID-19: Management and challenges. *Lancet Gastroenterol. Hepatol.* **2020**, *5*, 428–430. [CrossRef]

57. Imig, J.D.; Ryan, M.J. Immune and inflammatory role in renal disease. *Compr. Physiol.* **2013**, *3*, 957–976. [CrossRef]
58. Lely, A.T.; Hamming, I.; van Goor, H.; Navis, G.J. Renal ACE2 expression in human kidney disease. *J. Pathol.* **2004**, *204*, 587–593. [CrossRef]
59. Fan, C.; Li, K.; Ding, Y.; Lu, W.L.; Wang, J. ACE2 Expression in Kidney and Testis May Cause Kidney and Testis Damage After 2019-nCoV Infection. *MedRxiv* **2020**. [CrossRef]

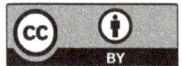

© 2020 by the authors. Licensee MDPI, Basel, Switzerland. This article is an open access article distributed under the terms and conditions of the Creative Commons Attribution (CC BY) license (http://creativecommons.org/licenses/by/4.0/).

MDPI
St. Alban-Anlage 66
4052 Basel
Switzerland
Tel. +41 61 683 77 34
Fax +41 61 302 89 18
www.mdpi.com

Tropical Medicine and Infectious Disease Editorial Office
E-mail: tropicalmed@mdpi.com
www.mdpi.com/journal/tropicalmed

www.ingramcontent.com/pod-product-compliance
Lightning Source LLC
LaVergne TN
LVHW070457100526
838202LV00014B/1738